T0204240

GROW YOUR PUPS WITH BONES

The BARF Programme
For Breeding Healthy Dogs
And Eliminating Skeletal Disease

DR. IAN BILLINGHURST

Published by
Ian Billinghurst

'GROW YOUR PUPS WITH BONES'
P.O. BOX WO 64 BATHURST 2795
N.S.W. AUSTRALIA

'Grow Your Pups With Bones'
First published in Australia 1998
By Ian Billinghurst
Third printing

This book is an Australian product
Design and Typesetting by Ian Billinghurst
Illustrations by Ian Billinghurst
Edited by Dr. Jane Stevenson and Rick Billinghurst
Photography by Roslyn Billinghurst

Printed in Australia by SOS Printing Pty Ltd
PO Box 411 Alexandria 2015, N.S.W. Australia

ISBN 0 9585925 0 0

Also written by Ian Billinghurst
'Give Your Dog a Bone' - 1993

To order further copies of either book , address all enquiries to ...
Dr. Ian Billinghurst
P.O. Box WO 64 Bathurst 2795
N.S.W. Australia

Phone 02 6334 2009
Fax   02 6334 2140
e-mail   barfdiet@ix.net.au

Contents

Part Three
Bones Build Bones

Note to Readers

The following information is supplied on the understanding that it is not designed to take the place of your veterinarian. Its aim is to supplement your veterinarian's advice and guidance. Diagnosis of a medical or surgical condition in your dog can only be carried out by a veterinary surgeon. The author of this book cannot be responsible for any decisions any reader may make with regard to feeding or treating their dog[s]. Any application of the recommendations set forth in the following pages is at the reader's discretion and sole risk. It is strongly advised that the reader at all times seeks out the best veterinary resources available, in order that informed decisions on the care of dogs is obtained at all times.

– Acknowledgements –

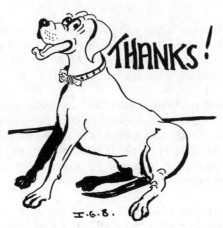

Grow Your Pups With Bones has been written with the assistance of many dogs. Some of these dogs have been my patients. Others have shared their lives with me. Many I have never met. However, without the help of all of them, I could not have written this book. Particular thanks are due to Ellie and Cillie, the two dogs in my life right now. They continue to be two of my best teachers.

I would also like to thank my clients - past and present - and the many other dog owners who have contacted me over the years, seeking advice, offering comments and telling me about their dogs. Their input has shaped my thinking and therefore this book.

To all those people who purchased, read, and applied the principles outlined in my first book **Give Your Dog a Bone,** let me say thank you one and all for your support, feed-back and encouragement.

For their editing skills, critical insight and helpful advice, I would like to thank Dr. Jane Stevenson - veterinary surgeon, and Rick Billinghurst - my brother.

Finally, let me say that I could not have written **Grow Your Pups With Bones** without the loving help and support of my darling wife Roslyn, and our family. Thank you.

How to use this book

If you are anything like me when you get a new book, you will start at the end and work your way backwards. Sometimes I just open a book at random and start reading from anywhere. Alternatively, you might read the table of contents and see what interests you.

However,**Grow Your Pups With Bones** has been organised in a sequential way. Each chapter is built on the foundation of preceding chapters. The book begins with the BARF diet which sets the scene for the rest of the book. This growth of ideas is particularly important in Part Three which deals with skeletal health and disease in pups. On that basis, I would suggest that you treat **Grow Your Pups With Bones** like a novel.

Start by reading Part One which tells you all about the BARF diet. It is only after you are familiar with the BARF diet that you will receive full value from the rest of the book. Having read and understood the BARF diet you may then choose to read either part Two - which is about feeding for breeding - or move straight into Part Three which is about skeletal disease in pups.

If you find a section that is difficult for any reason, don't worry. Just keep reading. Any difficult stuff is only there for the sake of explanation and completeness. Push your way through it. The forest will very soon open out into a cleared area which is the important bit. The bit that tells you what you have to do to have a healthy dog.

You will not find an index in this book. Grow Your Pups With Bones is not designed as a text book where you 'look things up.' If at any stage you do require specific information, the table of contents and the headings throughout each chapter should help you find the information you need. Also, don't be afraid to mark this book. As you read the book, do so with a pen or a highlighter in your hand. Mark those sections you may wish to find again - for whatever reason.

May you enjoy this book and have healthy dogs.

Ian Billinghurst
August 1998

INTRODUCTION

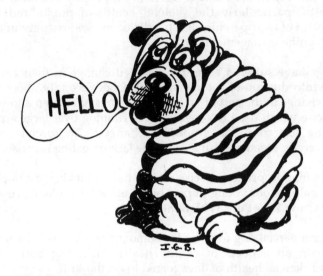

Grow Your Pups With Bones has been written to explain the vital role that diet and exercise plays in two critical aspects of our dogs' health. Firstly their ability to ...

REPRODUCE

and secondly their ability to ...

GROW - WITHOUT BONE AND JOINT PROBLEMS

The need to write this book has become increasingly apparent to me over the last few years as I witness the reproductive and skeletal health of the modern dog continue to decline, despite the wealth of knowledge and dollars poured into the canine health industry.

Grow Your Pups with Bones has been written to show you that skeletal health failure and reproductive disease - do not have to be. That fixing these problems is 'super-easy!'

1

Since the 1930's ...

... the health of the dog in the western world has gradually declined. This decline in health, particularly the skeletal health of pups and the reproductive health of their parents, has paralleled marked changes in two vital aspects of canine management.

Firstly, our dogs have suffered an unprecedented change in their eating habits with the introduction of commercial dog food. Secondly, there has been a gradual change in the sort of exercise our dogs have been allowed. Our dogs' exercise which used to consist of free running over large areas, play and eating exercise, has gradually changed to forced and inappropriate exercise together with a complete lack of eating exercise.

The switch to an inappropriate exercise regime has had its biggest impact on the skeletal health of our young pups. This factor will be fully discussed in **Part Three of Grow Your Pups With Bones.**

The switch to commercial dog food as the standard way to feed dogs has seen a decline in all aspects of canine health including both the **reproductive and skeletal health** of dogs forced to eat the stuff.

This decline in general health, reproductive and skeletal health has been marked and outstanding, yet nobody has been willing to make the obvious connection between the gradual increase in degenerative disease and the very obvious cause - our dogs' awful and inappropriate diet.

There is a mass of research ...

... commissioned by pet food manufacturers and carried out by independent bodies, which demonstrates that pet foods are responsible for a wide range of degenerative diseases, including reproductive problems and skeletal diseases such as Hip and Elbow Dysplasia. A mass of clinical experience supports this research.

The vets involved in this research acknowledge that the diseases caused by pet foods are rarely linked to their cause by the public or by vets in practice. This is because such damning research has not become common knowledge within the veterinary profession.

The result is that the veterinary profession accepts pet foods without question. We refuse to critically examine these products. We ignore all evidence which shows them to be defective. Instead we accept as a matter of blind faith that commercially produced scientifically balanced pet foods are so good and so health producing that they are beyond criticism. When it comes to these products our heads are well and truly buried in the sand!

There is another reason we accept these products so uncritically

It is because our profession, in fact the entire pet industry, has become dependent on both the products and their manufacturers.

Pet food manufacturers fund our breed associations and our dog shows. They subsidise the production and training of guide dogs. They give money to our professional associations, our magazines, and our universities. They support our conferences and our building funds. They carry out research into our patients' diseases, and pay vets and others to carry out that research. They teach our young vets about nutrition and fill our waiting rooms with their product. This boosts our incomes, and if we sell enough of it, we benefit with kick-backs. The icing on the cake is that their products provide us with patients. Sooner or later.

In other words, this stuff we vets sell and recommend is of great benefit. To us! We sell it, bank the profits and enjoy the kick-backs. We no longer have to be experts in nutrition. It brews up a crop of new patients. Our clients will never know that our recommendations caused their pets' ill health. We receive accolades from the public for providing such a useful service, and we remain credible in the sight of our profession for following [rather like sheep] the currently accepted practice. Without question - of course!

However, if we can get our patients off the stuff ...

... and switch them to a biologically appropriate programme of diet and exercise, their health problems begin to disappear. Daily I receive letters attesting to this fact and my clients continually show me dogs that have gone from poor health to brilliant health.

This return to health includes the disappearance of ...

... reproductive problems - which begin to melt away ...

... and orthopaedic bone disease in juvenile dogs - which simply fail to show.

Grow Your Pups With Bones has been written so that dog owners, breeders, vets and anyone else who is involved with the production and raising of puppies can know how simple it is to raise dogs with very few reproductive problems and sound skeletal systems.

When our dogs' health fails in these two areas, it is almost always because of our failure to feed a biologically appropriate diet, and in the case of growing pups particularly, the failure to use biologically appropriate exercise.

When dogs are switched to the Bones and Raw Food Programme of diet and exercise - as outlined in Part One of **Grow Your Pups With Bones** - health problems in those two areas disappear.

By making such remarkably simple but profound changes to their dogs' diet and exercise regime, readers of **Grow Your Pups With Bones** will quickly discover what so many other dog owners now know. The peace of mind, the dollar savings and the great pleasure to be derived from the stress-free production of large numbers of healthy pups which can and will grow into sound adults, totally free of skeletal disease.

Please note

In all my years as a practising vet, not one client has told me that switching their dog[s] from a properly formulated bones and raw food type diet to a commercial dog food has resulted in any long term, sustained and noticeable improvement in their dogs' health. However, I want to make it clear from the outset that if such a product could be found, a commercial dog food which had been demonstrated in properly controlled trials to outperform a dog's biologically appropriate diet - over a lifetime - then I would be the first one to endorse it.

To date this has not happened. On the contrary, daily I receive testimony by word of mouth, by mail, by telephone and by e-mail that dogs switched from commercial dog foods to a biologically appropriate diet based on bones and raw foods show dramatic, continuing and sustained improvements in health.

I also continue to receive testimony concerning the decline in health seen over generations of dogs that have changed from a biologically appropriate diet to a diet based on commercial pet food.

If you would like to eliminate reproductive problems or skeletal disease - including problems such as Hip and Elbow Dysplasia - from your dog[s] or from your breeding programme, I strongly advise you to read, mark and digest the contents of this book. Follow the programme outlined in the book and you too will experience a radical change - for the better - in all aspects of your dogs' health including their reproductive and skeletal health.

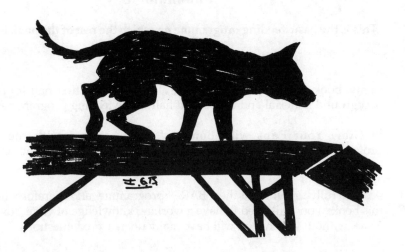

HOW 'GROW YOUR PUPS WITH BONES' IS ORGANISED

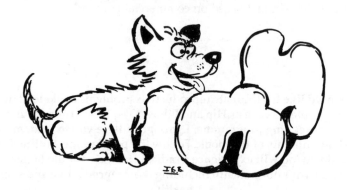

PART ONE – THE BONES AND RAW FOOD ['BARF'] PROGRAMME

This is the basic feeding programme on which the rest of the book is based.

So read it first.

In my book, **Give Your Dog a Bone**, I devoted the first half to essential background material and the second half to the feeding programmes.

In **Grow Your Pups with Bones** I have started with the feeding programme which is essential background knowledge for the rest of the book.

Also, to fully understand the "BARF" programme and therefore the rest of this book, you will need to have a working knowledge of **Give Your Dog a Bone**, without which you will have many unanswered questions.

6

PART TWO - FEEDING FOR BREEDING

This section is written for breeders, and any other concerned members of the canine world, including vets. If you are willing to admit that our current breeding programmes are not 100% perfect, that there is room for improvement, then you are ready to read FEEDING FOR BREEDING. Read it and take the plunge. Switch the animals in your care to the BARF programme and follow the simple commonsense guidelines outlined in PART ONE of this book.

You will be astounded by the rapid and immediate improvement in the health of dogs switched to the BARF programme. You will also need patience. Much of the damage which we are now seeing has taken generations of sub-standard nutrition to evolve. It will take several generations to remove. Don't be discouraged. By sticking to the programme, you will eventually produce dogs that reproduce easily and consistently into old age. You will see pups that become long-lived healthy adults, without bone or joint disease.

PART THREE - BONES BUILD BONES

This section is vital reading for anybody who has anything to do with pups. Particularly dog breeders and puppy owners. Its message is simple. **Bone disease in young dogs is preventable**. Pups of any breed, including the giant breeds, can be raised to have sound bones and joints, no matter how many genes they may have inherited for problems such as Hip and Elbow Dysplasia. By following the simple guidelines outlined in this section, the vast majority of the bone and joint problems in pups will simply disappear!

PART ONE

THE BONES AND RAW FOOD ['BARF'] PROGRAMME

CHAPTER ONE

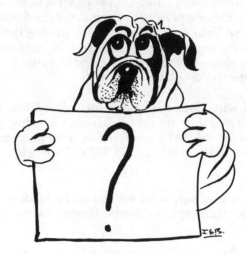

WHAT IS
THE 'BARF' DIET?

"To barf", as you may know is a slang expression which means - "to vomit." Most dogs are quite happy to eat vomit. It is actually natural for a dog to eat vomit. For example, weanling pups lick their parents' mouths as a signal that they are hungry and want to be fed. That instinct remains with our domestic dogs.

Next time your dog attempts to lick your mouth - realise what he or she may be asking you to do! However, I am not suggesting you need to go that far for your dogs, although some of my critics have levelled that accusation against me!

'BARF' is an acronym for 'Bones And Raw Food.' Hence the 'BARF diet' or the 'BARF programme.' This expression is not my invention. I have no idea who first used it, although I suspect it has come out of America.

However, no matter who invented it or where it came from, I am very grateful to its inventor because the word or expression BARF is a great shorthand way of presenting some vital dietary information.

The BARF diet as presented in **Grow Your Pups With Bones** is a simplified, more streamlined and more prescriptive version of the dietary programme I proposed in '**Give Your Dog a Bone.**' Since writing that book, I have received innumerable suggestions, questions, criticisms and experiences which have helped shape this present book and in particular have pointed strongly towards the 'BARF' diet.

The BARF diet is what dogs have eaten for several hundred thousand years, so it follows that they are very much used to eating it. In fact they actually require to eat the BARF diet if they are to become and remain healthy. And I do mean EVERY DOG OF EVERY BREED requires to be fed this way.

The BARF diet is precisely what we should be feeding our breeding animals to optimise their reproductive health and maximise their healthy longevity.

The BARF diet is the diet we should be feeding our growing pups to massively reduce the incidence of Bone and Joint disease and to promote truly healthy growth.

There is an important post script or PS to the BARF diet. PS stands for Plus Supplements. The supplements we add to the BARF diet are based on the modern concept of healthy life extension, using anti-oxidant vitamins and minerals together with phytochemicals, herbs, and similar products, all of which have life extending and health enhancing properties.

For a full explanation and introduction to the concept and philosophy of whole raw foods for dogs - i.e. - the BARF diet, I strongly suggest you read my first book **Give Your Dog a Bone.** That book, although it does not use the expression BARF, explains about the BARF diet in detail. Why and how it produces extreme health, why it is essential that the food be raw, the importance of bones, and much more. It also points out the consequences of feeding cooked and processed foods to our pets. Particularly commercial pet food.

The consequence of not feeding our dogs the BARF diet is a decline in their health. That decline in health includes problems such as dogs filled with cancer, dogs racked with arthritic pain, dogs unable to breathe or move because of heart failure, dogs that are vomiting, dehydrating and wasting away because of kidney failure.

Where the BARF diet is adopted, most health problems disappear.

In this book my concern is two-fold. Firstly to teach anybody who has anything to do with breeding how to use the BARF diet to vastly improve their whole breeding programme, and secondly to show the owners of growing pups how to produce healthy pups - free of bone and joint disease.

Let me stress from the outset that ONLY YOU can provide this sort of nutrition for your dog[s]. There is absolutely no one else that can do this for you. Certainly not a dog food company.

By adopting the BARF diet - you are becoming totally responsible for your dogs' health - and healthy they WILL become. My aim in all my writings is to return this power to you - the individual dog owner.

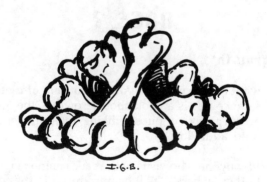

I.G.B.

CHAPTER TWO

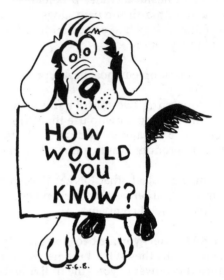

IS THE 'BARF' DIET SUITABLE FOR GROWING AND BREEDING DOGS ?

Diets for 'growth'

At this point I want to discuss with you the concept of diets for 'growth.' Why do that? Because this is a book about growth - the growth of pups inside their mum, the growth of pups drinking their mother's milk, and the growth of pups into adult dogs.

In today's world, anyone who visits vets, reads canine magazines, or talks to breeders and other 'experts,' will be introduced to the concept and the apparent need for special 'growth' foods for dogs. **The commercial dog food programme says that puppies, pregnant bitches and lactating bitches need 'growth foods,'** while adult non-reproducing dogs require a 'maintenance food' which is an entirely different product.

Special foods, 'designed for growth', have become part of the processed pet food programme. That programme says that foods designed for growing animals must have more nutrients that support growth compared to diets designed to maintain a grown animal in good health. It also says they must contain better quality nutrients.

This contrasts with the BARF programme, where top quality ingredients are used in all diets, and where there is much less difference between the various types of diets.

Since publishing **Give Your Dog a Bone** I have spoken with many dog owners and breeders who have been concerned that the BARF diet may not be suitable for growing, lactating or pregnant dogs. In other words that it is not suitable as a growth type of food. These are people who have been 'educated' to believe in the concept that dogs require vastly different foods as they pass through the various life stages.

We have to ask ourselves - "is the simple and apparently obvious concept of growth foods for dogs as laudable, useful, and worthwhile as it appears to be?"

Is such a concept part of basic undeniable 'truth,' or is the concept of special foods for growth yet another way we have been programmed to think by the pet food companies? Is it another device to convince us to follow the pet food programme?

Is this concept producing health or sickness? Does the concept of 'special growth foods' have a place in diets based on more biologically appropriate foods? How necessary or relevant is this concept for growing dogs when using the BARF programme?

Common sense tells us that our dogs' ancestors have grown and reproduced using the BARF diet without the 'benefit' of special foods for several hundred thousand years. In other words, our dogs' ancestors have grown properly, survived and reproduced on the same basic foods, no matter what stage of life they were at.

There is abundant evidence that the modern 'growth' foods - particularly the 'growth' foods for puppies - are part of the cause of the skeletal disease we are seeing at an ever increasing rate, in the larger and giant breeds of dogs. See Part Three for a full explanation.

'Growth' diets are a modern concept

It has to be appreciated that the concept of 'life stage foods' has come about because of the inadequacies of processed foods. When using the BARF diet, such 'modern wisdom' may largely be abandoned.

Those breeders and owners who genuinely implement the BARF method rapidly discover that it works brilliantly with little or no modification for all life stages.

They quickly discover that it may be fed to growing, pregnant or lactating dogs, or dogs at any other life stage, and produce exceptional results. Not only that, they also discover that it is far superior to any of the commercial products - and that includes the 'super premium foods.'

How life stage foods came to be

In the 1940's and 1950's when pet food manufacturers realised the potential profit to be had from pet foods, they also realised they had to produce a product which contained every nutrient [according to current knowledge] a dog required, all in the one product.

They had to produce the sort of product that vets would recommend and that people would continue to buy. **They were in fact attempting to copy the natural diet.**

Unfortunately they failed to reproduce that natural diet

There are many reasons why the commercial pet foods have never been close to a dog's natural diet. Those reasons include the fact that they are based on grain and that they are cooked. For a full explanation of the deficiencies of commercial dog food, please read **Chapter Three in Give Your Dog a Bone.**

One of the reasons that commercial pet foods fail to produce healthy dogs is that they do not follow the 'balanced over time' concept. That is, they do not consist of a series of products which when fed over a period of time will create a balanced diet. See **Chapter Six in Give Your Dog a Bone.**

Pet food manufacturers knew they could not sell a programme consisting of a number of different products. They knew they had to produce a single product that 'contained everything a dog needs.' That is why pet food manufacturers introduced the 'never heard of before' concept that every meal should be complete and balanced. In addition, the products they produced were also designed to cater for the needs of all classes of dogs, from growing puppies, through to old age and everything in between.

The product they developed became the 'general purpose' dog food. It is still the most popular dog food sold. It is the middle of the road product sold in supermarkets. This general purpose dog food is cheap [compared to the modern super premium dog foods] and it is widely available.

For this 'all purpose' product to be able to be fed to all classes of dogs AND be complete and balanced at every meal, the manufacturers had to make sure it contained sufficient nutrients to supply the extra needs of growing, pregnant, lactating and working dogs. This meant extra protein, minerals and energy in the form of fat had to be added to these foods.

When this 'complete and balanced all purpose' dog food is fed over a lifetime to the average desexed pet at home - which is a very common occurrence - the excessive levels of calcium, phosphorus, protein, salt and calories it contains results in the development of kidney disease, heart disease, obesity and many other degenerative diseases.

When this 'complete and balanced all purpose' product is fed to the growing puppy, particularly puppies of the giant breeds, it has the potential to cause skeletal problems such as Hip and Elbow Dysplasia. This is because it contains too much fat, protein, and calcium.

During the 1970's and 80's, a number of pet food manufacturers became aware that the all purpose pet food was the basic cause of a number of health problems such as skeletal problems in growing pups and also heart and renal disease.

That was the impetus for several of these pet food manufacturers to develop ...

... The 'life stage' foods

15

The 'life stage' foods are produced in an attempt to remedy the problems caused by the 'all-purpose' pet food. The new life stage foods include:

1] commercially produced 'maintenance' foods - These products are designed to maintain the non-active adult. These products have lower levels of protein, minerals and calories compared to all-purpose foods, working dog foods and growth foods. They are based on very poor quality materials. You can gauge this by the price. These are the foods which like the all purpose foods help lay the foundation for modern veterinary practice with its ever growing list of complicated degenerative diseases.

2] commercially produced 'working dog' foods - These products are designed [obviously] for working dogs - they have higher energy levels - that is , they contain more fat, although some manufacturers use misleading advertising. They advertise these products as being higher in protein. Manufacturers do this because they fear the public's negative reaction to the idea of extra fat. It should be noted that thirty years ago in Australia, working dogs kept on working well into their teens. Today they are lucky to be able to work past seven years of age. There is little doubt that this drop in longevity is because their diet has changed from a basic BARF type programme to commercial pet food.

3] commercially produced 'senior' foods - These products are designed to meet the needs of older dogs with failing kidneys and hearts and a weakened digestive system, which unfortunately are the legacy of a lifetime spent eating biologically inappropriate processed pet foods. The senior foods are more digestible and have lower levels of salt, phosphorus and protein. What they do not have is high levels of anti-oxidants and other life extending nutrients.

4] commercially produced 'prescription' foods - These products are designed to treat a broad range of diseases which - ironically - are caused by the other processed pet foods. The diseases these prescription foods treat are caused by the whole range of commercial dog foods, from the cheapest to the dearest, including both the all purpose products as well as the super premium foods!

5] commercially produced 'growth' foods - These products are designed to promote the **growth of puppies** and cater for the needs of **pregnant and lactating bitches. Commercially produced 'growth' foods ...**

- **are usually made from better quality base ingredients** compared to the very poor ingredients many manufacturers use in the 'maintenance' type foods.

However, that does not mean these commercially produced growth foods are to be recommended!

They have an enormous number of inherent flaws, not the least of which is the presence of high levels of - the dangerous to health - heat damaged polyunsaturated fatty acids.

The reason I have given you that information on the origins and nature of the commercially produced 'life stage' dog foods is so that you will begin to understand the simplicity, the superior nature and much greater health producing powers of the BARF diet.

The BARF diet, by comparison to the modern products, remains very much the same for all classes of dogs.

The BARF diet is always based on the same healthy high class foods. These foods are all equally digestible and equally healthy no matter what class of dog is being fed.

The BARF diet is in fact the healthy equivalent of that original 'all purpose' pet food; the product that the pet food manufacturers were trying to copy from nature.

However, where the commercial programme failed to produce such a product, the BARF diet succeeds beautifully. It CAN be fed to all classes of dogs with great confidence; instead of promoting disease like the commercially produced 'all-purpose' product, it actually promotes health and prevents disease.

The BARF diet can also fulfil all the requirements of the 'life stage' products. All you need do is vary the proportion of the different components of the diet. By doing so, you can very easily produce your own life stage foods - using the same basic ingredients. The BARF programme is indeed flexible and versatile!

When constructing a BARF diet for growth ...

... **all you need do is increase the total amount fed, and what you do feed should contain more structural material** - the mineral and protein foods, and perhaps some more energy foods. Exactly how you do that will be explained in detail as you continue reading **Grow Your Pups With Bones.**

However, just to put you in the picture, the simple change required is usually just an increase in the raw meaty bone component of the diet, and a decrease in the amount of vegetable material fed.

Let me emphasise that there is no change in the quality of the food that you use in the BARF programme. For a growth type of diet you feed the same HIGH QUALITY food you would normally use for the diet of a non-reproducing, non-growing, non-working dog.

Also note that when you construct a BARF diet for the growth of a puppy of one of the the giant breeds, you may well be reducing, not increasing, the levels of fat, protein and calcium in that diet! That is, you may well be decreasing the raw meaty bones and increasing the vegetable component of the diet in order to slow the growth rate of that giant breed puppy!

The excessive levels of protein, calories, and calcium in so many of the commercially produced - so called - 'growth foods for puppies' continue to be a major cause of skeletal problems in many of our larger breeds of dogs.

Even lactation, which is the most demanding time in a nutritional sense, requires very little change when using the BARF diet.

What I want you to take away from this chapter is CONFIDENCE.
I want you to be confident that **the BARF diet is superior to**
any commercial pet food programme, and
will definitely cater
for the needs of growing, pregnant and lactating animals.

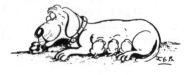

CHAPTER THREE

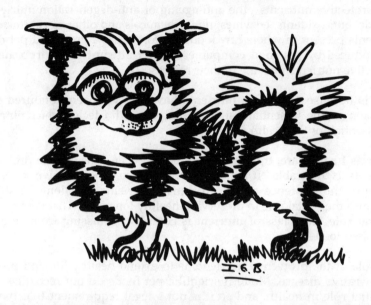

THE NUTRIENTS WHICH SUPPORT GROWTH

In the last chapter I discussed with you the concept of 'growth foods.' In this chapter we shall briefly examine the nutrients which support growth.

The nutrients which support growth are exactly the same nutrients as required for 'maintenance.' That is - proteins, minerals, vitamins, fats, carbohydrates - and also - the protective nutrients such as anti-oxidants, enzymes, phytochemicals [the masses of anti-ageing chemicals found in plants] and other anti-ageing nutrients, many of which probably remain undiscovered.

Growth diets should contain high levels of the protective nutrients

The protective nutrients - the anti-ageing or anti-degeneration nutrients - include anti-oxidants, enzymes, phytochemicals and other as yet unknown nutrients present in whole raw foods. Unfortunately, processed pet foods as produced by pet food companies do not attempt to incorporate the protective nutrients into any of their recipes.

That is because protective nutrients have not yet been honoured with inclusion on the 'essential' list by the 'experts' who decide which nutrients are essential for the health of our dogs.

So far as I am aware, those 'experts' do not even consider the protective nutrients as 'desirable.' It is possible those same experts may not even be aware of the existence of the protective nutrients, let alone be able to recognise their vital role in preserving healthy longevity! That is why, as a general rule, this class of nutrient is completely missing from modern processed foods.

The role of the protective nutrients is to extend healthy life and prevent degenerative disease. Modern scientific pet foods do not recognise their essential role in health, and so it is not a legal requirement that they be present in any pet foods. Their presence is vital to both the short and long term health of your dog[s]. These nutrients are a vital and essential component of the BARF programme. In fact they are present in abundance in the BARF programme. Their presence is part of the reason that dogs raised on the BARF programme develop healthy bones and joints and have very few reproductive problems.

Just remember that when you follow the BARF programme, most of these protective nutrients are 'naturally' present. Those which are not, are readily available from a health food store, or even the supermarket.

Let us now take a brief look at the other growth-supporting nutrients.

Proteins for growth

Proteins contribute most of the structural or building materials for growth. Growing pups, pregnant bitches, and bitches suckling a litter of puppies all need extra protein for growth or milk production, on top of their requirements to maintain their body in good order. That is the reason modern comercially produced 'growth' diets are designed with extra protein. The better ones contain protein of superior quality. Good quality proteins have a high proportion of the essential amino acids. For more information on the essential amino acids, please consult Chapter Five in **Give Your Dog a Bone.**

The BARF diet by comparison with the commercial programme contains superior quality proteins at ALL times.

The most logical source of good quality protein is raw meaty bones. Chicken pieces including the wings, necks, and carcases are excellent. Chicken pieces contain plenty of first class protein which is found in the skin, the flesh, the bone, and the marrow. This high quality protein is easily digestible. The BARF programme feeds this superior quality protein to ALL classes of dog, whether they are growing or not.

Chicken pieces can form the basis of a Bones and Raw Food Programme for both cats and dogs. This is because by themselves they are almost a balanced diet for both these species. They contain B complex vitamins, fat soluble vitamins and are an excellent source of bone, with all the valuable factors that bones contribute. They also contain high levels of the Omega-6 essential fatty acids.The marrow also contains high levels of blood forming nutrients.

With lamb off-cuts it is often necessary to remove the fat. Young beef bones - for example ox-tails - are excellent eating for all dogs. Just note that both lamb and beef have lower levels of essential fatty acids compared to chicken.

The larger beef bones make 'great chewing' for all breeds, but be careful of the **older** harder bones, as these are the ones most likely to damage teeth. However, that does not mean your dog should miss out on these bigger bones. Make sure the ones you give your dog[s] are from a young animal.

These big bones are a valuable source of cartilage. Cartilage is an essential protein-based nutrient for joint growth in dogs. More recently it has also been recognised as an anti-degeneration and anti-ageing food, becoming widely used in the treatment of some forms of cancers in humans.

This is another one of those 'recently discovered' reasons that dogs raised and maintained on the BARF diet are so healthy and rarely develop any of the degenerative diseases such as arthritis or cancer.

For more details on protein and bones refer to Chapter Seven in **Give Your Dog a Bone.**

Other sources of concentrated high quality protein include cottage cheese - an excellent source of branch chain amino acids - and best of all - whole raw eggs.

You can also achieve a balanced protein with all the essential amino acids using a combination of approximately equal amounts of grains and legumes. See Chapter Twenty One in **Give Your Dog a Bone.**

A word of warning: too much protein in a growth diet for puppies of the giant breeds has been shown to be a major underlying cause of such problems as Hip and Elbow Dysplasia.

Uitamins for growth

The important message so far as vitamins are concerned is - be prepared to supplement. A 'growth' diet most definitely requires high levels of vitamins. Those vitamins must be supplied at the third level - the 'vitamins in abundance level' - as described in **Give Your Dog a Bone.** This means high levels of the B group, vitamin C, and the fat soluble vitamins, A, D, E and K.

Please note that these vitamins are present in large amounts in fresh whole raw foods. That is, fruit and vegetables and raw organ meats and raw meaty bones. Also in nuts, legumes and grains.

Vitamins are required for basic bodily processes, and to support the extra work of growth, reproduction and lactation.

It is important to fully understand the role of vitamins in canine health, so for more details on vitamins and their functions in the BARF programme, consult both Chapter Five in **Give Your Dog a Bone** and the relevant chapters in **Grow Your Pups With Bones**. One example of the care required when supplementing with vitamins is the danger of adding too much vitamin A to a pregnant bitch's diet.

Want to know more about vitamins and growth? Good. Keep reading and do not be concerned; all will be made clear so read on!

Fats required for growth

Growing, pregnant and lactating dogs need extra energy and the most concentrated form of energy is fat. That fat MUST contain high levels of the essential fatty acids. Fats are part of the basic structural materials that make up every membrane of every cell in your dog's body. Raw chicken fat has high levels of the Omega-6 group of essential fatty acids. The Omega-3 group are best obtained from raw cold pressed linseed oil or fish oil. They are also present in green leafy vegetables.

If the Omega-3 group of essential fatty acids are not at sufficiently high levels in the diet of a pregnant bitch or a young pup, there will not be full development of the brain or the retina of the eyes of puppies.

That is one reason why foods rich in the Omega-3 group of essential fatty acids such as fish oil or cold pressed flax seed oil must be part of the pregnant and lactating bitch's diet. Those oils must also be part of the diet fed to puppies from weaning onwards. It is in the latter third of pregnancy and the first couple of months after birth that the puppies' eyes and brain are developing and growing rapidly.

When feeding foods high in these essential fatty acids, you must supplement with vitamin E to prevent them becoming rancid and therefore poisonous - in the dog's body.

Care is also required because there are occasions where adding extra fats to a growth type diet can cause major problems. The occasions I refer to involve pregnant bitches and growing pups - particularly pups of the giant breeds. Want to know more? Good. Keep reading. All of this shall be discussed in detail.

Before leaving the topic of fats, do be aware that all cooked and processed foods contain damaged fats. Any fat that has been heated above 160 degrees centigrade is by definition damaged, and will damage your dog. This means that the so called super premium foods with their high levels of polyunsaturates are the most dangerous products of all in this respect.

Minerals for growth

All dogs need minerals as part of their diet, but growing dogs have a need for higher levels. This is particularly true of diets designed for growing pups and lactating mums. However, great care is required because there are occasions where adding extra calcium to a 'growth' type diet can cause major problems. The occasions I refer to involve pregnant bitches and growing pups - particularly pups of the giant breeds. You don't understand? You want to know more? Good. Keep reading. You will not be disappointed. This too shall be discussed.

In the meantime, be reassured. If you feed plenty of raw meaty bones as the basis of the diet you feed to your dog - of any age or breed or life stage, there is no way you can feed too much calcium.

Growth diets should be RAW!

In common with any other biologically appropriate diet for dogs, let me remind you that the best type of growth diet is a raw food diet. So long as the bulk of that growth type diet is raw, then most of your dog's enzyme and anti-oxidant needs will be met. This is a major reason why processed foods have such a poor success rate, not only as growth diets, but in all modern feeding situations.

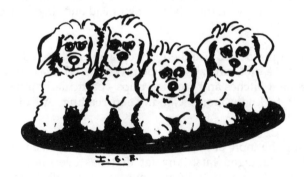

I. G. R.

CHAPTER FOUR

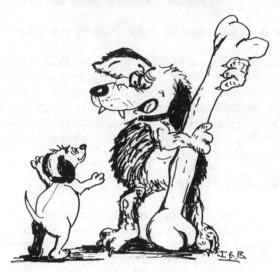

WHAT YOU WILL NEED
TO PRODUCE THE BARF DIET

The first thing you will need is a supply of raw meaty bones ...

These raw meaty bones will form the basis of the BARF diet. I strongly suggest you source some chicken or possibly turkey waste. Turkeys are probably more available for some people in the United States. The following remarks apply equally to chicken, turkey or even duck scraps.

The waste will include wings, necks, backs - whatever. It will also include carcases or frames. The frame is what is left when most of the flesh has been removed from one of these birds. It consists of bone, cartilage, fat and a little bit of flesh. The ratio of flesh to bone, cartilage, and fat is ideal in wings, backs, necks and frames. Other scraps and waste need to be evaluated and used intelligently to achieve the required balance of these components, according to the needs of the animals you are feeding.

Sometimes whole birds will become available for you. That is fine, but don't feed them all the time. There is not enough bone and too much flesh.

Where do you get these raw meaty bones?

The individual dog owner will either buy them from a butcher or similar, or join with a breeders' or owners' buying co-operative - which I am about to describe. In addition, be on the look-out for companies and individuals who have begun to produce, supply, package and distribute this sort of food for our pets. They are the new age pet food companies. However, if you do decide to use their services, be a good consumer and evaluate their products and claims carefully!

Forming a co-operative

It is a good idea to form a co-operative with other breeders or dog owners and buy your raw meaty bones in bulk. You will need to find a chicken or turkey processing plant that will sell you their scraps. You will be competing with pet food manufacturers to buy these scraps, but in so doing you are turning a waste product into healthy rather than harmful food for your dogs. Use a processor whose slaughtering and processing methods are hygienic and who will supply this material fresh, in bulk, free of harmful chemicals of any description, and at a reasonable price..

Make sure the birds they process have not been raised on a diet chock full of hormones. If you cannot be sure, it may be worthwhile looking to some organic source.

Someone may wish to start a business

This is happening a lot all over Australia. It is happening in the UK. America is an ideal country for starting a business of this nature. Such a business can be as little or as big as your imagination can make it. It usually starts with one person or family buying the chicken or turkey scraps and packaging them into convenient sizes and grades - e.g. 2 lb [1 kg] lots of necks etc.. They store the product in freezers and arrange its distribution to other members of the co-operative or buyers' group. The benefits they receive in profits - even with a modest mark up - have the potential to be enormous. If they supply a consistently worthwhile product the demand will skyrocket. The person or group who runs this business will also benefit from very cheap dog food.

There may be one of these businesses near you. They will advertise in all the popular pet magazines so be on the look-out for them, but also - as I have mentioned - scrutinise such businesses carefully.

You also need a supply of larger bones ...

And/or 'off-cuts' from a butcher. Not the old really hard ones, of course. While our dogs are happily gnawing away at these larger, rougher and less meatier bones, a number of functions vital to their health are being performed. Those bones are cleaning the dogs' teeth and massaging the gums. Something modern foods cannot do and that owners should not have to do. They also provide what I call eating exercise. An isometric form of exercise where most of the dog's body is used and stressed in a healthy way for extended periods as it rips and tears at the bones. This is important at every stage of a dog's life from about three weeks of age onwards. Bones also satisfy a psychological need that dogs have to eat in this way. They are very calming for a dog - rather like an all day sucker or a healthy 'cigarette' for dogs.

When actually consumed as opposed to merely gnawed and sucked at, bones are nutritionally valuable. For your dog they are a source of high quality proteins, fats, fat soluble vitamins and also cartilage, which is so essential for joint health. They are your dog's most important source of minerals - and that includes calcium. They supply many blood forming elements including iron from the marrow. As you can see - bones are SO important!

You need a source of offal ...

Such as liver, kidney, brain, heart, etc., etc.. All fresh and raw. These may be cut into convenient sized pieces and stored in the freezer. They must have come from a reputable source - having passed through a meat inspection process. If you can obtain offal from battery raised chickens or turkeys - there will be no problem with parasites. Offal, particularly in its raw state, is a valuable source of nutrients, including high class protein, essential fatty acids, minerals, vitamins and so on. Very important food for your dog.

You need a source of vegetable material ...

Vegetables play a vital role in the health of dogs, and the importance of using vegetables to ensure your dog's health cannot be stressed enough. The omission of vegetable material from the modern dog's diet is the biggest nutritional error we make, apart from our failure to feed raw meaty bones. The lack of vegetable material - of the right kind - is one of the greatest contributors to the modern dog's ill health - including the inability to maximise and optimise fertility.

What vegetables should you be feeding?

The answer to that is very simple. Any of the vegetables. Whatever vegetables are in season. WHATEVER YOU CAN LAY YOUR HANDS ON. Green leafy vegetables, such as silver beet, spinach, celery, members of the cabbage family, capsicum, root vegetables such as carrots and sugar beet, and whatever fruit is in season or you can get hold of, including such things as tomatoes, apples, oranges, pears, mangoes, grapes, bananas - whatever. The wider the variety the better. Each different fruit and vegetable contributes a different set of nutrients.

Fruit should preferably be well ripened to over-ripe. It is an excellent source of simple sugars - the non complex carbohydrates. These supply instant energy as opposed to the slowly released energy from complex carbohydrates. The raw fruit contains health promoting factors usually destroyed by heat. As a source of sugar fruit also contains the element chromium which ensures the sugar is used properly and does not become a cause of sugar diabetes. The fruit also contains healthy fibre.

If you have only one or two dogs you may get enough from household scraps and fruit and vegetable peelings which you supplement with extra fruit and vegetables you buy specifically for the dogs. If you have more than one or two dogs I suggest you go ahead and buy fruit and vegetables specially for your dogs. Some breeders buy the pulp from a commercial source, such as a fruit juice producing factory.

Always make sure the vegetables and fruits that you use have been washed thoroughly to remove chemical sprays etc., because you DO want to use the outside bits. They are usually the most concentrated source of vital nutrients.

Dried fruits and vegetables are an excellent source of concentrated simple sugars, fibre and chromium. The most healthy ones are the ones without added oil - the sun dried ones. The dried fruits have a role to play in treating and preventing constipation because they are a concentrated source of fibre.

Vegetable material MUST be suitably processed ...

All the vegetable material will need to be processed before it becomes useful to your dog[s] as food. By that I mean totally crushed. Not cooked and not grated. I cannot emphasise enough the fact that all the vegetable material must be presented to your dogs in a RAW and totally broken down state. For this you will need a blender and a juicer. Both need to be robust machines. They will be getting a lot of work. For the "seriously keen to use the BARF diet" person, you should buy very strong domestic units, or better still, the commercial type. You will need a very strong blender when making some puppy and/or invalid foods from chicken pieces with bone.

You will recall that when I introduced the concept of the BARF diet, I said you did not have to vomit for your dog. While that is true, let me point out that what I am describing here, in many ways fulfils that role for your dog.

Much of the vegetable material [vegetable material means vegetables and fruit], you will put through the juicer. The juice is saved to be drunk by the family [humans] or the dogs. If it is being saved for more than a few hours - freeze it. If it is to be used in the next couple of hours refrigerate it. Other vegetables, and fruit in particular will go straight into the blender. To ensure the blades pick this material up - add some of the previously saved juice.

You will want to vary the moisture content of the vegetable mix depending on how you are presenting it to your dog. It can be presented as a 'soup' type meal or as a more solid patty or lump or 'cake.' You will do this by varying the proportions of pulp and juice from the juicer to the blended material from the blender. The pulp from the juicer is dry, the juice is obviously very moist and the blended material is somewhere in between.

You will need minced meat ...

... from chicken, beef, pork, lamb etc. It must be fresh with no chemical preservatives in it. Be very suspicious of any commercially prepared pet mince. If it is straight mince, make sure it is lean. If you are making it from the necks, wings, carcases etc. it will obviously have some fat in it - and the bones. You can make this on a small scale using chicken wings and necks etc. by breaking up the raw material with a cleaver and then finishing the process off in your blender. If you need large amounts and you don't have the necessary equipment you may choose to employ some commercial organisation to do this for you. In Australia, many people get their butcher to do this for them.

Please note ...

... it is important that the mince you use be free of preservatives and other foreign chemicals, as well as being freshly and hygienically sourced and minced. To ensure that is so, do shop around for your raw materials very carefully. Pet shops have been known to keep adding a little more preservative to their mince every day until it is sold. If you buy it after a week or so of this treatment, you have bought a dangerous product.

You will need a source of health promoting oil ...

Genuinely never been heated at any stage and kept away from light and oxygen. What you are looking for is - **cold pressed - under nitrogen - in the dark - nutritional grade** linseed and/or hemp oil. You can also use olive oil [in addition - not in place of these]. The olive oil must also be cold pressed and extra virgin. This is the only oil you can buy from the supermarket and be confident that it is a healthy oil. You will also need Cod liver oil. It too must be a product that has never been heated at any stage and one that has been kept away from light and oxygen. Cold pressed and fresh. Buy from a health food store with a good turn-over of product.

When you feed your dogs the healthy oils that I am recommending, you must also feed appropriate anti-oxidants. That is, vitamin E, vitamin C, the B vitamins, zinc, chromium, selenium, magnesium etc. At this point - human grade supplements are to be recommended. Bones, kelp, possibly brewer's yeast, fresh vegetables and offal will all help.

Storing these oils

All of these oils must be stored in the refrigerator [or the freezer] - at all times - in light proof, air tight containers. The Cod liver oil, flax and Hemp seed oil must be used up within 6 to 8 weeks of being opened. I would suggest you buy them directly from the manufacturers where possible. Butter is OK, or better than OK if it has come from raw milk, but the oils I am recommending - cod liver, linseed and hemp - are far superior because of their high content of the essential fatty acids, the Omega-3's and the Omega-6's.

These health promoting oils - in their fresh raw unadulterated state - are vital for your dogs' health. They are missing from all modern processed foods - or if added, have been transformed by heat, light and oxygen into a dangerous form by the time they reach you and your dog[s].

The oils you should not feed to your dog ...

Do not use old oils. They are rancid and dangerous. Never ever use oils that have been used for cooking - they are even more dangerous. Do not use ordinary vegetable oils from the supermarket. They have been heat treated and are dangerous. Never use margarine. It is a product containing many artificial chemicals - a danger to your dogs' and your own health. Do not buy your oils from any place where they have been sitting out on a shelf, not refrigerated, not in light proof containers, and not in air proof containers. If they smell rancid or taste bitter when you open them - do not use them. Note well, it is in this heat affected and therefore dangerous form they are presented to you in all the super premium dog foods.

You will need a source of healthy bacteria ...

That is - good quality, low fat yoghurt from the supermarket or Probiotics from the health food store.. These are essential for bowel health and for general health. Vital for newborn pups particularly where they or the bitch have been treated with antibiotics.

You will need a source of various vitamins ...

To maximise your dogs' health, and in particular to maximise their fertility, you will most definitely need to supply extra vitamins. These include the multi-B vitamins, vitamin E and vitamin C - preferably in powder form, to mix through the other foods. You may freeze any of the vitamins with the exception of vitamin E. It may be that freezing harms this vitamin. Until there is definite information on this, add vitamin E to your food mixes when they are just about to be fed, but not to food that you intend to freeze.

You will need a source of good quality Kelp powder [or tablets] ...

Kelp is absolutely vital as a source of minerals. The sea is the storehouse of every mineral present on earth, and kelp contains them all. It is the perfect mineral supplement, and this includes selenium and iodine. The selenium is a vital immune-system-stimulating and anti-ageing nutrient. Iodine is essential for maintaining your dog's metabolic rate. It is a vital ingredient for reproduction and growth of puppies. The only safe form in which to supply it is kelp which can safely be fed in abundance. Iodine is often in very short supply in modern soils due to overcropping and modern fertilisers. It can also be lacking in places like Australia where it has been leached out of the landscape over time. The result is that iodine is absent or in short supply in many modern foods.

You will need eggs

Try and find a source of good quality, preferably organic and free range - hens' or ducks' or whatever - eggs. They are a cheap source of top quality protein, vitamin A, and minerals. If you can get free range eggs, these also contain good levels of the essential fatty acids.

You will need a source of honey

Good quality, preferably cold extracted - honey. An excellent source of simple sugars - the non complex carbohydrates, providing instant energy as opposed to the slowly released energy from complex carbohydrates. Useful in many different circumstances with breeding adults and growing pups. The good thing about honey is that it keeps.

Always have some honey on hand. **Raw honey contains health promoting factors usually destroyed by heat. As a source of sugar it also contains the element chromium which ensures the sugar is used properly and does not become a cause of sugar diabetes.**

You will need a source of milk

Ideally it will be raw milk from a reputable source - that is - from disease free goats or cows. Failing that, use pasteurised, long-life or powdered milk. Liquid milk can be frozen if required.

An optional requirement is grain

That is, 'feed' grain, such as wheat, or corn or barley etc.. There are two ways to use this as dog food. Firstly, it may be fed when it has been freshly sprouted - in this case you treat it as any other vegetable material. The second way is to 'process' it in the following way: it has to be both crushed and soaked. The grain must be soaked in water or raw vegetable juice or milk for at least twelve hours - overnight for example. It can be soaked first and then crushed by a food processor/juicer, or it can be ground into flour and then soaked. The grain that has been processed in this way can be added to a vegetable meal where extra concentrated calories - but not fat - may be needed. Rolled oats may be fed in place of the other grains using the soaked and crushed method, but because rolled oats has been heat treated, it does not have the same nutritional benefits as living grain.

The question of bacteria and parasites in raw foods

This issue has been covered in **Give Your Dog a Bone.** The hydatid problem being dealt with in Chapter Nine, and the question of bacterial contamination with such bacteria as   E. Coli, Salmonella and Campylobacter jejuni being discussed in Chapter Seven on page 135.

However, let me stress with regard to the question of bacteria, that these organisms are ubiquitous. Especially E coli. Human faeces is full of it. Leave food out in a warm place all day and whammo - Salmonella poisoning. Where did it come from? The food handlers. Do you cook chicken for your family at home? If so you handle raw chicken. If you handle raw chicken you are handling all three of those bacteria. It would be impossible not to.

Do realise we have all consumed these three and countless other bacteria as shall your children - and hopefully your dogs - over time.

You doubtless have antibodies in your body to all of these bacteria. In all probability, so do your dogs. If we and our dogs are to become resistant to these bugs we have to 'contact' them. The only individuals who MAY need protection from these bugs are those with AIDS.

A dog's immune system is designed to handle those three bacteria and many more. It is much more adept at this than our immune system. Dogs are amongst other things scavengers by nature. They actually thrive on bacteria-ridden food in their natural state. However, when you 'cotton wool' the dogs of an entire nation - AS IS HAPPENING IN THE UNITED STATES FOR EXAMPLE - that is, feed them nothing but heat sterilised food, you are depriving them of the opportunity to develop an immune response to these and many other organisms.

That is why in America there is the unusual situation of dogs sometimes not being able to mount an attack on these particular bacteria. They are immune deficient in that they have no natural immunity to these organisms, having never come across them before. In addition, their immune system is also compromised because the heat sterilised food they eat is not capable of building a healthy immune system in the way that a biologically appropriate raw whole natural diet is able.

With respect to parasites that may be present in some meats in some countries, first let me say that I shall not attempt to cover this question in detail. That would require a whole book.

However, **there are two simple principles which may be safely employed where there is any possibility of parasitic contamination of your dogs' food.**

The meat and bones you use should:

1] either be sourced from those species that do not carry that particular parasite, or ...

2] they should be sourced from farms that guarantee freedom from the parasites in question. Farms which grow the so called 'specific pathogen free stock.'

CHAPTER FIVE

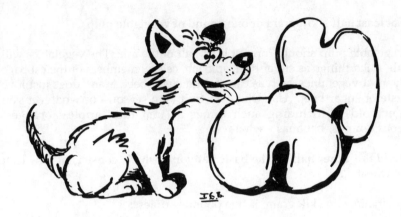

THE BARF DIET

Once you have all the material as described in Chapter Four,   feeding your dogs a healthy BARF diet becomes absurdly easy.

The two basic foods that you will feed will be

1] the Raw Meaty Bones and
2] the vegetable mix - or patties - which contains just about everything else.

HEALTHY PATTIES FOR YOUR DOGS

We devised these when one of our own dogs would not eat vegetables. Since that time they have become the second arm of the BARF diet - the first arm being the raw meaty bones.

The patties are based on half raw crushed vegetables and/or fruit, the other half being raw lean minced meat.

To make one kilogram or two pounds of basic patty mixture

Take at least half a kilogram or one pound of vegetable pulp ...

The vegetable pulp should form at least half of the mix. The vegetables will include such things as silver beet, spinach, celery, members of the cabbage family, root vegetables such as carrots and sugar beet. Many dogs just love the taste of sugar beet. Use whatever fruit is in season - or whatever you can get hold of including such things as tomatoes, apples, oranges, mangoes, grapes, bananas - whatever.

Now add the other half of the basic patty mix which consists of raw lean minced meat ...

Approximately one kilogram or two pounds - or less.

This raw minced lean meat should only form at the most half or preferably less than half of the patty mix. It can be virtually any lean mince - beef, buffalo, chicken, rabbit, turkey, lamb, pork, kangaroo - whatever. It may be minced chicken or turkey wings or necks, in which case, because wings and necks contain bones, the mince will be more fatty and will of course contain the all important bone.

To the mixture of vegetable pulp and raw lean mince we add such things as

Yoghurt - low fat and plain - say half a small tub.
Eggs - raw and preferably free range - about three.
Flax seed oil - 2 or 3 dessert spoons
Raw Liver - a quarter of a lamb's liver
Garlic - 1 or 2 cloves
Kelp powder - 2 or 3 teaspoons
B vitamins and vitamin C - a mega dose - see **Chapter Five in Give Your Dog a Bone.**

You may also add other healthy food scraps - such as small amounts of cooked vegetables, rice, cottage cheese etc.. Do note however, that these should make up no more than 25 % of the total patty mixture.

Also note that food scraps of this nature are more likely to be available for individual dogs in families rather than to large numbers of dogs in a breeding or boarding kennel.

IMPORTANT

It is ESSENTIAL that your dog eats everything you have put in the mix, so MAKE SURE THE WHOLE LOT IS MIXED INTO ONE HOMOGENEOUS MASS THAT YOUR DOG[S] CANNOT SEPARATE AND THEREFORE PICK AND CHOOSE the bits they do and don't want.

Any surplus not fed on the day - should be formed into patties, frozen then thawed out and used as required. Add the vitamin E just before you feed the patties. E.g. for a 25 lb dog, give 200 i.u. daily.

These patties can be fed when your dog is most hungry. If that is at night - for example - then feed the raw meaty bones in the morning. If you are feeding only once a day you may alternate these two meals. The raw meaty bones one day, the patties the next.

Feed your dog cod liver oil every day, e.g., for a 25 kg dog, give 3 to 4 ml daily.

You can make as much or as little patty mix as you like

Let me emphasise that the above healthy patty recipe may be scaled up or down. It all depends on how much you need, how much freezer space you have for storing it, how much you want to make and freeze ahead of time and what sort of equipment you have to produce it.

Modifying the BARF diet

The basic BARF diet **may** need modification - depending on whether you are feeding the male stud dog, puppies, teenage dogs, young bitches before they come on heat for the first time, empty bitches between cycles, bitches coming on heat, bitches being mated, bitches in the first half of pregnancy, bitches in the second half of pregnancy, bitches just prior to giving birth, bitches that have given birth, bitches in early lactation, bitches in mid lactation, bitches in late lactation, bitches when the pups are being weaned, bitches when the pups have been weaned and dry bitches. All of this will be discussed in the relevant chapters. Other factors influencing the composition of the BARF diet include the need for individual animals to gain or lose weight, and the presence of varying disease problems such as allergies, diabetes, cancer, arthritis etc. etc..

FOR DETAILS CONCERNING ...

... The BARF programme for puppies

Please turn to Chapter Twenty Two in Part Three of **Grow Your Pups With Bones.**

... The BARF programme for Pregnancy

Please turn to Chapter Four in Part Two of **Grow Your Pups With Bones.**

... The BARF programme for lactation

Please turn to Chapter Seven in Part Two of **Grow Your Pups With Bones.**

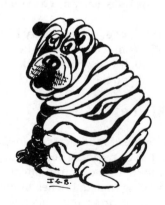

PART TWO

FEEDING FOR BREEDING

INTRODUCTION

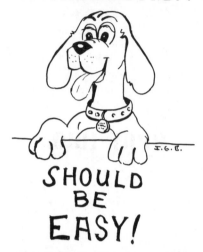

SHOULD BE EASY!

Dog breeding can be fraught with difficulty

Talk to any vet who works for breeders and you will wonder how it is that any pups are born at all. A major headache seems to be getting bitches pregnant. Sometimes it is because the male is impotent or does not produce sperm. More commonly it is because we have difficulty deciding when it is **she** should be mated. Then there seems to be an increasing need for artificial insemination because of some other problem with either him or her.

However, the problems do not stop there. **She** seems to have no end of problems including bizarre patterns of cycling, infections of the reproductive tract, failure to conceive, foetal resorption, abortions, small litters, assisted births, caesarean sections, pups born weak and sickly, pups born dead, post partum haemorrhage, retained after-births, poor milk supply, toxic milk, no milk, mastitis, fading puppy syndrome, birth defects such as cleft palates, holes in skulls, no brains, the intestines hanging out, deformed limbs, eyes missing etc....... The list is seemingly endless.

Quite apart from the problems associated with getting pups on the ground, between 15% and 40% of all puppies born do not make it to three months of age.

When breeding problems arise - as they inevitably seem to ...

It is tempting to believe that many of them are either inherited or due to a 'build up of disease' in the kennels. While that is often the case, and even if it is, ninety nine times out of a hundred, EVERY one of those problems disappears when the kennel is switched to a BARF diet. This is because most of these problems have their origins in a depleted immune system which leads to both a build up of disease in the kennel, and a greater susceptibility to disease. It gets worse. What is being fed may also have allowed a genetic weakness to surface as disease.

What I want you to fix firmly in your mind is the good news

Practically every one of the problems faced by dog breeders can be fixed by switching the dogs in their care to the BARF programme. This is because most of the problems encountered while breeding dogs are caused by poor food choices for breeding stock at all stages of their lives.

Most of the poor food choices involve processed foods, despite the fact that these nutritionally inadequate products are praised by both vets and breeders alike as the 'only way to feed dogs.' They are the basic cause of so many breeders' woes, particularly the dry foods. And no, I don't only mean the cheap ones, I also mean the highly expensive 'super premium' foods.

When breeders can be persuaded to switch diets ...

... to take their dogs off the commercial product and start on the BARF programme, over a period of time, the vast majority of the breeding problems I have mentioned begin to disappear. Much to their amazement and relief.

For example, kennels with a history of caesareans and assisted births find that the incidence of these drops dramatically when they switch their dogs to the BARF programme. But be warned. Some problems do not disappear overnight. This is not a programme for the impatient person craving instant results.

You will have to be patient

Many changes do occur suddenly. Changes such as the over-all health of the bitch, the puppies and the stud dog. The incidence of gross malformations of puppies will drop sharply, and eventually disappear entirely.

Problems such as infertility and chronic infections improve only slowly and still require the assistance of antibiotics and other drugs. But improve they do as the depleted immune system returns to health.

Bitches with problems, particularly older bitches that have been on commercial dog food for most of their life, can take more than a year or even longer to become sufficiently healthy to produce a healthy trouble free litter. Unfortunately, even the best of diets may not be able to change the results of a lifetime of poor quality food. In many cases, particularly where the problem involves either an infertile male, or a bitch that is over five or six years of age, it will be more prudent to start again with younger healthier stock and feed them correctly from the start.

Many breeders who begin and stick with the BARF programme, report improvements which take place over several generations, indicating the long term effects of both good and bad nutrition.

The important message I have is that it is possible to make most reproductive problems disappear. Permanently. You can produce big litters of healthy robust pups with very little hassle - AND - a bitch that breezes through the whole procedure with no problems - emerging the picture of health.

Never forget the male dog

If you are having problems getting bitches into pup, do investigate the fertility of the male as one of the first things you do. Modern feeding practices can raise a magnificent looking male with not a single sperm in sight. See Chapter One of Part One for more details on this important topic.

What are your aims as a breeder?

What are you aiming or shooting for as a breeder? I don't mean your genetic aims, I can only guess at those; I mean your aims in terms of puppy production and bitch health? The answers are pretty simple. You will be shooting for maximum fertility, an easy birth with your bitches remaining healthy and fully fertile.

By maximum fertility ...

... I mean you will want a fully fertile male. A male that can continue his stud career well into his old age.

You will want your bitch to come on heat, strongly and regularly, every 7 months or so, be able to conceive easily, to carry the pregnancy through with no resorption or abortions or toxaemia and produce a good-sized litter of pups which are robust, vigorous healthy pups of even size with no abnormalities. You will want her to do this well into old age.

By old age I do not mean six years of age. I mean nine years for a giant dog, and twelve to fifteen years for one of the smaller breeds such as a poodle.

Note that you are shooting for the optimum number of pups ...

... for your particular breed. Born with a birth weight ideal for your breed, that go on to be healthy adults. You are not aiming for the maximum number of pups. When there are too many pups, they are usually too small and fewer survive.

You will want her to give birth with ease – no assistance required

Obviously, if you have a breed or a line of dogs where the pups' heads are actually bigger than the birth canal, then no diet on earth can stop the need for a caesarean section; except one that caused severe stunting which would never be a good idea.

Apart from that, numerous breeders have discovered and are discovering that switching to the BARF diet has entirely eliminated the need for both assisted births and caesarean sections.

Without milk there are no pups

You will want your bitch to produce ample milk of good quality and be able to raise her whole litter with no losses, all in excellent health. No fading litters, no milk fever or Eclampsia; ready to go again next time she cycles.

The quality and quantity of milk produced by a breeding bitch is totally dependent upon diet. Feeding for milk production starts prior to mating - about three generations previous - and is continued during pregnancy. More of that in Chapter Seven - Feeding the Lactating Bitch.

In a nutshell, mating and conception should be followed by 63 days of healthy pregnancy, which terminates in an easy birth of healthy strong and vigorous puppies, who will go on to be healthy adult dogs.

That is what all breeders aim for, but which few attain. Very rarely will a breeder be able to say ... "Yes, my breeding programme is just like that - trouble free - no problems - everything always goes smoothly, plenty of healthy puppies, and a superbly healthy bitch that is able to produce large litters of healthy pups well into old age."

If you cannot say yes to all of that but would like to, be assured you have right now the opportunity to find out how your breeding programme can be exactly like that. So keep reading!

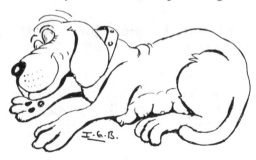

CHAPTER ONE

BASIC NUTRITION

FOR HIM

AND HER

AND THE KIDS

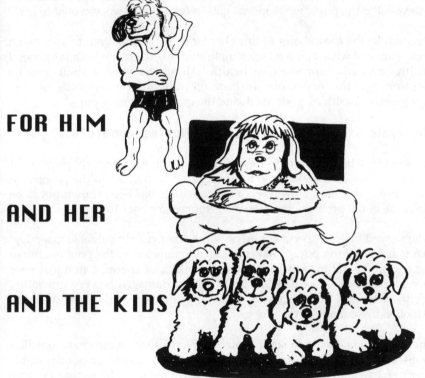

This chapter is here to tell you that HE IS IMPORTANT!

It is not uncommon for breeders to focus their attention on the female dog when it comes to special diets and super-nutrition. Sometimes **she** is plied with various supplements and extra fresh food - and rightly so - while the poor old male dog is spared very little thought. It is just assumed he will do his job, with nothing special in the way of nutrition being required.

If you need to learn about the nutrition of the male stud dog ...

... and if you have one, that means you - this is the chapter to read. I am devoting this one chapter to him, but he still has to share it with mum and the kids, because much of the information in this chapter applies equally to them. Do note that the whole of Part Three of **Grow Your Pups With Bones** is devoted to the pups, while mum gets most of Part Two devoted to her.

Meanwhile, the central aim of this chapter is to inspire you to take much greater care of what you feed your male stud dog to ensure both his general health and his reproductive health. Along the way, I shall also be mentioning the enormous impact of individual nutrients on the reproductive health of your bitch and the growth of young pups..

The male stud dog is a much neglected creature

Particularly when it comes to reproduction. If there is a fertility problem, it is common for all the attention to be focussed on her, when the problem is quite often with him. However, once the female has been shown not to be the cause of the problem, then the focus must come back to him.

When asked to do a 'sperm count' on some 'particularly valuable male dog' that is not fathering pups, I never cease to be amazed by the poor quality of the semen. Sometimes there is a complete lack of sperm. Often just very low sperm counts. Occasionally I see lots of damaged or very unhealthy sperm with very low activity. I am also amazed at the lack of libido exhibited by so many of these dogs.

The question is - **why do some male dogs have such an enormous fertility problem?** Why do they have a low libido, or no sperm, or poorly viable sperm, particularly when their owners assure me that "he is always given the best of everything." The answer turns out to be very simple. Just as it does with most female infertility.

These dogs are **not** given the best of everything. Far from it. Almost one hundred percent of these male stud dogs are infertile because they have not been, and are not being fed properly. Despite the protests of their owners to the contrary.

Unfortunately, as breeders come to rely more and more on commercially produced pet food to feed their dogs, the problem of both male and female infertility is becoming increasingly common.

A common complaint from breeders with valuable but useless male dogs goes something like ... **"how do street dogs that nobody cares for, get bitches pregnant, while stud dogs with all the 'advantages' of vets and scientific food and drugs etc., fail so miserably?"**

The answer is simple. The dog on the street produces healthy viable semen and has a high libido because of its broadly based, relatively nutritious, and relatively healthy diet.

The street dog feasts on raw [and cooked] meaty bones and numerous scraps which have come from all sorts of foods including green leafy vegetables, fruit, organ meats, dairy foods, eggs and so on.

The street dog is fortunate enough to lack the 'advantage' of a steady diet of artificial synthetic foods with their narrow spectrum of nutrients, their damaged fats and proteins, their high chemical and grain levels, their high levels of artificial calcium, salt and sugar, their low levels of natural anti-oxidants, enzymes, available micro nutrients and phytochemicals etc. etc..

And by far the worst food ...

... so far as its ability to support reproduction is concerned, is dry dog food. Yet the dry dog foods are the most popular, especially when it comes to the large and giant breeds. Convenience is most of the explanation. Cost is the other part, although not so far as the super premium brands are concerned. They are incredibly expensive, considering what they are made from.

Although the smaller breeds are not immune from it, male infertility is found most commonly in the larger breeds. This is because the larger breeds are fed on an almost solo diet of dry dog food. For that reason I will discuss infertility, particularly male infertility, largely with reference to dry dog foods.

For both male and female infertility and poor puppy growth ...

... **poor quality dry dog foods** are an almost foolproof recipe. They contain excessive calcium, salt and grains; poor quality protein; low levels of the vitamins A, D, E and K, the B group, and vitamin C; are lacking in available minerals, particularly zinc, and contain practically no essential fatty acids. The fats they do contain are heat damaged, and once the bag of dog food is opened, the fats it contains may quickly become rancid.

However, do realise that infertility in either sex, or poor puppy growth, can be the result of **any** bad diet. That can include ANY type of commercial pet food, or a badly formulated home made diet such as one based on copious quantities of cereals, or an all meat diet, or any diet over supplemented with calcium.

It has become part of 'basic known truth' that dry dog foods are the 'best' way to feed large dogs. Part of that supposed 'truth' is that "you have to add lots of extra calcium to a large dog's diet." It is widely believed that larger dogs need a more calcium rich diet - while they are growing - for their bones. Nothing could be further from the truth! For more details on feeding calcium to pups, see Part Three Chapter Eight - 'The Calcium Dilemma.' The 'need' to feed dogs this way has produced a very simple and foolproof method for producing male infertility.

The best way to be certain of low to non-existent fertility in your male dog is to feed him a cheap, poor quality dry food for the whole of his life, beginning when he is a puppy. To make absolutely sure, add lots of extra artificial calcium. This is a well-known recipe, widely used by owners of larger dogs, who as a group seem 'driven' to produce infertility of both males and females, and most particularly the males, using this method.

To ensure success, make sure the dry dog food is a very cheap one, add only calcium to that diet. No fresh foods, no liver or eggs or kelp or crushed vegetables and no other vitamin or mineral supplements. No essential fatty acid supplements.

This diet has a multitude of deficiencies - all capable by themselves of producing infertility and poor growth. Chief among these is a zinc deficiency. I will fill you in on the details of this zinc deficiency, including how it causes infertility, later in this chapter.

To convince you to adopt the BARF diet ...

... and NOT to feed any of your reproducing or growing dogs with commercial dog food - I want you to read, digest and consider the following vitally important nutritional information.

Essential fatty acids and your dogs' fertility and your puppies' growth

Essential fatty acids are involved in every facet of reproduction and growth. To raise healthy, highly sexed, highly fertile dogs, both male and female, and healthy puppies that have freedom from skeletal disease, the diet you feed them must contain adequate levels of the essential fatty acids. The Omega-6's and the Omega-3's. Ideally, these fats must NOT have been damaged by heat.

Because they are all cooked, **it is impossible for ANY processed food to contain undamaged and therefore healthy essential fatty acids**. Apart from that, most processed foods are woefully deficient in the essential fatty acids anyway. If essential fatty acids have been added, as with some of the super premium brands, those added fats are heat damaged. They may also be rancid, or the product may contain chemical anti-oxidants such as BHT, BHA or ETHOXYQUIN - all known carcinogens. **There simply is no way ANY of these products can supply the essential fatty acids in a healthy way.**

- **Essential fatty acids are a vital part of every cell membrane in every cell in a dog's body. That is why essential fatty acids must be present in the diet to ensure that both sperm cells and egg cells are normal and healthy. These cells of reproduction, particularly the sperm, consist largely of cell membranes.**

- The essential fatty acids play many key roles in the central nervous system. **They must be present if your pup is to grow a normal brain and have normal vision.**

- The brain is an exceedingly concentrated collection of cell membranes. **Pups deprived of adequate levels of essential fatty acids never develop to their full mental capacity and can be nervy and unpredictable.**

- It is highly probable that diseases such as **progressive retinal atrophy will appear much earlier in susceptible animals fed these commercial dog foods with their low levels of essential fatty acids and other vital nutrients.**

- **Essential fatty acids must be present for normal hormone production and function.** As you would realise, hormones play an essential role in both the growth of your pup's skeleton and in reproduction. To function normally, hormones require an adequate supply of essential fatty acids - not damaged in any way.

- Essential fatty acids must be present in full quantity and proper balance if the cells of the growing points in growing bones are to grow and develop normally. Every skeletal disease we see in growing dogs involves these cells.

There are literally thousands more situations where essential fatty acids play key roles in metabolism. That is why modern foods with their heat damaged fatty acids or their almost complete lack of essential fatty acids are a major cause of disease, including reproductive and growth problems in modern dogs.

By contrast, the BARF diet contains high levels of cold extracted, non rancid, undamaged essential fatty acids, stabilised by vitamin E.

The Omega-6's come from chicken and the Omega-3's come from green leafy vegetables, cod liver oil and flax or hemp seed oil.

If you are not using the BARF diet and you are not supplementing with these oils, the information on brain, vision and reproductive health is ample reason for doing so. HOWEVER - there are many more reasons to use the BARF diet - so keep reading.

Uitamin A, fertility, and growth

Vitamin A is a vital factor in many functions associated with the growth of pups, and the reproductive ability of mum and dad. The diet must also contain plenty of available zinc together with good quality protein. Without adequate levels of zinc and good quality protein, the vitamin A cannot be released from the liver to perform its many functions.

Vitamin A - Does your feeding programme supply adequate levels?

- In reproduction vitamin A plays a vital role in maintaining libido - in both HIM and HER.

- Vitamin A must be present to prevent both testicular and ovarian degeneration and to maintain hormone levels, particularly testosterone levels in males.

- Vitamin A plays a vital role in producing large numbers of perfectly formed healthy active sperm.

- **Vitamin A helps maintain healthy eyes** and skin, and all internal linings of your dog's reproductive, gastrointestinal and urinary tracts.

- **Vitamin A levels need to be present in adequate amounts to support the activity of the adrenals** in their role of producing bodily cortisone - the anti-stress hormone which plays a vital role in dealing with the stress of reproduction. For example, the stress a male stud dog undergoes when it is asked to perform repeatedly throughout the breeding season.

- **Vitamin A is required to keep your dogs healthy through its many effects on the immune system,** particularly its role in keeping the thymus fully functioning. This is an essential role in immune system health in both growing pups and breeding adults.

- **Vitamin A plays many roles in growth. Of particular interest is its role in proper dental development and bone growth.** Without adequate vitamin A together with zinc and good quality protein, pups will never develop their bones to full strength and proper development.

- Think of the countless pups raised on poor quality dry dog foods with their poor quality protein, their low levels of vitamin A, together with their excessive calcium which makes the zinc unavailable! And we wonder why our pups develop such poor dental and skeletal health, requiring canine orthodontics and skeletal surgery!

You can make sure of your dogs' vitamin A levels ...

... by **supplementing daily with cod liver oil** as recommended in the BARF diet. This will ensure excellent levels of vitamin A plus vitamin D and some of the essential fatty acids, particularly the Omega-3's.

Apart from ensuring plenty of zinc and good quality protein are present in the diet of a male stud dog, so that vitamin A can be released from the liver, **I suggest your male stud dog receive vitamin A supplementation at the rate of 200 i.u. per kg of dog per day. This can be increased for periods of 1 to 2 months to 500 i.u. per kg of dog per day when he is being used on a constant basis.**

Please note that where you have been supplementing your female dog with vitamin A, do not supplement it during the first two thirds of pregnancy. For the details on why this is so please see Chapter Four.

Vitamin C – for health, growth and reproductive performance

Vitamin C helps detoxify commercial dog food with all its carcinogens and biologically inappropriate chemicals. It helps protect against our modern world, so full of environmental pollutants. It helps destroy dangerous free radicals in the body.

Vitamin C assists in the formation of blood cells and helps blood transport oxygen to the cells. It assists in the uptake of iron from the digestive tract. It is vital for the health of a dog's immune system.

Vitamin C is strongly recommended for the pregnant mum - it helps her give birth easily - and it helps with milk production in the lactating mum.

In the male dog, vitamin C is required in high concentrations in seminal fluid to protect the sperm from the harmful effects of oxidation. If it is not present in adequate amounts, failure to conceive can be the net result.

Commercial dog food contains no added vitamin C. Not only that, because they are such poor products, they do little to stimulate a dog's liver to produce its own. Unless you supply a dog fed on commercial dog food with supplementary vitamin C, you can be sure that low vitamin C levels will be another nail in the coffin so far as your male dog's ability to reproduce is concerned.

Vitamin C is the major anti-stress vitamin, and both reproduction and growth are very stressful times. That is why it must be present in adequate amounts for your male stud dog to perform to his maximum potential.This is also true of your female. In fact supplementing mum, dad and the kids with vitamin C can only be of benefit at all stages of life.

The dose rate I suggest as a minimum is 50 mg per kg per day. If you can divide that up and give it in 2 or 3 separate doses - so much the better.

I strongly suggest your male stud dog be supplemented with vitamin C at the rate of 50 mg per kg per day, which can be safely doubled or tripled during periods of heightened sexual activity. Supplement with vitamin C - even when you are feeding your male dog properly - on the BARF diet.

Growing pups should be supplemented at a similar dose rate. That is, 50 mg per kg per day. Vitamin C is vital for normal bone growth. Supplementing with vitamin C has proven of benefit in certain situations of poor diet, in helping to prevent skeletal disease such as Hip and Elbow Dysplasia. For further information on vitamin C and bone growth - see Part Three.

The bottom line is - do supplement Him, Her AND the Kids with vitamin C. For more information on vitamin C and its role in your dog's healthy life, refer to Chapter Five in **Give Your Dog a Bone.**

Vitamin E for growth and reproduction

The earliest described role for vitamin E was its role in reproduction. It has long been known as the fertility vitamin.

Research has taught us that vitamin E performs most of its beneficial functions because it protects the polyunsaturated fats within an animal's body from becoming rancid. Those rancid fats cause major degeneration within the body. It is able to do this because it is a major anti-oxidant. **In this role vitamin E is a major 'age fighter.'**

As an anti-oxidant, vitamin E protects the fats in all the membranes in each and every cell of an animal's body. This includes such cells as sperm and eggs, and the nerve cells in the brain and spinal cord.

Because of this role in keeping fats in the body from going rancid, **it is absolutely essential that vitamin E should be added as a supplement whenever you add polyunsaturated fats such as cod liver oil or flax seed oil to the diet.**

Vitamin E plays a vital role in the health of the immune system, along with other anti-oxidants such as **vitamin A, vitamin C and the minerals zinc and selenium**. This group of nutrients must be present to ensure the healthy growth of all bodily systems in growing pups, including the immune and skeletal system.

I also strongly recommend that group of nutrients to all the 'mad swabbers of reproductive tracts' out there in 'canine breeding world.'

People who 'just have to swab,' and then use antibiotics to kill the very normal bacteria present in their bitch's reproductive tract, would be far better employed stimulating their dogs' immune systems by feeding the BARF diet including all these vitamins and minerals.

Vitamin E is also involved in the formation of the genetic material - DNA - passed on by both the sperm and the egg.

Vitamin E is essential for the health of the micro-circulation within the body and this includes most particularly the circulation within the male dog's testicles.

Vitamin E has a generally protective effect on the dog's body by protecting against the deteriorating effects of ageing, which can drastically reduce libido and healthy sperm [and egg] production.

Vitamin E also helps prevent the destruction by free radicals, of vitamin A in a dog's body.

In other words, vitamin E has a major role to play in keeping both your male and female dog sexually healthy and active. Part of that role involves healthy testicles and ovaries, and healthy - normal - hormone production.

Animal studies have implicated a lack of vitamin E in early termination of pregnancy by miscarriages or abortions.

Many studies have shown vitamin E to increase fertility in both male and female animals. It increases libido.

In male dogs, adequate vitamin E will help both prevent and cure an inflamed prostate together with zinc and vitamin A.

Because dry dog food - in fact most commercial dog food and most home cooked food as well - is low in vitamin E, it is little wonder that male dogs fed this food often have reproductive problems. More so of course when they are on a solo diet of the dry stuff. These comments apply equally to female dog fertility.

For all of the above reasons I strongly suggest a vitamin E supplement for all male [and female] stud dogs at the rate of 15 i.u. per kg per day - as part of the BARF programme. This level of supplementation can be doubled during periods of stress, which includes intense sexual activity, or where an infectious process is present.

Vitamin D for growth and reproduction

Conventional wisdom says that if your dogs spend plenty of time in the sun, there should be no problems with them receiving adequate quantities of vitamin D. However, a combination of dry dog food, dark skin pigmentation and a heavy hair coat can result in a vitamin D deficiency.

This is because dry dog foods often contain rancid fats and a lack of vitamin E. The rancid fats destroy the vitamin D and the lack of vitamin E allows the destruction to happen.

The lack of vitamin D can be a major factor in the production of an unhealthy skeletal system, resulting in Rickets in young dogs or Osteomalacia in the older dog. For more information on this problem see Part Three.

There is some evidence to suggest that a lack of vitamin D is involved in the production of 'swimmer' puppies.

The simple solution is to feed the BARF diet which recommends that cod liver oil - which contains vitamin D - should be fed daily. Other good sources of vitamin D include free range eggs and liver. Because vitamin D is ABSOLUTELY essential for all aspects of growth and reproduction, make sure your dogs get it somehow!

Uitamin K for growth and reproduction

Vitamin K plays an essential role in clotting of the blood, it is an anti-oxidant, and it is essential for protein formation in a dog's body. In other words it plays at least one vital role in both growth and reproduction.

Most dogs obtain sufficient vitamin K by direct absorption from the bowel where it is made by bacteria. Dogs with continual bowel problems needing the use of sulpha drugs - and these are very common with dogs fed cooked and processed foods - may not manufacture enough of it. That short-fall will be made up by the BARF diet with its high level of green leafy vegetables and liver.

The B complex group of uitamins for growth and reproduction

These are all found at very low levels in commercial dog foods. As you read through the list, remember, that all the B vitamins are totally non-toxic. What does that mean? It means that you can only do your breeding stock and your growing puppies a whole heap of good by supplementing them with a super abundant supply of the whole range of B vitamins. As you read on you will also learn that extra amounts of specific members of the B group can be supplemented with great benefit where particular dogs have specific needs.

Because of the general calming effect of the B vitamins, dogs receiving insufficient will be very 'nervy,' for example, those dogs being fed dry dog foods. Such dogs will also show low energy levels, because the B vitamins are involved in energy production from proteins, carbohydrates and fats.

That is why the B vitamins are vital for such energetic pastimes as being a mum or a dad or for being a growing pup. In other words - DO supplement all your dogs with the whole B complex.

The individuals in the B complex ...

Vitamin B1 or Thiamine

This vitamin is essential for normal healthy growth including mental health. **A deficiency of vitamin B1 early in life results in reduced sexual development.** Not a great start for a stud dog, and obviously a potential problem in both sexes. **This problem is highly possible in dogs fed a solo diet of dry dog food with its exceptionally low levels of the B vitamins.**

There is evidence to suggest that a lack of this vitamin could be involved in the fading puppy syndrome, however, if supplementing young pups via a lactating mum, it is essential to supplement with ALL of the B vitamins, not just this one. B1 is present in a wide range of nuts, fruits and meats. For example - a good natural source is pork and also oranges.

Note that the high sugar content of commercial pet foods and human breakfast cereals - and passive smoking - depletes body reserves of B1.

For energy and calm, make sure your male dog receives the B complex with extra B1 if necessary.

Vitamin B2 or Riboflavin

This is another essential vitamin for all of the above reasons, including growth and fertility - in both males and females. **Vitamin B2 or Riboflavin is also vital in helping to produce gushing quantities of milk.** Keep that in mind for the appropriate occasion. Milk is an excellent source of B2.

Vitamin B3 or Niacin

This vitamin is essential for the health of the reproductive system in both males and females, and plays a major role in the growth of pups, including normal skeletal growth, and helps with the absorption of food from the digestive tract.

Low levels of B3 will result in your male [and female] dog suffering from weak orgasms. In other words, this vitamin helps maintain a high libido.

Other nutrients involved in this orgasmic function include vitamin B6 - found in bananas and chicken for example - and the amino acid histidine. It is certainly worthwhile supplementing extra of all of these during the breeding season.

Vitamin B3 along with B1 and B6 has a major calming affect on the brain. This is very useful with highly nervous dogs. B3 is useful in the relief of arthritis. This will benefit the older male dog in his quest to father puppies.

Meat - especially chicken - and also liver are both excellent sources.

Uitamin B5 or Calcium Pantothenate

This vitamin is the vitamin that confers staying power. On that basis it is essential if you are to own a healthy virile strapping male dog. It has many roles to play including the promotion of longevity, dealing with stress via the production of natural cortisone, conferring that tremendous staying power through its involvement in energy metabolism, and a role in sexual libido through its role in producing the neurotransmitter called acetylcholine.

Like the other B vitamins , B5 is in desperately short supply in all dog foods, particularly the dry variety. Vitamin B5 like the other B vitamins is destroyed by heating.

I would strongly recommend you supply extra vitamin B5 to your male stud dog, particularly during the breeding season. About 10 to 20 mg per kg per day.

Uitamin B6 or Pyridoxine

This vitamin plays a major role in allowing animal bodies to absorb the minerals iron and zinc and vitamin B12. **A lack of vitamin B6 helps produce anaemia, arthritis, poor appetite, nausea, and toxic states in the bitch during pregnancy. Here we see the production of cleft palates or possibly even stillbirths in the pups.** Pregnant bitches must receive extra vitamin B6, before during and after pregnancy.

B6 along with B1 and B3 plays an important role in calming and regulating the brain. Once again, the commercial dog foods cannot be relied upon to supply this vitamin. Hyperactive, irritable, nervy dogs switched from the commercial dog foods and fed the BARF diet are almost instantly calmer and stay that way. Bitches whose nervous state will not allow pregnancy, benefit from supplementation with these vitamins. If you have such a bitch, I would also strongly suggest she be supplemented with the herb Hypericum or St. John's Wort.

Without adequate B6, your breeding dogs will lose appetite, drop weight, become anaemic, have poor immunity and show a decreased libido due to a lack of orgasmic activity, and may produce birth defects or dead pups. That sounds pretty shocking! It is however, what we see constantly in dogs and bitches fed the awful processed foods!

The answer? Feed the BARF diet and avoid these problems. Supplement to be certain. **B6 is found in most fresh whole raw foods including most vegetables [broccoli, Brussels sprouts, cauliflower, sweet corn, potatoes], and most meat - especially chicken - then beef, pork, lamb and fish. If these products are part of your feeding programme - no worries!**

Biotin

Biotin is an essential nutrient involved in the production of a healthy thyroid gland, healthy adrenals, and healthy ovaries and testicles. All of these organs are intimately involved in both growth and reproduction. Biotin needs the presence of vitamin E to remain viable. Naturally, most commercial dog foods, particularly the dry type have low levels of both of these.

Fortunately your dog's body is able to make this vitamin in the intestines. Unfortunately, antibiotics will interfere with this process. Many modern dogs fed on processed pet foods suffer severe drops in immunity leading to infectious disease which requires long term antibiotic therapy. This will interfere with Biotin production and absorption from the bowel. Young pups are particularly susceptible to a lack of Biotin due to prolonged use of antibiotics.

Let me encourage you to avoid the need for long term antibiotics by feeding the BARF diet. Egg yolk, brewer's yeast, and liver are all good sources of Biotin, as is a complete vitamin B supplement.

Folic Acid

The lack of folic acid causes major problems in breeding dogs. In males it is vital for sperm formation. In females folic acid is absolutely vital for the proper development of the foetus. Insufficient can result in abortions, malformed pups, retarded pups, or dead pups. Yes you read that right. Folic acid is one of those nutrients which is almost non-existent in processed foods whereas the BARF diet supplies it in abundance. The presence of folic acid is one of the many reasons breeding dogs fed the BARF way have been quietly reproducing without problems for years. The lack of folic acid is one of the many reasons why dogs and bitches on the commercial programme have had numerous problems for years.

Research has shown that dogs which have a high folic acid intake all year round - usually from natural sources - perform far better in the reproduction stakes than those who are given supplements only at the time of reproduction. Folic acid is present in abundance in green leafy vegetables!

In other words, to ensure all your dogs receive plenty of folate, switch them to the BARF diet - and keep them on it!

Vitamin B12

This vitamin is present in most whole raw foods of animal origin, for example milk, eggs [the yolk only] and meat. Of the meats, lamb is the best source followed by beef and fish, with chicken and pork having very low levels. The very best source however is liver which has forty times as much B12 as lamb and sixty times as much as egg yolks.

B12 is another brain food and it also plays an essential role in skeletal health, both in young pups as they grow, and as dogs age. It also has a vital role to play in blood formation.

Vitamin B12 has many roles to play in reproduction. **Its most direct role in fertility is the part it plays in the production of genetic material - DNA and RNA.**

While it is very rare to see an outright deficiency of this vitamin, **the literature is full of reports involving the improvement in health of dogs supplemented with extra B12.**

This is understandable because our dogs' ancestors received vast amounts of vitamin B12 as a result of their feeding habits. The BARF diet! Dogs of all ages must receive adequate quantities. That does not mean feeding commercial dog food. It does mean feeding the BARF diet.

That is why with our modern dogs, much benefit is to be gained from supplementing with extra B12 - either as an injection or orally - in the months prior to the breeding season. Giving it all year round will be fine as well!

Choline

This nutrient which is found in abundance in egg yolks - as part of the sulphur containing amino acid methionine - and also in all unrefined oils in small amounts including flax seed oil, forms part of all cell membranes, including of course the sperm and the egg. It requires the presence of vitamin B12, Folacin and essential fatty acids before it can become part of these membranes.

Unfortunately choline is woefully deficient in many commercially produced dog foods, particularly the dry dog foods.

Choline is also essential for its role in the brain where it is part of the neurotransmitter acetylcholine. Its role here is probably why supplemental choline has proved of immense benefit in stimulating sexual activity and interest in the male dog whose interest in sex [libido] has declined. When giving supplemental choline it is best given together with the whole range of B group vitamins, vitamin E and the essential fatty acids.

MINERALS FOR REPRODUCTION AND GROWTH

FIRST – the most important one – ZINC

A lack of zinc, particularly in dry dog foods ...

- if bad enough can decrease the growth rate of puppies, even to the point of causing a permanently stunted dog.

- will prevent the full and proper development of a puppy's nervous system.

- will contribute to anaemia.

- will help produce Osteochondrosis which can lead to bone and joint problems such as Hip and Elbow Dysplasia in growing puppies and/or arthritis in the older dog.

- will contribute in a major way to skin problems.

- will result in a poorly functioning immune system.

- will result in a bitch that performs poorly in the reproductive stakes.

- <u>is responsible for more male dog infertility than any other nutrient deficiency.</u>

- **Zinc is the nutrient which ensures that your male dog is fertile. It is why human fathers to be are urged to eat lots of oysters which are a rich source of zinc. The zinc will not only help with the sex drive, it also ensures there are plenty of healthy sperm.** As mentioned earlier in this chapter ...

... The ultimate recipe for male dog infertility ...

... is a lifetime diet of dry dog foods plus massive calcium supplements.

This very common method of raising dogs has been shown to have a directly damaging effect on male fertility. The zinc deficiency such a diet produces results in testicular degeneration, poor sperm production and a lack of motility in the sperm.

The infertility caused by these diets is not due to a complete lack of zinc in the food. The zinc IS there. The problem is, your dog cannot absorb it.

This inability to absorb the zinc which is present is due to the massively excessive calcium levels in most dry dog foods, and the very high cereal levels, with their phytic acid. The calcium and the phytic acid both attach themselves to metals such as zinc and chromium, selenium and iron. They tie these metals up, making them unavailable to our dogs. It gets worse. Many dog breeders and owners, particularly those with the larger breeds, compound this problem by adding even more calcium to their dogs' diets.

The larger breeds are the ones most likely to be fed this almost exclusive diet of dry food and calcium supplements as they grow.

Even if that zinc deficient diet had all the necessary essential fatty acids, the high quality protein and the missing vitamins added to it, **the lack of zinc would still result in a complete and irreversible lack of sperm production in any dog raised on it.**

Also note that the lack of sperm production does not require a complete lack of zinc.

The growth of testicles that look normal but do not produce sperm occurs at zinc levels that will support maximum growth rate. In fact the dog may have normal libido. That is why we have so many beautiful looking male dogs, completely unable to father a single litter!

Male dogs raised on such a diet have a permanent inability to produce sperm

In these cases of infertility caused by a lifetime zinc deficiency, there is no going back. The damage is permanent. You will have to start again with a brand new puppy; only this time - feed it correctly!

The bottom line with zinc deficiencies, as with all the other problems inherent in commercial dog foods, is that you must get your dog off those awful foods, and stop feeding them extra calcium. Instead, switch your dog to the BARF diet. Realise that calcium supplied as raw meaty bones will enhance - not reduce - your dog's zinc supply!

To ensure plenty of zinc in your growing or adult dogs' diet, you may add such foods as herrings, cow's milk, liver [particularly pork liver], beef or lamb meat, particularly lamb shanks, [chicken has about as much zinc as lamb or beef] and egg yolk. Peas are also a good source of zinc, as are carrots and cabbage and cooked oatmeal porridge.

If you feel the need to supplement with extra zinc ...

... you can use any of the zinc supplements. With a veterinary product - follow the directions. If you have a zinc supplement designed for humans - the dose for a 20 kg dog is half the dose rate recommended for a child.

Let me warn you at this point ...

... be very careful when adding extra zinc. Too much can be just as bad as too little. Excessive zinc can have disastrous effects, equally as bad as the problems you are trying to solve. It will prevent the absorption of other minerals such as copper and iron, and it will decrease the growth rate. It can also cause a depraved appetite or no appetite at all, and may cause diarrhoea, liver problems, and if really excessive - drowsiness and paralysis.

In other words - do not overdo the supplementation of zinc. On the other hand, feeding extra zinc in zinc rich foods is perfectly safe.

Sulphur

Dog foods, based as they are on cereal grains, with or without soy protein, will be low in methionine and other sulphur-containing amino acids. This is another reason these foods contribute to growth problems in puppies, joint problems in older dogs, and reproductive problems in male dogs. A lack of sulphur in the diet also results in low levels of the amino acid taurine, the lack of which is a major contributor to epileptic seizures. **Methionine, an amino acid, is the best form in which to supply sulphur. Methionine is found in eggs.**

I think you would agree that poorly grown male dogs which have joint problems and poor fertility are not exactly the perfect male stud dogs everybody is looking for. I guess this is one more reason not to raise your dogs on these awful commercially made products.

Onions and garlic contain sulphur, but with these you have to be careful for the following reasons.

It has been documented that too much onion - raw, cooked or dehydrated - will cause a haemolytic anaemia in susceptible dogs. Usually small dogs. The literature suggests that excess garlic can also cause anaemias. I have fed both of these to my own dogs for years without adverse effects, as have many of my clients together with many other people I have spoken with over the years. I know of no trials which can put a figure on just what is a toxic dose of either of these substances.

Dogs that eat eggs, chicken, dairy foods, muscle meat, and red or green peppers, will get plenty of sulphur. Feed these as part of the BARF diet.

Magnesium

All dogs require magnesium for normal bone growth, energy production, heart function, muscle contraction, protein synthesis, and proper nervous function. For example, dolomite, which is a compound of magnesium, is very calming. Magnesium also takes part in countless essential chemical reactions within the body.

High levels of supplementary - artificial - calcium will depress the uptake of magnesium and can result in Osteochondrosis - the first stage of skeletal disease in young dogs. This is often seen as an over-extension of the carpal joints and can be mistaken for a calcium deficiency.

Once again, to ensure your dogs have correct levels of this mineral, feed the BARF diet. Apart from bones which are an excellent and safe source of magnesium, it is also safely found in milk, nuts, whole grains - sprouted or crushed and soaked overnight - in green vegetables as part of the chlorophyll molecule, in seafood, kelp and dolomite. Note at this point that of all the mineral supplements fed to dogs, dolomite would be one of the safest.

Manganese

This essential trace mineral is necessary for a myriad of functions in your dog's body including reproduction, growth and development, and also for muscular strength, which is important at all stages of reproduction, and obviously very much so for a male dog.

Manganese is essential for the production of the hormones produced by the thyroid gland. These hormones set the body's thermostat and underpin its entire metabolic functioning. They are vital for both growth and reproduction.

The only way to be sure you are supplying the correct levels of this nutrient in the correct form is to feed the BARF diet, and include liver, egg yolk, cereal bran [not essential if you are feeding the other items], green leafy vegetables - especially spinach and parsley, nuts and seeds and whole grain cereals suitably prepared by sprouting or crushing and soaking overnight.

Selenium

This mineral is vital for the well being of all dogs. Many soils and many diets, including most commercial diets, are deficient in selenium. It plays an essential role in the anti-oxidant defence mechanisms of all mammals - and that includes our dogs AND us! Without adequate selenium degenerative disease of ALL kinds occur early in life.

Selenium may well be present - usually at very low levels - in modern pet foods. Unfortunately, it may often be completely unavailable because of the chemical complexes it forms with the added calcium in these foods. These complexes form when these foods are cooked as part of their processing.

A lack of selenium and vitamin E have been implicated in fading puppy syndrome - and this factor alone should be another nail in the coffin of your desire to feed commercial dog food which can be so low in both selenium and vitamin E.

The role of selenium in growth and reproduction is to ensure healthy growth and long lived normal functioning with minimal deterioration. In reproduction, that means both male and female dogs will continue to reproduce normally without problems into what is now considered 'advanced old age.'

As part of the BARF diet, selenium, vitamin E and the sulphur containing amino acid - methionine - will protect your dogs from the rapid deterioration - the rapid ageing - which is a feature of our modern dogs, where we now consider the dog of five to six years of age to be entering 'old age.'

Selenium should be supplied together with vitamin E and sulphur

Methionine, an amino acid, is the best form in which to supply sulphur. Both methionine and selenium are found in eggs.

Foods rich in selenium include brewer's yeast, garlic, liver, eggs, fish, meat, brown rice and other whole grain cereals - suitably prepared by either sprouting or crushing and soaking overnight.

Iodine

Iodine is required for the normal healthy functioning of the thyroid gland. Thyroid hormones are responsible for normal growth and reproduction. Dogs fed modern commercially prepared diets with their multitudes of problems, risk the possibility of an iodine deficiency. Insufficient iodine will result in slow growth, obesity and poor reproduction in both sexes.

The excess calcium in commercial dog foods, or modern homemade diets supplemented with excessive calcium, can depress the functioning of the thyroid gland, thereby depressing the functioning of both the male and female dogs' reproductive ability.

Kelp - the safe iodine supplement

Excessive iodine can be harmful. However, insufficient iodine will result in both reproductive and growth problems. To ensure safe and adequate iodine levels in the diet, add a level teaspoon of kelp powder to your 20 kg [44 lb] dog's diet daily. Sensible supplementation of iodine using kelp in this manner will do no harm and will in fact do positive good for both growing and breeding dogs. In addition, by supplementing with kelp in this way, you are ensuring that every trace mineral your male stud dog and your bitch could possibly require is being incorporated in their diet at safe and adequate levels.

Iron

A deficiency of iron will result in anaemia. That means fatigue, poor growth, poor reproduction, and great susceptibility to disease. Dogs with lots of fleas or a heavy hookworm infestation will become anaemic very rapidly. Once again, it is the dogs on the poor commercial diets which develop these parasitic infections much more easily. On top of that it can happen that the extra calcium and the phytic acid in some dog foods will bind with the iron in the product thus making it unavailable for your dog. This is particularly so in the dry dog foods.

As you can see this is another great reason for adopting the BARF programme.

The foods which you can incorporate into your BARF programme for both your male stud dog and your bitch to ensure they both receive their share of iron include lean red meat such as beef or venison, green leafy vegetables, whole grain cereals - suitably prepared by sprouting or crushing and soaking, liver and other organ meats, dried fruits, legumes and molasses. The other excellent source is bone marrow. Yes, dogs that eat lots of raw meaty bones will not want for iron!

People who live on the land and kill their own beasts often save the blood and freeze it. This is an excellent food to add to the patty mix in the BARF programme. It is rich in iron and so many other highly valuable nutrients. It may be used in place of liver in the patty mix.

The final word on iron is that vitamin C must be present in your dog in adequate amounts to ensure healthy uptake of this mineral. This is another great reason to supplement with vitamin C.

Copper

Most foods fed to dogs contain plenty of copper and dogs do not need a lot. However, copper may become deficient where dogs are fed high calcium mostly processed cereal diets. That is, poorly made dry dog foods. This would be made worse by an owner who was supplementing that product with heaps of calcium.

A copper deficiency will lead to problems with anaemia, growth and reproduction. The best source of copper is liver and brains, particularly where these are derived from young animals, e.g. lambs.

Dogs fed the BARF diet will not suffer a copper deficiency.

Uigorous fertile male stud dogs are so easy to produce!

All you have to do is feed the BARF diet,making sure that the foods you use for HIM are slanted towards male fertility.

Just in case your memory is like mine and you cannot remember everything that I have mentioned in this chapter which will benefit HIM - [and her, together with the pups] - let me present to you the ...

... BARF diet supplemented for fertility

As usual this diet will be based on a broad range of raw meaty bones. These are a must as the basis of any fertility diet for dogs.

A broad range of green leafy vegetables comes next. They will be crushed and formed into patties.

The vegetable patties may contain such important foods as: brewer's yeast [leave out if the brewer's yeast has any tendency to make him itchy]; cottage cheese; **kelp**; whole raw fish - or failing that sardines in spring water; **a complete multi B supplement**; **yoghurt** - fresh, natural and low fat - in fact any whole raw dairy products from a healthy disease free source and can include goats and or sheep etc. products; **eggs** - raw and preferably free range and organic; cold pressed stored in the dark under nitrogen - **flax seed oil**; **a vitamin E supplement**; **cod liver oil**, and/or shark or fish oil - also fresh and unrefined and non-rancid; **organ meats** such as liver, blood, brains, heart, kidneys, thymus etc.; **vitamin C**, zinc and selenium supplements; dolomite powder - especially for an old toothless dog which cannot eat bones easily; garlic; small amounts of cooked brown rice; molasses.

Note the importance of essential fatty acids

The so called Omega-6's and the Omega-3's. When supplying these essential fatty acids in the diet - as you must always do with the BARF diet - do supplement with vitamin E. The rate is 15 i.u. per kg of dog per day - or thereabouts. This amount of vitamin E can be doubled with increased oil supplements or in times of increased stress.

For a twenty kg [44 lb] dog supply approximately half to one dessert spoon of flax seed oil daily. The amount given will depend on how fat or lean the dog is and what sort of oils have figured in that dog's eating history.

As a general rule, fat dogs will receive less flax seed oil, thin dogs will get more, and dogs with a history of a good diet will need less. Please make sure your flax seed oil is from a reputable source. That it was 'cold pressed' in the dark and stored in a freezer or refrigerator until opening. Do make sure that after you have opened it you continue to store it in the dark, in a refrigerator until it is used. Always use it fresh and throw it away if it is not used up in six to eight weeks.

Hemp seed oil is an excellent source of essential fatty acids. It contains the ideal balance of Omega-6's to Omega-3's - that is - 3 : 1. If you can obtain a supply of this valuable oil, then use it in place of the flax seed oil.

Note the importance of eggs!

The humble egg is indeed a wondrous fertility food. And if you think about its role in producing a whole chicken or duck or turkey - or whatever - that is hardly surprising. The egg contains so many nutrients vital for fertility. These include high class protein, essential fatty acids [particularly free range organic eggs], biotin, vitamin B 12, choline, zinc, the sulphur containing amino acids, and selenium.

In other words, you really don't need to give it a great deal of thought - just feed that male stud dog and the breeding bitch plenty of eggs. Of course they are also excellent food for the pups.

'Priming HIM up' for breeding

You must start 'priming him up' some two months prior to the breeding season. This is the time to begin supplementing with the fertility foods because that is how long it takes for sperm formation. If you are not doing so already, begin to add the following to his program. Plenty of eggs for all the reasons already mentioned and particularly because eggs play a major role in fertility. Cod liver oil. Kelp powder. Extra flax seed oil and extra vitamins such as vitamin C, the B group and vitamin E. Whole fish, including herrings or sardines. Liver, brains, kidneys and heart.

Continue feeding this way throughout the breeding season, particularly if your dog is in high demand and undergoing intense periods of sexual activity.

Of the B group, do ensure extra B3, B5, B6, folacin and choline is part of the regime, particularly if your male stud dog [or your bitch] is beginning to get on in years.

Make sure HE [and she] gets plenty of sunshine, and failing that, plenty of cod liver oil. Do ensure they both receive an abundance of green leafy vegetables. Also, if they have been treated with antibiotics lately, it is an excellent idea to add yoghurt, liver and extra egg yolks to the programme.

Let me emphasise that when your male dog is working hard, that is, giving daily services, do make sure you keep this high powered fertility diet going. That way you will never be disappointed with his performance, and he will be able to keep producing 'gallons' of healthy fertile semen well into advanced old age. Not only that, he will be healthy enough in his muscles, bones and joints to carry out his duties naturally without the need for artificial insemination. So many of our older stud dogs are too arthritic, too fat and too low in libido to do their job without that sort of help.

Do team that excellent diet with plenty of aerobic exercise. Keep HIM lean and his muscles hard.

If you are buying or leasing an older male dog for use as a stud dog ...

... then make sure you get him started on the BARF diet for fertility as soon as possible. This is particularly so if you are attempting to convert a 'dried dog food and calcium male' into something worthwhile. Do make sure that he is being fed this way for at least two months - and six months would be a safer bet - prior to the period you need him.

In fact if he has been raised on dry dog food and calcium supplements, do make sure he is fertile before buying or leasing him. When did he last sire a litter? Does he have sperm in his ejaculate? Are the levels of sperm in his ejaculate greater than two hundred million?

Also be aware that any huge stresses - such as an illness, a huge dog fight, or a period of intense sexual activity on a poor diet - are all prescriptions for infertility, in the two to six, or even twelve months that follow such a happening.

If you have just acquired a new male puppy – a future stud dog ...

- ... start feeding him the BARF diet for puppies as described in Part Three Chapter Twenty Two.

- Make sure that he receives extra vitamin B1 along with a complete B vitamin supplement for healthy testicular development.

- **Make sure he receives adequate zinc in his diet** by feeding him plenty of raw meaty bones together with such products as herrings, cow's milk, liver - particularly pork liver - beef or lamb meat, particularly lamb shanks, [chicken has less zinc than lamb or beef] and egg yolk. Peas are also a good source of zinc, as are carrots and cabbage and cooked oatmeal porridge.

- Do not feed artificial calcium supplements.

- Do not feed a grain based diet.

- Do not feed an all meat diet.

- Do feed plenty of vegetables.

Mating factors

Timing of mating is vital. The sperm must be in the reproductive tract BEFORE or at the time of ovulation, and no later than about two days after ovulation.

For all practical purposes assume that the eggs will only survive for about twenty four hours after ovulation. On the other hand the sperm may be considered good for about three to five days.

Ideally we want the sperm waiting in the female reproductive tract - ready for the eggs to be shed.

In practical terms that means with natural mating she should be mated every second or third day from when she will first accept him until such time as she refuses his advances.

This is usually easy to achieve in nature. When a bitch is on heat, more than one dog will help her become pregnant. This also happens out on the streets of our cities and suburbs where a steady line-up of suitors ensures she always becomes pregnant.

However, in controlled breeding situations - i.e. modern dog breeding - there is only one male involved. This means we have potential problems.

She may not like him. He may not be very fertile. We may not get the timing of mating right.

In an attempt to overcome such problems, some novice breeders with their own male will simply leave her with that male for the duration of the 'heat period.' That will be OK if she likes him and if he manages to get that semen in before she ovulates OR in the day or two after ovulation.

However, if she is a late ovulator but an early acceptor of his advances, he may actually exhaust his semen before ovulation and fertilisation can occur. This will happen if he is allowed to mate her more than two or three times a day. In other words, if she is to be mated every day, only allow one mating per day. A normally fertile male can make sufficient sperm to keep up with one mating per day, but not too much more.

Finally let me say that so long as we feed HIM right with the BARF programme for fertility, ensuring HE produces viable semen and has some libido left, no matter how old and decrepit HE becomes, between vaginal cytology and progesterone tests [to determine when SHE ovulates] and A.I. [to get HIS semen in HER reproductive tract at the correct time] , we should be able to use HIM well into old age to get HER pregnant.

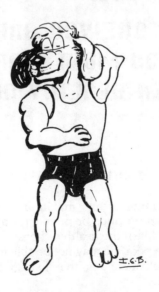

CHAPTER TWO

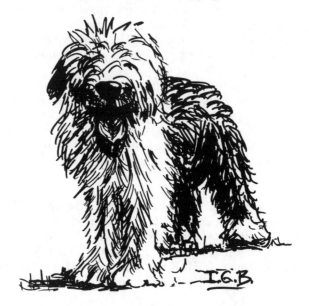

BEFORE YOU BREED
YOU MUST START
WITH HEALTHY DOGS

Never try and breed with unhealthy animals

Maximally healthy parents means maximum fertility. Poor health of breeding stock can mean no pups or pups with problems. If you had to decide which one should be more healthy, choose the bitch. However, if the health of the male is too poor, he may not be able to produce viable sperm. If you are going to have a male dog, then I suggest you also maximise his health. See Chapter One.

You should start thinking about the health of your breeding dogs well before they are due to be bred. That means feeding them properly for as long as possible prior to the time of breeding.

Ideally, both parents should be raised in such a way that they are fully fertile. Modern breeders have 'perfected' a technique involving dry food and calcium supplements which produces a perfectly healthy looking male which is totally infertile. Chapter One deals with this important topic in detail.

If your bitch has been on a poor diet ...

... prior to breeding - like most bitches these days - you can expect at the very least, decreased conception, decreased number of live births, and the pups that are born will have decreased vigour, muscle tone and ability to survive. Puppies born to mothers raised on a poor diet will have defective immune systems and will remain immune deficient for life.

In other words a poor start is a catastrophe. Some breeders never realise how poorly they have been faring until they adopt the BARF programme and see the amazing difference.

Preparing for breeding ...

Should begin about three generations prior to breeding. To accomplish this your breeding stock should have been born of healthy parents who were themselves born of healthy parents. However, you have to start somewhere, so if you have not done so already, start optimising your breeding stock's diet, and therefore their health, right now. Get them off that processed food, or that badly done home produced diet and switch them to the BARF programme NOW.

If there is any doubt about the fertility of your male dog ...

... get him to your vet and have his semen checked - now! It is surprising just how many males are infertile. No sperm in their semen. Most breeders assume it is hereditary. In fact it is commonly due to a zinc deficient diet and is irreversible if that is the case. See Chapter One for more information on this vital topic.

If you are not one hundred percent sure about your bitch's health ...

... take her to your vet for a full physical examination. This includes a check of her vagina for abnormalities.

Make sure SHE has been vaccinated against the major viral diseases such as parvovirus, distemper, hepatitis etc.. Either homoeopathically or conventionally. It is essential that she can pass a high level of immunity to her pups. They need to be protected from these diseases while their own immune system is developing. She will pass this temporary immunity to them across the placenta before they are born , and via her first milk - her colostrum - in the twenty four hours following birth.

Many people are concerned about the risks associated with vaccinating dogs. They are particularly concerned about multiple live vaccines and the practice of yearly boosters. As they see it, the risks of vaccination include causing the disease those vaccines were meant to prevent, and causing other problems by damaging the immune system.

My experience, over 20 plus years as a veterinary surgeon, tells me that where a dog follows the BARF diet, there appears to be very little risk of damage by the vaccines, and much to gain by vaccinating dogs to prevent these awful diseases. Where problems are seen, the dogs in question have been fed a sub-standard diet - a commercial diet - instead of following the BARF programme. Their immune systems were not capable of dealing with either the disease or the vaccines.

Do make sure SHE is free of external parasites such as fleas, lice and mites - including ear mites. If these are present in any numbers it indicates that SHE is unhealthy - not one hundred percent ready to be a parent. **You will not see a BARF dog with a huge burden of fleas.**

It gets worse. A flea burden further damages health by producing anaemia and a tapeworm infestation. This further reduces HER fertility. Kill the fleas - on her and in her environment. Kill the tapeworms, have her blood checked for anaemia and most important of all - FIX THE DIET!

76

Ear mites are a common problem in puppies. These pups usually come from long established breeders who produce large numbers of pups. Ear mites can be eliminated. It is not hard, it just requires persistence. Treat every dog and cat on the place with insecticidal ear drops together with ear cleaning drops every 3rd day for a month.

Do make sure SHE is free of intestinal worms and heartworm. Hopefully SHE has been on a regular intestinal worming programme all her life, and has - if necessary - been on a preventative programme for heartworm. If there is any doubt about heartworm, have her checked for it. If SHE has not been wormed in the last three months - do so.

Your vet can run some very simple blood tests ...

... to see whether SHE is anaemic, and whether her blood proteins are up to normal healthy levels. Do have these tests done, they are very simple, but are one of the quickest, easiest and most reliable ways of predicting whether or not your bitch will be successful at producing a healthy litter.

If SHE is ready for breeding her packed cell volume should be greater than 40 %, the haemoglobin should be greater than 10 %, and the plasma protein should be greater than 5 %. Values below these levels indicate poor nutrition.

Poor nutrition will produce anaemia in the following ways ...

1] SHE is anaemic because her diet is low in the blood-forming nutrients.

2] SHE is anaemic because her diet has allowed or caused some other problem to surface - such as a flea burden - which will need to be investigated and corrected before breeding. Do note that poor health caused by a poor diet attracts parasites such as fleas.

If your bitch is found to have low values for any of these tests, she will almost certainly have problems. But do not worry. Switch her to the BARF diet, plus supplements as explained in Chapter One. In particular add some extra liver, and her health will improve. A sure indicator will be a rise in those blood levels.

HER weight is vital

To maximise HER chances of reproductive success, SHE must be at her ideal weight at mating, not differing by more than 10% either way. Bitches either under or over weight by more than ten percent when bred can have difficulties becoming pregnant, holding pregnancy, giving birth, feeding pups etc. etc.. For this she must be individually assessed. Breed averages will not do. Take your vet's advice on this. If she is not close to her ideal weight, adjust her food intake so she will be at her ideal weight when mated.

A simple way to determine her ideal weight is to record or find what she weighed as a young slim mature adult. This information is often retained in her veterinary records. It is the weight where you can feel but not see her ribs. The weight where she has a pronounced waistline.

The grossly overweight bitch ...

... is not hard to recognise. She has difficulty moving. She becomes puffed very easily. She looks fat.

However, in the case of a breeding bitch, just a little bit overweight can make all the difference between a trouble free time and difficulties. If you are not sure, do see your vet because many people get so used to looking at slightly fat animals, they lose the ability to make this judgement. A good rule of thumb is that you should be easily able to feel the ribs but not see them, and if you look down at her from above, there should be a definite hour-glass figure.

An underweight, undernourished, unhealthy bitch ...

... is not hard to recognise. She 'looks poor.' She does not 'look good' because she has very few fat stores, and she has visible loss of muscle mass. She looks bony. She will appear mildly to severely dehydrated. This is recognised as tight inelastic skin. You pick the skin up and instead of snapping back instantly, it returns only slowly to its normal state. Such a bitch will be anaemic which is easily recognised as pale gums, although if she is also dehydrated, this can give a false colour to the gums.

Her coat will be sparse with washed out colour. It will be staring and dry, instead of being thick, colourful, and lustrous. She will not have a lot of energy. Her eyes may be slightly dry, perhaps slightly sunken and may contain mucus. They may be a little red. There will almost certainly be other health problems as well.

Of course not all dogs will fit this extreme picture, but this will give you some idea.

A healthy bitch ...

... will be slim, full of life with pliant elastic skin, have a shiny lustrous full coloured coat, a light covering of fat, with well developed muscles. She will be bright of eye, alert, inquisitive, have healthy pink gums, and be bounding with energy, ready to work or play all day long.

Does your bitch need vaginal swabs before mating?

Wild bitches don't have vaginal swabs and yet they reproduce beautifully! The practice of swabbing bitches prior to mating has no scientific or logical validity. It defies common sense. And yet we continue to do it.

In the wild, not one single vaginal swab is taken prior to mating. No antibiotics are given as routine prior to mating. If we could swab those wild vaginas, we would find many of the so called pathogens found in our own bitches - and yet the wild dogs continue to happily reproduce. The truth is, our own bitches are no different. Those vaginal swabs are mostly a waste of time, money and resources.

Why are we picking on the female? Why is her vagina to blame and why is the male's prepuce considered blameless in this matter - without ever testing it? If we have to swab anything, it would be more logical to swab the male. He is the one that encounters a wide range of bitches.

The vagina and the prepuce are warm, moist, dark, secreting places; perfect for growing bacteria. They are home to a whole range of bacteria which live in both places without causing any problems. It would be most unlikely to swab them and find nothing. However, the presence of pathogenic bacteria in the absence of any evidence of infection is not a reason to administer antibiotics.

On the other hand, the indiscriminate use of antibiotics may well result in problems, Particularly in bitches raised and maintained on commercial dog food. Antibiotic administration has been heavily linked with the fading puppy syndrome.

If your bitch has a uterine infection, that is a totally different matter

If your bitch has had infections involving her reproductive tract, or is diagnosed as having an infection, **recognisable by obvious clinical signs such as a frank pus-filled discharge,** then of course she MUST be treated with the appropriate antibiotic, and this SHOULD involve a vaginal swab.

However, do not just rely on the antibiotics to fix the problem. Without the help of your bitch's immune system working at full strength there is no way any antibiotic can help your bitch beat the infection and produce healthy puppies.

You MUST strengthen your bitch's immune system

Do this even if she does not have an infection! The simplest way to strengthen her immune system, if you have not done so already, is to switch her to the BARF diet. While ever you have her on a commercial dog food - and that includes the so-called 'super premium' dog foods - you are compromising her immune system.

Make sure you use the BARF diet plus the supplements and other additives which are immune system enhancers. These will include The B complex, the herb Echinacea, cod liver oil, vitamin E, zinc, and vitamin C, all of which are brilliant immune system stimulators.

Note, do not use cod liver oil or any vitamin A supplement during the first six weeks of pregnancy. For an explanation - see Chapter Four.

Yoghurt or probiotics are essential

If your bitch does require to be treated with antibiotics, you must also feed her probiotics - either as the pure bacterial supplement, or as low fat live culture yoghurt. The use of probiotics or yoghurt as a source of probiotics is important for her own bowel and general health, and also for the survival of the pups.

The use of these beneficial bacteria during pregnancy and throughout lactation will save you much heartache. **They greatly reduce the chances of your pups developing the fading puppy syndrome** which often follows the use of antibiotics either in treating the bitch or treating the pups themselves. If the pups have to have antibiotics at any stage, it is essential that they receive daily yoghurt or probiotics during that time and for several weeks after.

By the way...

... I know that most of you breeders will continue to swab. That is fine - it's your money. I just think it is better for you to know the facts. At least you can be a bit more knowledgeable and intelligent about what you are doing. But please, if you are using antibiotics - do use the yoghurt or the probiotics. If you are not sure, ask your vet. Most vets now stock or are able to obtain special animal probiotics. Alternatively, see your health food store.

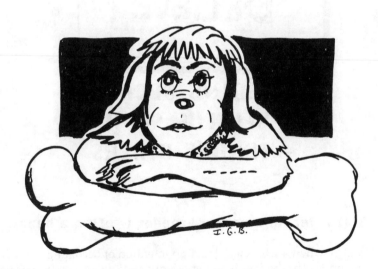

CHAPTER THREE

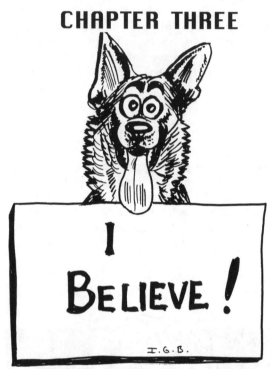

BREEDING SECRETS
–BELIEVE SOME
– IGNORE OTHERS

That first litter by a novice breeder is often a beauty ...

... particularly when the owner[s] had no intention of becoming 'breeders.' It often begins with the family pet suddenly and unexpectedly becoming pregnant. SHE breezes through the whole process with ease. No problems conceiving, no problems giving birth, no problems feeding the pups. Just the way it should be.

The problems start later ...

... usually after that novice breeder has been breeding for some time. Time enough for the new breeder to have talked to more experienced breeders.

Those conversations invariably include the idea that despite it appearing to be simple, breeding is in fact very difficult. That although as a novice they did well, things will not always be that easy. Then comes the advice. Mountains of it. Much of it is dietary advice. As a rule, established breeders can be reluctant to share their secrets. If for some reason they do share - be warned - what they tell you can often be misleading. **It is usually when the novice attempts to follow this free dietary advice that things start to go wrong.**

The truth behind those 'secrets'

The 'secret nutritional tricks' discovered and used by long time breeders have often taken years of trial and error to come to light. Those 'secrets' are commonly the nutrients missing from previously inadequate diets.

To be effective, such 'tricks' or 'secrets' have to be interpreted and used in the context of the entire management programme from which they sprang.

Sometimes the secret is a particular brand of pet food. Mostly the novice is not told about the supplements used along with that food. Alternatively the novice may be told about some of the the supplements but not the food. Which ever way it goes, you can be certain the whole management programme is not revealed.

So be aware when an experienced breeder hands you a 'secret dietary trick.' It is rarely the whole story. When the novice attempts to use that 'secret' along with half a dozen other 'secrets' they have been given, the outcome is commonly failure.

The thing is, if what you are doing is successful, don't meddle with it - "if it ain't broke - don't try and fix it!"

But why does the novice breeder so often succeed?

Let me say right from the beginning - it IS more than beginner's luck. If we return to those novice breeders and examine their recipe for success, we find that it involves a very simple formula - with the following ingredients.

Youth, family food, naive food, playful exercise, shelter and love. What do I mean by all of that? It is very simple. let me explain ...

- **Youth:** the younger the dog, the more healthy its reproductive organs are likely to be.

- **Family food:** with a growing family, the type of food scraps which become available to feed the dog include food scraps designed to support the growth of young children. Wholesome, healthy, fruits, vegetables, meat and eggs etc.

- **Naive food:** includes raw meaty bones. Most people realise that dogs eat bones. If those people have not been 'educated' to think differently, they will feed bones to their dogs. Sadly, in today's world, such 'uneducated' people are becoming harder to find. Particularly in the cities and suburbs. In the Australian country areas, and doubtless in other rural centres all over the world, commonsense feeding of dogs continues as it always has done. Here the dogs remain healthy, never needing to see the vet. Often they are not even vaccinated. Most vets are unaware that such healthy dogs exist!

- **Playful exercise:** is the joyful exuberant play seen when loving dogs and loving owners simply enjoy playing together on a daily basis. This form of exercise is the foundation of health, particularly where there is plenty of room for the dog to really stretch out and run. It is most important that dogs are not forced to participate in long boring walks. Particularly growing pups.

- **Shelter and love:** come naturally in a loving caring family environment. As the pregnant bitch is closely observed in such a situation, her family respond to her increased needs automatically, without giving it a second thought.

'Serious' breeding is different – so it seems

When people start to 'seriously breed,' they often change just about everything which made their project initially so successful. They change the food, the exercise, the accommodation and the attitude towards their dogs.

No longer do they use the secrets of success used by the novice breeder. They now use the secrets of failure tried and tested as true - by the more experienced folk.

- The healthy food is abandoned. Now they feed their dogs like all the other breeders. They feed the commercial stuff.

- Their youthful dogs age rapidly with that awful food.

- The exercise changes from family play to long boring walks.

- The dog is no longer a member of the family. It lives outside in a cold draughty kennel.

- Problems are no longer attacked with common sense. The 'wisdom' of other breeders is employed.

Unfortunately it does not stop there. **'Serious breeders' increase their problems by adding the following ...**

Modern Infertility – much of it is due to ...NOT BREEDING!

A major cause of infertility in modern bitches is the practice of waiting until the bitch is 3 or 4 years old before breeding her.

The other equally dangerous-to-fertility practice is where bitches are not bred every time they cycle. They are bred every second or third cycle for example. This may be fine in theory, and great politically, but biologically - it is unsound. A disaster.

The practice of not breeding early, and not breeding at every season, when combined with the abysmal commercial diets results in many breeding problems and much infertility.

What are our reasons for delaying breeding?

I guess there all sorts of reasons, including:

- the need for a bitch to get her 'title'

- or we say she is 'too young' to breed by which we usually mean that we believe she will have an immature attitude towards the pups.

All of that may well be; however - let us consider the natural situation and look at those wild bitches.

Wild bitches are born to breed

When a wild bitch first cycles - she is mated, and if the seasons are good, she is kept 'barefoot and pregnant' for the rest of her days.

Wild bitches do not have periods when they are not bred - except when the seasons are poor.

However, the barefoot and pregnant approach does not only happen in the wild. Although it is much less common than it used to be, over my twenty plus years in practice I have observed the results of this barefoot and pregnant philosophy played out in the wilds of Australian suburbs on numerous occasions.

Our bitches are born to breed!

Rosie was one such dog. Owned by a young and growing family, she was kept 'barefoot and pregnant' from the day she first came on heat. The 'dads' lived next door and up the street. Rosie loved them all, and produced litters of seven and eight pups every six to seven months.

As she got older, the interval between litters increased gradually, but she continued without problem for at least ten years, at which time I lost track of her. In that time she produced close to 100 live pups with no problems that ever required my attention, and virtually no losses of pups.

Let me stress, this was not an isolated case. I have known many such bitches. They all produced around a hundred pups - over a lifetime. They all remained in superb health - with a minimum of fuss.

Again, it is not my intention to enter into a discussion regarding the morality of this scenario. You can make your own judgments on that. What interests me and is instructive for us, are the biological facts. Why it is that these family pets can 'out-gun' almost any bitch living in a breeding colony?

What was Rosie's secret?

The answer is simple and relates in part to the secrets used by novice breeders.

The novice breeders' diet

The 'wild bitches of suburbia' have invariably been fed a wide variety of foods, including lots of bones, both cooked and raw, some commercial dog foods - but usually not a lot - and lots and lots of 'left-overs' from a young and growing family. Not a lot of junk food, just wholesome cereal and milk, meat, egg and vegetable scraps.

Their meals were not so much regular as constantly irregular. These bitches helped out at family barbecues, at picnics and at every meal time, always eager to have a little bit of what ever was going. When they needed more, they asked for it and got it. Their food did not stop at bones, meat and vegetables. All sorts of fruits were part of their diet. However there is more to it than feeding: they were also kept 'barefoot and pregnant.'

What is wrong with 'Barefoot and Pregnant'

Why don't we breed our bitches every time they cycle? One reason is convenience, but most commonly it is to 'give them a rest.' The belief is that a bitch cannot remain healthy if kept continually pregnant and also that the practice of breeding at every season is morally wrong or cruel or politically incorrect - or something.

However, I am not here to discuss the cruelty or political correctness aspect. What interests me are the lessons we must learn from all of this.

MODERN bitches DO have a problem with 'Barefoot and Pregnant'

It certainly is true that when bred twice a year, many modern bitches suffer a decline in health and a decline in fertility. However the low level of health, the inability to be successfully bred season after season is not inevitable as is commonly believed. The health of these 'puppy factories' suffers because they are being fed a poor diet which cannot sustain that level of activity. Of course I am putting this all down to diet on the assumption that the kennels are hygienically maintained, the dogs are all vaccinated and wormed and exercise is adequate. If these things are also done poorly, which sadly can be the case, the health of these poor bitches declines even more quickly!

The benefits of continual pregnancy ...

... are well demonstrated by Rosie. The first part of Rosie's secret recipe for fertility was her diet, but the second and equally important part is that she was kept pregnant from the start. We create enormous fertility problems by commencing   breeding late in a bitch's life, and only breeding intermittently as is so often the case these days. The problems result from some basic reproductive physiology which I shall now walk you through.

The hormone progesterone is the problem

When a bitch is pregnant she produces the hormone progesterone. Progesterone maintains pregnancy. It has the job of keeping the internal lining of the uterus in a thick reproductive state. The longer the internal lining is kept in that state, the more likely it will develop an irreversible age related degenerative disease called cystic-endometrial-hyperplasia. This is a chronic inflammatory disease of the internal lining of the uterus. It causes infertility by preventing implantation of the fertilised egg. That sounds as though keeping her pregnant would be a bad idea? Not so!

The average bitch cycles or comes on heat every seven months. Every time she cycles and ovulates, she goes   through the motions of pregnancy, whether she is actually pregnant or not. She is always hormonally pregnant after cycling. She does this because whether she is pregnant or not she produces   progesterone and continues to produce it until it is time for her to give birth. It is the sudden cessation of progesterone production which is one of the triggers for birth.

By keeping her pregnant you limit progesterone production

If she is pregnant, progesterone production stops after 63 days. It is when she is not pregnant that progesterone production goes on and on and on.

That is because there is no sudden cessation of progesterone production. After the 63 days are up, it continues to be produced at a declining rate for a total of 90 to 120 days.

By allowing a bitch to actually become pregnant - as she is designed to do - you limit the time that her uterus is under the influence of the hormone progesterone, and so you give her the greatest chance of remaining fertile longer.

If you couple that with the BARF programme - which involves the sort of diet which will enable her to remain healthy despite the fact of being pregnant twice a year - her chances of remaining fertile and healthy into old age are remarkably increased.

What happens when we delay breeding until later in life?

This an example of that universal law - 'Use it or lose it.' When a young bitch is not allowed to fall pregnant, her body becomes used to not being pregnant. As time goes by pregnancy becomes more and more difficult. Her body believes that puppy production is not to be.

If you are serious about maximising the breeding potential of a bitch, from a biologically correct point of view, early pregnancy and continual breeding combined with an appropriate diet and exercise regime is vital.

Let's deal with the feeding bit in a little more detail ...

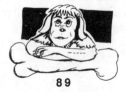

CHAPTER FOUR

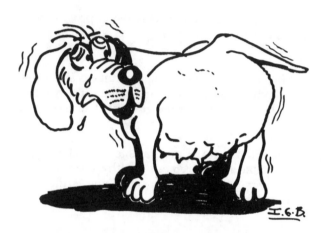

WHAT DO WE FEED HER DURING PREGNANCY?

The answer is - the BARF diet! If you have not read Part One - the BARF diet, go back and read it NOW. Having done that - read on ...

A successful pregnancy is a well-prepared-for event

The success or otherwise of any breeding exercise will depend on what your bitch has been fed throughout her life. During pregnancy she will draw upon nutrients deposited in her body long before she became pregnant. It is her past nutritional history which is going to have a dramatic impact on whether your bitch becomes pregnant, holds the pregnancy, and goes on to produce a large healthy litter with no birth problems and plenty of milk.

If your bitch has a history of being kept on a poor diet such as commercial dog food, or a poor home made diet such as an all meat diet, there will be major problems. She may not even become pregnant. If she does, she may abort or produce deformed puppies. Keep that in mind when you begin your breeding programme.

Does that mean a pregnant bitch needs a special diet?

Pregnancy is a special time. A dynamic state with many changes and much growth occurring inside the mother's body over a very short period of time.

Is this a time when a mother's nutritional needs change dramatically?

If your bitch has been on a very good diet throughout her life - right up until her pregnancy - the BARF diet - then for at least the first two thirds of pregnancy - the answer is NO. She remains on the basic BARF diet.

It is only during the last third of pregnancy you will have to increase the amount of food fed, because that is when the pups do most of their growing.

That food may have to be just a little bit more concentrated. By more concentrated I mean that it should contains a greater amount of the nutrients essential for growth. That includes extra protein, extra vitamins, extra essential fatty acids and extra minerals, with the exception - surprisingly - of calcium.

Bitches that have been kept on a poor diet throughout life ...

... and are not fed with greater concentrations of growth nutrients in the second half of pregnancy become very hungry. That hunger is a signal that she lacks those growth nutrients. In an attempt to get more nutrients for the growth of her puppies, that bitch will eat vast quantities of food which may not help the pups to grow properly. For example, if the food is high in calories such as fats and carbohydrates, but low in proteins and vitamins, she will simply become fat.

In other words, in that vital second half of pregnancy, you must feed a diet which has been designed to allow growth to occur. The BARF diet will do exactly that.

WARNING - two common errors made by breeders

One of the most common mistakes made by breeders is to over feed during pregnancy. Although pregnancy is a time of growth, if your bitch was fed properly prior to pregnancy, her nutritional requirements during pregnancy remain pretty well unchanged. Certainly she does not need heaps and heaps more food. Just a little bit more towards the end of pregnancy.

Over feeding in pregnancy will result in a fat bitch. She will have difficulty giving birth. Underfeeding during lactation will result in a poor milk supply, puppies that do not grow well, and a bitch that comes out of lactation dangerously underweight with severely compromised health.

However, do not go to the opposite extreme. Do not underfeed during pregnancy, because no matter how good her previous diet has been, a poor diet during pregnancy will result in fewer live births and the ones that are born will lack vigour due to nutritional depletion. Their muscle tone and their ability to survive will be greatly decreased. So please - do not slack off during pregnancy, but do not over feed.

The second common error that people make with their breeding bitches is to underfeed them in lactation. But we shall talk about that in Chapter Seven.

The simple solution? Continue feeding the BARF diet!

Nutrition at mating time

Not only should your bitch be close to her ideal weight at mating, she should also be gaining weight at this time. She should be on a 'rising plane of nutrition.' This will help her fertility immeasurably.

When you know your bitch is close to coming on heat, due on in about two to three weeks time, temporarily increase both the amount and the quality you feed her. By increasing the quality of the food fed, I mean that it should contain a greater amount of the nutrients essential for growth.   That includes extra protein, extra vitamins, extra essential fatty acids and extra minerals.

In practical terms that means less vegetables, more chicken wings, more liver, more flax seed oil and more eggs. Add extra supplements including kelp, cod liver oil, vitamin E, multi B and vitamin C.

This more concentrated food is particularly important prior to coming on heat. It may not be possible to get a lot of food into her round the time she is mated. Some bitches will eat at this time while others refuse.

Ideally she should have been slightly on the lean side - about 5% below her ideal weight - and very active, for about one month prior to coming on heat. When fed extra food for a short period just before mating, she will be gaining weight at the time she ovulates and conceives. Her body responds to this increase in nutrition with brilliant hormone production, and a maximum number of healthy eggs shed and a maximum number fertilised.

Try and time it so at the time of mating, she is at her ideal weight - blooming with 'condition.'

What you are doing here is telling her body that good times are coming and this is an excellent time to reproduce. This is why very thin bitches, or bitches that are losing weight due to a poor diet, often fail to conceive.

Will this produce too many pups?

Definitely not. Bodies are much too clever for that. Although your bitch produces far more embryos than she needs, her uterus will pick and choose the best and healthiest among them to grow and become puppies. The others, the ones for whom there is no room, are simply reabsorbed.

If you follow this method of feeding at mating time, you have done everything possible to produce the optimum number of puppies, with a very good chance that they will all be healthy.

Please note ...

... cod liver oil should not be fed during the first two thirds of pregnancy. The high levels of vitamin A can be dangerous to foetal health in that period. However, let me stress that it is essential to feed cod liver oil prior to pregnancy, and then again at the end of pregnancy and most particularly during lactation.

To ensure that the optimum numbers of pups are retained by her uterus, keep that high plane of nutrition going for seven to ten days after mating, tapering it off gradually, so that at fourteen days after mating, she has returned to her normal diet. Normal both in quantity and quality. The only supplement you will leave out at this time will be cod liver oil.

Let me repeat the message that it is important not to overfeed your bitch during this first two thirds of pregnancy. The puppies are not growing much during this period and it is important that you do not get mum too fat. An obese mum is not a healthy mum, and **obesity is anything greater than 15 % over her ideal weight.**

During the first third of pregnancy ...

SHE does not gain a lot of weight. The puppies are not growing much, and there is only a small amount of growth of the uterus and the mammary glands, together with a minor increases in fat stores. In fact, most of any increase in weight consists of foetal fluids.

However, do be aware that although mum is not gaining much weight, there is a whole lot going on at a microscopic and biochemical level as those tiny embryos start their incredible journey towards being puppies. Also realise that this incredible period which is the beginning of a number of new lives is not anything that cannot be handled by your bitch's bodily reserves combined with that basic healthy BARF diet.

In other words, if your bitch has been on a healthy BARF diet prior to being mated, she simply continues on that diet.

If you have chosen to feed her a more concentrated growth type of diet during this first half of pregnancy - a diet with increased levels of energy and proteins - do not overdo it. Excessive calories at this time will simply produce needless obesity.

Fat bitches have difficulty giving birth, partly because of the fat obstructing the birth canal and partly due to their lack of exercise during pregnancy which results in poor muscle tone in uterine and abdominal muscles.

Let me repeat, the diet you were feeding your bitch before she became pregnant - the BARF diet - is fine to feed for the first half of pregnancy.

9 4

The only thing I would stress at this time is to keep up the kelp, the vitamin E, the multi B and the vitamin C. Particularly the vitamin C. It has been found that extra vitamin C during pregnancy aids in an easy delivery. No need for caesarean sections.

Let me stress once again, it is important not to overfeed her at this time. She must be kept slim and active.

Pregnancy Diagnosis

- Ultrasound may be used - by skilled operators - from as early as 21 days till late in pregnancy.

- Radiographs are best employed during the last third of pregnancy when the foetal skeletons are becoming mineralised.

- The palpation or feel method is best employed at about thirty days.

By the palpation or feel method, at about twenty eight to thirty days, your vet can feel or palpate the presence of the two pregnant uterine horns. Each horn feels like a string of golf balls or marbles, depending on the size of the bitch.

After another week to ten days has passed, those 'rounded balls' all join together to form a sausage like structure - which is mostly fluid - making diagnosis by palpation much more difficult until late in pregnancy when the pregnancy is usually pretty obvious.

False pregnancies

Observation in early pregnancy is not reliable as a means of deciding whether your dog is pregnant. This is because all bitches go through the hormonal cycle or motions of pregnancy following a heat period - whether they are in fact pregnant or not. They show mammary gland enlargement and even abdominal enlargement to varying degrees. They can look quite pregnant even when they are not. Occasionally bitches   will take themselves through the birth process at the appropriate time.

Some breeders find that bitches going off their food at some time between the third and the fifth week is a fairly reliable sign of pregnancy: that is, these bitches have ...

... Morning sickness

It is not uncommon for bitches round about four weeks into their pregnancy to go through a period of 'morning sickness' when they voluntarily cut down on their food intake. They usually will only eat very plain food in small amounts at this time. It is believed that this happens to stop mum from eating anything that could damage the foetus at a critical stage of its development. As I mentioned previously, this particular signal is used by some breeders as a reasonably reliable method of diagnosing pregnancy.

Warning

Be careful not to unduly stress your bitch with foods foreign to her during her pregnancy. This is particularly so during the third, fourth, and fifth week of pregnancy when most of the vital internal organs are forming in those little puppies.

If you have at this time suddenly decided to switch her to the BARF diet, she may object to all these 'strange' foods which you are suddenly thrusting upon her; she may stop eating altogether and be very distressed. That would be worse than a bad diet of commercial dog food.

It is important to get your bitch used to and very happy about eating natural foods well before she becomes pregnant. The trick is to have her eating all these wonderful foods from the day she comes into your life.

At what stage in the pregnancy do we start to feed our bitch more food?

It is usual to feed more food during the last half of pregnancy. It is simply a matter of gradually feeding more food to keep pace with her increasing weight. This is particularly so during the last third of pregnancy. If you have been feeding her the BARF diet - there is not a great deal that you have to change. Just a bit more of the same.

It is during the last third of pregnancy that the pups do most of their growing. If she has not done so already, now is the time that she may begin to demand more food.

As a general rule of thumb, you will increase the amount of food fed each week, beginning at about week six, by 5% to 10%, so that by week eight she is having up to one and a quarter to one and a half times what she had in early pregnancy.

It is most important that you do not try and stuff all this food into your pregnant bitch in just one sitting. As the pregnancy proceeds, and the puppies grow inside their mum, there is less and less room inside her to accommodate the extra food that she and the pups need. That means we either have to increase the nutrient density of the food or feed smaller meals more often. In practice we do both.

Over the last three to four weeks of pregnancy, gradually reduce meal size and increase meal frequency so that by week eight your pregnant bitch is having three or four meals a day, with each meal being about half to a third the size of what it was when you were feeding her once a day.

To increase the nutrient density of the food you will increase gradually the more concentrated foods such as meat ,eggs, liver, kidneys, brain, flax seed oil, etc. These are the nutrients which promote growth. You reduce her raw meaty bones - the chicken wings and chicken necks - to about 25% of her overall diet, and cut out the big bones altogether.

You will feed less vegetables and fruit. That means the patties will now be about 25% vegetables and fruit, with the rest made up of meat, eggs, liver, kidneys, brains etc..

To assist this building process, add extra supplements including kelp, vitamin E, multi B and vitamin C. You may begin to include a small amount of cod liver oil once again.

No matter what the breed, large or small, it is important to increase the nutrient density of the food, to increase meal frequency and to reduce meal size. For example, although the small breeds produce fewer pups than the larger breeds, those pups can take up a lot more room inside their mum than the pups in one of the giant breeds.

Carbohydrates and pregnancy

Modern research tells us that SHE has a special need for carbohydrates towards the end of pregnancy. What is the rationale for this?

First let me say that the requirement for a bitch to be fed extra starchy foods towards the end of pregnancy is rarely a problem in bitches fed the BARF diet.

Mostly this relates to the smaller breeds. Bitches who have not been fed a BARF diet, but have been enduring a mostly meat diet all their lives. A high protein diet. These bitches, particularly Chihuahuas, can suffer from hypoglycaemia [low blood sugar] and give birth to fewer live pups.

Suitable forms of complex carbohydrates in this case include cooked brown rice, whole grain bread, boiled whole potatoes, sweet potatoes, pumpkins etc., or rolled oats soaked in either milk or water. These will probably form about 20% of the overall diet during the last two or three weeks of pregnancy.

Two healthy ways to feed grain to your dogs ...

... firstly you can sprout them and feed them like any other vegetable, and secondly you can completely crush the uncooked grain, soak it overnight and then mix it with other raw totally crushed vegetables. Those raw totally crushed vegetables can include potatoes, pumpkin, sweet potatoes etc..

Note: never feed green potatoes. They contain solanine - a poisonous alkaloid.

WARNING - Do not feed a pregnant bitch extra calcium

Particularly during the last third of pregnancy.

One of the biggest mistakes made by breeders, both experienced and inexperienced, is to feed great heaps of calcium to their pregnant bitches in the hope of preventing milk fever. Please do not do it! Instead of preventing problems you are more likely to create them. If you ignore this advice then you must be prepared to continue with heavy calcium supplementation all through lactation.

It has been observed that pregnant dogs in the wild, towards the end of pregnancy, eat lots more of the organ meats rather than bones. They eat concentrated foods, rich in essential fatty acids, proteins and vitamins. Foods that are low in calcium. Foods such as heart, liver, kidney, brains and so on. On the other hand, after they give birth, these new canine mums add bone eating to their menu once again.

The cessation of bone eating prior to whelping tells us two important things

Firstly - as we have already discussed - the need to feed high protein concentrated food towards the end of pregnancy, bearing in mind that this is not so true where a bitch has been fed a high protein diet all her life, as is common in the smaller breeds.

Secondly - the time to add EXTRA CALCIUM to the diet of a breeding bitch - if you are going to add any at all - is after the whelping - not before.

The thinking behind the practice of feeding loads of calcium during pregnancy is that it will prevent milk fever or Eclampsia.

However, by feeding extra calcium during pregnancy you are more likely to cause Eclampsia than prevent it. In addition that extra calcium can cause soft tissue calcification and other birth defects in the pups. For further information concerning Eclampsia, please turn to Chapter Six.

Getting close to whelping or giving birth

During week nine, the pups do not grow much in weight but they do a lot of finishing or developing type growth. During this last week of pregnancy, as your bitch comes closer to whelping, gradually reduce the total amount of food fed, so that a couple of days before she is due to give birth, she is receiving about half of that increased amount you were feeding during week eight. You will also increase the amount of vegetables and flax seed oil, almost totally eliminating the bones, and much reducing the meat and offal. You are now feeding a slightly laxative type of diet.

As she gets close to giving birth, you might only be feeding a quarter of what she was having in week eight. At the same time, gradually reduce the vitamins and other additives proportionately to her reduction in total food intake.

In those final few days before giving birth, she will draw on many of the nutrients stored in her body. Her bodily reserves. These reserves include amongst other things, the calcium stores in her bones. She will continue to do this for the first three or four days after the puppies are born. That is why it is so important that she has been properly fed to this point.

The birth or whelping process

A few days before whelping the bitch often appears as if she is sagging, with her belly and mammary glands hanging closer to the ground. Her mammary glands become enlarged and pink. Milk can usually be expressed at this time.

She normally starts nesting about twenty four hours before she is due to give birth.

Do not be surprised if she goes off her food in the last twelve hours before she whelps. On the other hand, not all pregnant bitches do this ... so like most things in life, there are very few hard and fast rules, just greater probabilities of certain things happening.

When the bitch is ready to give birth, she completely stops her production of progesterone. This initiates the birth process. It also causes a sudden and temporary drop in the body temperature from its normal 38.5 degrees Celsius to around 37 degrees Celsius for a few hours. This occurs approximately eight to twelve hours before she whelps.

This temperature drop is a reliable indicator of the impending birth process. That is why it is a very good idea to monitor her temperature as the predicted time of her whelping approaches. Take her temperature every three or four hours and keep a record. By monitoring her in this way there will be no surprises. You will have a very good idea of when she is due to whelp. This becomes very important if for some reason she is unable to give birth normally.

Another common feature around the time of whelping is for the bitch to completely empty her bowels before giving birth. The reason for this is so there will be maximum room in the birth canal. The puppies do not want to be competing with a large lump of faeces as they struggle to be born.

The 'Afterbirths'

During the birth process, an 'afterbirth' - or placenta - will usually be passed after each pup. The pup's placenta is the organ through which it obtained nourishment during those vital 63 days of pregnancy.

As the pups are born, the bitch will normally clear the tissues which encase the pups, licking the pups vigorously to stimulate breathing, and when the after birth is passed will eat it.

Eating the 'afterbirths' is fine, normal and natural. It provides her with much needed top quality concentrated food, which will carry her through the next several days when she may not feel like eating and she may not wish to leave the pups.

Assisting with the birth process

If the bitch has not removed the sac from the pup within one to two minutes, do interfere and remove it, otherwise the pup will asphyxiate. Having said that let me add that it is very wise to interfere as little as possible. Most bitches that have too much help learn not to do anything themselves and make very poor mothers.

So many bitches have problems giving birth

What should be a [relatively] simple process - somewhat akin - forgive me ladies - to shelling peas, becomes a protracted agonising affair. A process requiring veterinary attention ranging from oxytocin and calcium injections to get the process underway - through assisted deliveries - all the way to the need for caesarean sections.

Most people who have experienced such problems with their bitches, find those problems disappear when they begin to feed their bitches the BARF diet.

I have two other tips which when combined with the natural diet will help your bitch give birth more easily.

The first of these is to feed vitamin C throughout the pregnancy. For a 20 kg bitch feed at least 500 mg twice daily.

The second tip is to feed red raspberry leaf tablets during the last third of pregnancy. For a 20 kg [44 lb] bitch, give two tablets daily.

Which method will you choose for your bitches?

Just recently some very good clients of mine had their little Chihuahua bitch Evie give birth to seven healthy puppies - right on time, without assistance - in the space of only a few hours. They had done exactly as I had suggested throughout the pregnancy. They fed the BARF diet, they gave the raspberry leaf tablets and they gave the vitamin C. They kept her slim and active.

That very same day I had to perform a caesarean section on another Chihuahua bitch ... called Bonnie. Bonnie is the same age as Evie. Bonnie like Evie was giving birth for the first time.

The only major difference between these two bitches was that the young lady that could not give birth naturally and had to have a caesarean had been fed on commercial dog food throughout not only her pregnancy but her entire life. She did not receive any supplements such as raspberry leaf tablets or vitamin C during her pregnancy. She had never eaten any form of fresh uncooked food in her entire life.

From that little story you must draw your own conclusions. For me it illustrates beautifully - or perhaps cruelly would be a more apt word to choose - my constant experience: that the dogs which have reproductive problems are the ones being fed those awful commercial dog foods. Particularly when that is all they are fed. When no fresh food of any description at all is offered to these poor creatures.

Now of course such a coincidental happening by itself proves nothing in a scientific or statistical sense. However, I know which method I would choose to feed my dogs!

CHAPTER FIVE

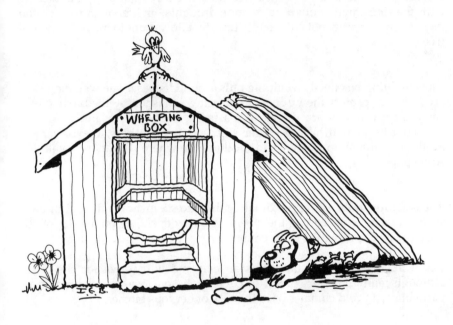

THE WHELPING BOX

For those readers who have not come across the concept of the whelping box, it is a box, room, or area, which has been specially designed and set aside to accommodate the whelping bitch and her litter. The whelping box aims to provide shelter, warmth and safety for the pups.

Unfortunately our traditional whelping box often provides more problems than it solves.

The basic idea is that the pregnant bitch whelps in the whelping box and then raises her litter in it.

That means the whelping box should be of sturdy construction and be large enough to accommodate the bitch and the puppies up to the time of weaning. It is normally constructed in such a way that it can be heated, with the sides high enough to exclude draughts, high enough to keep the pups from escaping, but sufficiently low to allow mum to move in and out freely.

The whelping box needs whelping rails around its base. The whelping rails are there to protect the puppies from being squashed by the bitch. Many early puppy losses are due to pups being squashed by mum. This is particularly so with a large litter size, young mothers, inexperienced mothers, clumsy mothers, bad mothers, or where there are weak and sickly pups.

The whelping rails are approximately three to six inches wide and three to six inches above the base of the whelping box, depending on the size of the bitch the box is designed to accommodate.

One wall of the box usually has an exit and entry area for the bitch, although many breeders prefer to completely enclose the whelping box, particularly in cold climates or in the case of nervous bitches.

Is this whelping box the best we can manage for our bitches and their pups?

Many breeders experience enormous problems with whelping boxes.

- So often these boxes fail to protect the pups from being **squashed or suffocated.**

- **In these boxes the temperature can be very hard to control.** Sometimes the pups are too hot, and sometimes too cold.

- **Often these boxes are too open and draughty, or they are too enclosed** and too humid. The draughty ones promote viral problems through chilling, whilst the humid ones provide a perfect environment for breeding bacteria.

- **Mostly these boxes can be very difficult to keep clean and dry**, and after being used for several litters have an enormous build-up of disease-causing pathogens. Pneumonia and bacterial mastitis is common when these unsanitary conditions are combined with overcrowding, high temperatures and high humidity. However, it gets worse.

- **Pups raised in whelping boxes often start their lives with a few weeks of unhealthy exercise.** They spend their first three weeks of life sliding around on newspaper. Newspaper, which is cold, hard and slippery. Newspaper which denies pups any possibility of getting a grip. This is one of the myriad techniques owners have developed to 'encourage' the production of bone and joint problems.

- At their worst, these hard slippery surfaces are the beginnings of problems such as Hip Dysplasia, 'swimmers,' bowed legs and slipping patellas, all of which happen quite 'naturally' as pups slide around rather than walk around their whelping area, particularly when other common errors involving diet are employed. At the very least these unhealthy conditions are the beginnings of a badly built puppy with bone and joint looseness and weak muscles.

- Even thick towelling, although better than newspaper, can still be scratched up into folds which may suffocate the pups.

What are the characteristics of an ideal whelping box?

- The ideal whelping box will prevent pups from being squashed or suffocated.

- The ideal whelping box will keep pups at the optimum temperature - the bitch's body temperature - not cooking them, and not allowing them to become chilled.

- The ideal whelping box will allow healthy circulation of fresh clean air without being either too draughty, or too enclosed and humid.

- The ideal whelping box will be easily cleaned and not allow the build-up of pathogenic organisms.

- The ideal whelping box will be well drained, dry and not allow the build-up of fluids such as urine and uterine discharges.

- The ideal whelping box will provide excellent traction for young paws and legs, allowing pups to get a firm grip without sliding.

The urban whelping box provides most of these features

What is the urban whelping box?

- It is a hole the urban bitch digs under the house, usually in the most inaccessible spot.

- It is a hole the bitch digs in the earth behind the whelping box under a piece of tin leaning up against the whelping box.

- Or any other similar arrangement a bitch given her freedom will organise.

The urban whelping box is exactly the same whelping box as used so successfully by a wild canid such as a wolf or a dingo or a fox.

Both the urban and wild whelping box is a saucer shaped hole or depression a bitch digs in the earth.

Is this hole in the earth – the ideal whelping box?

- In my experience of many hundreds of these 'whelping holes,' there have been minimal puppy losses through squashing. The reason has to do with the natural curve of the hole, the natural 'give' in this material as opposed to the hard solidity of the 'whelping box,' the fact that the pups fall to the bottom of the hole, while mum is curled around one side of the hole, and the fact that mum can enlarge that hole away from the pups when she is in danger of squashing them. The bottom line is - those pups are rarely squashed!

- No matter how freezing and cold the temperature may be outside these whelping holes, the pups in them are always snug and warm - so long as the hole is sheltered from the rain, and the hole does not fill with water. They never become too hot nor do they become chilled.

- These whelping holes provide the perfect micro-climate for little pups - even when mum has to temporarily leave them. When mum leaves, all the pups tumble to the bottom of the hole in a tight little bundle. That little bundle of pups stays warm because it has a small surface area, and a layer of still air over the top to conserve warmth.

- There is no worry that a pup will stray away from the others and become chilled. If a pup does move away from the others, it will not go far, and when it becomes sleepy, it simply tumbles back down amongst the others.

- Because of the very open arrangement of these whelping holes, together with being below the level of their surrounds, there is always a healthy circulation of beautiful fresh air. Air that is moisturised, but not humid, and certainly never draughty.

- When this whelping hole becomes soiled, mum very simply digs another one, thus preventing any build up of pathogenic organisms.

- These whelping holes in my experience are always warm and snug and dry and very absorbent of vaginal discharges, urine and even diarrhoea. Once again, if these liquids start to build up, a fresh hole is dug by mum, or fresh soil is scraped in.

- Finally, these whelping holes provide excellent traction for young paws and legs, allowing pups to get a firm grip without sliding.

In summary, this simple depression enables maximum conservation of warmth, freedom from draughts and maximum puppy safety. It never becomes too humid nor does it become too hot. As exploring newborns, the pups are able to tumble safely back into mum's protectively curled body. That soil formed depression also provides great absorption for fluids which simply drain away. The soil base of this 'whelping hole' provides optimum traction or grip for young paws. Pups in whelping holes never have to move around on slippery surfaces.

Should you do this for your pups ?

If your current whelping arrangements are less than ideal, let me encourage you to try the whelping hole

As you can see, all you need is shelter, a well drained site and clean soil to provide the perfect environment for whelping and raising pups. Countless bitches from the beginning of dog time have whelped successfully in a hole they have dug for themselves. Countless bitches still do - forced by necessity, and protected, thankfully - by that same necessity - from being forced to raise pups in the hostile environment of the 'whelping box.'

If you cannot organise that simple hole in the earth for your bitches - and I bet you could if you tried - do as I do, provide your bitch with deep piles of aged, dust free, deodorised wood mulch and/or straw. A deep litter system for bitches.

The deep litter whelping hole

The bitch forms her 'whelping hole' in any of these materials with great safety, and warmth for the pups, and great traction for young paws and legs. The deep litter whelping hole enables maximum conservation of warmth. This hole mimics the natural situation where the wild bitch digs a bowl shaped hole in the earth in which to both deliver the pups and then to suckle them in those first three weeks when the pups are totally reliant on mum for their nutrition, their toilet functions and their temperature regulation.

In addition, these deep litter whelping holes provide great absorbency for all those unwanted liquids so prevalent at this time. The urine, and vaginal discharges etc..

When the bitch whelps in a whelping hole she has dug in deep litter, the hole is always exactly the right size. The straying struggling pups will always roll back down to mum who is lying protectively curled round them.

The pups never lack traction in this material, so they are developing healthy limbs and joints from the word go.

The wood shavings can be changed after each litter is whelped. While the litter of pups is on those shavings, mum can dig fresh holes as required. Each hole she digs is absorbent and beautifully clean and warm because it dries out quickly and helps conserve heat. This is all very close to nature.

As pups begin to walk, the soil or litter base base on which they live provides the perfect grip they require. This ensures optimum use and therefore development and strength of those little legs and their bones and joints. This gives every pup the maximum chance of developing a strong healthy body with minimal chance of developing such problems as Hip Dysplasia, bowed legs, slipping patellas, or becoming 'swimmers.'

My simple whelping box ...

... **was originally a wood shed which has since become my giant whelping box which is suitable for any breed.**

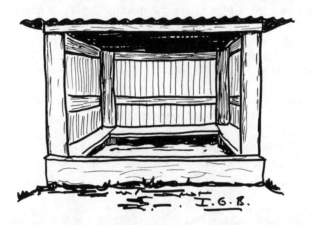

This shed is built on very sandy soil on the side of a hill facing north, so it has the perfect aspect - for the southern hemisphere - and great drainage. I have dug the soil out of the bottom of the woodshed to a depth of eighteen inches. The bottom is filled with wood shavings.

The depth of the wood shavings has been further increased by running a fifteen inch wide plank of wood across the front of the shed. This gives me a depth of shavings in excess of twenty inches together with about six to eight inches of board above the height of the shavings - sufficient to keep the pups from struggling out of that safe area too early in their life, but over which mum can quite easily jump. I have another rail round the base of the shed - see picture - which acts as a whelping rail. It also stops the pups as they grow from escaping too soon to the outside world.

The bitch digs her hole[s] wherever she wants to. As the pups grow, they crawl out of the hole and begin to dig their own holes. They have plenty of room to play. They can urinate and defaecate freely - those unwanted liquids and solids simply disappear into the shavings without contaminating the pup's environs. The pups enjoy the sun, they are sheltered from bad weather but always have fresh air. They can snuggle together or move apart as they want to, never too cold, and never too hot. They chew on bones, they fight over bones, they simply enjoy their life, just beautifully content. Mum moves in and out freely. The pups in this situation grow strong and healthy on their raw meaty bones and healthy play and eating exercise.

The wood shavings I use in my whelping box are produced for small animals such as guinea pigs or for the nesting boxes of free range laying hens. These shavings have been deodorised, had the dust extracted and are an almost perfect substitute for the natural earth which a wild bitch uses for her very safe, warm, clean and draught free saucer in which to whelp and feed her pups.

Can I challenge or perhaps encourage you to make similar arrangements for your pregnant bitches?

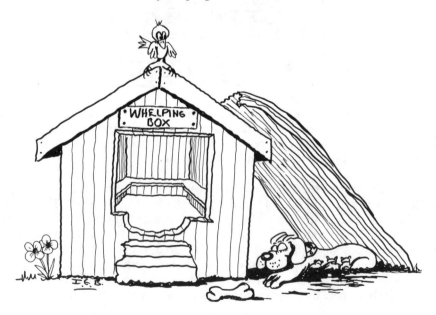

CHAPTER SIX

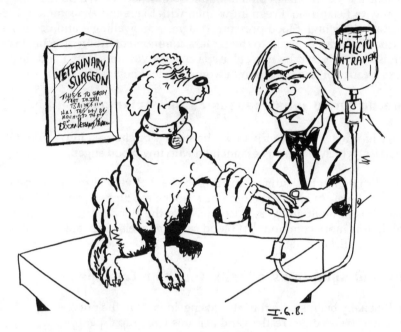

ECLAMPSIA OR MILK FEVER

Eclampsia is a condition of severe muscular spasms and high temperature that can occur in bitches in the period from before birth through to weaning of the pups. It most commonly appears in the two to three weeks following whelping, that is, when a bitch is at peak lactation. However, it can be seen before whelping, straight after whelping, or up to four to six weeks after whelping.

Eclampsia, which is commonly known as milk fever, goes under a number of other names including puerperal tetany, post parturient tetany and hypocalcemia.

The term Eclampsia is borrowed from human medicine...

... because the symptoms in bitches mimic somewhat the symptoms seen in women with Eclampsia. Pregnant women with the relatively common 'Pre-eclampsia' show high blood pressure, oedema - or swelling - and protein in the urine. This can proceed to the far less common condition of Eclampsia, which is characterised by muscular spasms, convulsions, coma and death. The exact cause of this condition in women is not known. However ...

... we do know what causes canine Eclampsia

The basic cause of Eclampsia in breeding bitches is **LOW BLOOD CALCIUM** which may also be combined with **low blood sugar**.

It is vital that blood calcium in any dog be kept at very strict and constant levels. The levels of blood calcium must not be too high, nor must they be too low. It is difficult and very uncommon for the blood calcium to become too high. It is more common that blood calcium levels drop, and when they do - we have Eclampsia.

Signs and symptoms of milk fever or Eclampsia

- It usually begins with the bitch losing interest in the pups.
- Then she becomes restless and nervous with rapid panting.
- This progresses to trembling and staggering.
- Untreated she will eventually go down and may then have violent contractions of muscle groups all over her body.
- This muscular activity causes a rapid and extreme rise in body temperature which can go to 41 degrees Celsius or more.
- The muscular spasms and convulsions if left untreated will eventually lead to coma and death.
- In some breeds the first you will know of the problem is when the bitch becomes aggressive towards the pups - for example with bull terriers.

Low blood calcium causes these signs and symptoms because one of the many roles of calcium is to stabilise nerve and muscle cells against continuous function or muscular spasm. That is, **low blood calcium causes the muscles to 'cramp.'**

But why have these bitches got low blood calcium?

When a bitch is lactating, it can be difficult for her to to keep a constant level of calcium in her blood, because the calcium is literally pouring from her blood into the milk.

As the bitch pours calcium into the milk, she must replace it. And where does she get that replacement calcium from? Two places - her food and her bones, and it is her bones she depends on most.

However, if there are not sufficient calcium stores in her bones, or if the hormones are not available to get calcium from her bones into her blood, her blood calcium levels will drop and she will develop Eclampsia.

In other words, Eclampsia can occur if the calcium stores in the bones are low, or if the hormonal system that withdraws calcium from the bones is not working.

That means to understand the cause[s] of Eclampsia, we have to understand why the calcium levels in the bones are low, and what has caused the hormone system to fail.

First, we will look at why the calcium levels in the bones are low

The cause is usually a lifetime of being fed a mainly meat, and therefore calcium deficient, diet. That is why the problem is seen more commonly in the smaller breeds. The smaller breeds train their owners to feed them a meat only diet; and usually cooked meat at that.

Not uncommonly a mostly meat diet will be fed over several generations in succession - each generation becoming more calcium deficient. As a result each generation becomes more prone to Eclampsia. When Eclampsia is seen to follow this family line, many vets and owners are tempted to believe **the problem is inherited. But of course, it isn't.**

However, the problem is not only due to a LACK of calcium in the diet. It is also due to CALCIUM LOSS. High protein diets have the effect of speeding up the removal of calcium from the body. This further depletes the calcium stores in the bones.

The end result of a bitch spending a lifetime eating a calcium-poor and calcium-depleting diet is a bitch that has very poor calcium reserves in her bones.

As you can imagine, when a bitch with such poor calcium reserves begins to draw on those reserves during lactation, there is simply not enough calcium to supply her needs. In this case not even switching to a bone-based diet will solve the problem. **Neither a BARF diet nor a commercial diet can supply her needs fast enough.** She will need a source of highly soluble, highly available artificial calcium such as Calcium Sandoz. Unless this is supplied constantly and in large amounts, her blood calcium will drop causing ECLAMPSIA.

Also keep in mind that because these dogs are being fed poor diets, they can also suffer other nutritional deficiencies; for example, if they are on a calcium deficient meat-only diet which can be low in vitamin D, AND they never get out in the sunshine, they may also be lacking sufficient vitamin D. Vitamin D plays a vital role in calcium metabolism, including the absorption of calcium from food.

However, there is more to this than a mere calcium deficiency. There is also a hormonal problem.

That leads us to the question ...

In what way is the bitch's hormonal system wrecked?

The problem is the failure by the bitch to produce the parathyroid hormone. This hormone takes the calcium out of the bones to keep the blood calcium levels normal. When breeders feed loads of artificial calcium prior to whelping, that is a signal to the parathyroid gland that parathyroid hormone will not be needed.

When that bitch starts to produce milk for her puppies, the parathyroid hormone is not released, the blood calcium levels drop and the bitch very quickly develops Eclampsia.

The only way to prevent Eclampsia in this situation is to continue feeding a very soluble source of calcium right through lactation.

This brings us to ...

... the 'recipe' used to 'produce' Eclampsia

- feed low calcium foods for a lifetime
- feed heaps of calcium towards the end of lactation
- stop the calcium supplements when she gives birth

- Please - let me urge you NOT TO DO THIS!

Now you are beginning to realise why ...

... Eclampsia usually occurs at peak lactation when the puppies are big and hungry, and not yet eating any solid food, but drinking plenty of mum's milk. This puts an enormous strain on mum's calcium reserves in her bones.

... Eclampsia is more common in bitches that have had several litters because the calcium reserves in the bitch's bones become a little more depleted with each successive litter.

... Eclampsia is more common in bitches with large litters because there is a much greater drain on the calcium reserves in the bitch's bones.

So how do we solve the Eclampsia problem?

1] Feed the BARF diet for a lifetime

Eclampsia is a problem which stems from a lifetime of poor eating habits. It is often a problem that began generations back, and may take several generations to resolve. However, the quickest way to resolve it is to feed a balanced raw meaty bone-based diet. The BARF diet.

The message here is, you must feed raw meaty bones - e.g. chicken wings, chicken necks, lamb off-cuts etc., as the basis of the diet [approximately 60% of the diet - or more] for all of the bitch's life, and continue to feed those raw meaty bones throughout pregnancy.

By feeding a bone-based diet for all of a bitch's life, you are ensuring excellent calcium reserves in her bones for lactation.

When her pups have been weaned, do continue to feed her a bone-based diet to ensure a healthy build up of calcium for her next lactation.

2] Do not supplement with calcium during pregnancy

Towards the end of pregnancy it is important to feed less calcium rich foods so that the bitch's parathyroids get the signal that they need to start working. That means feeding less bones and more meat, organ meats, healthy oils [e.g. linseed oil], and vegetables - as a source of carbohydrates and fibre.

3] Feed extra calcium DURING lactation, NOT before it

If you are going to feed extra calcium to your breeding bitches, do not feed it during pregnancy, feed it to them after they have whelped.

It is when the bitch is lactating that she needs heaps of extra calcium. There is very little calcium deposited in the puppies' bones before they are born compared to what they need and receive through the milk after they are born. Unfortunately, it is after the puppies are born that many breeders stop giving the calcium.

When the wild bitch starts eating after whelping, it has been observed that she chooses to eat masses of bones - and she will continue to eat bones throughout the lactation. She instinctively knows her best source of calcium. She knows what her body needs. **This is what YOU should be doing with your bitch[es].**

Many breeders prefer not to fix the problem

They prefer to live with it. This is because they consider it too much trouble to change the bitch's diet. They would rather carry on feeding their bitches with all meat diets, and supplement with calcium all through pregnancy and lactation.

In many cases that will work - to a point. It may stop the Eclampsia, but commonly these bitches end up with other health problems caused by that all meat diet. I have seen cancer, inflammatory bowel disease, various skin problems, sugar diabetes, and most common of all, kidney failure because of the all-meat diet with its high levels of protein and phosphorus.

If you have a bitch that suffers from Eclampsia ...

... she may always be susceptible to it. It is hard to reverse poor calcium storage in bones, particularly after several generations of calcium deficient diets. It may take a number of generations for the problem to disappear. The important thing, however, is not to give up. You can breed that bitch again, and she can be improved. You **can** increase the amount of calcium stored in her bones and you **can** improve the functioning of her parathyroid glands.

All you have to do is switch her to the BARF diet. However, even after switching that bitch to the BARF diet you must still be prepared to supplement her with calcium **during lactation** - not during pregnancy - and perhaps be ready to wean the pups early.

By starting a bitch that develops Eclampsia on the BARF diet, she WILL improve rather than deteriorate over successive litters of pups as the calcium stores in her bones and her general health improve. By keeping her offspring on the BARF diet, they will be better than her in respect to calcium stores and parathyroid hormone levels after whelping, and their offspring in turn will be better again. However, those bitches MUST stay on the BARF programme for this to happen.

This problem can be fixed in a kennel by firstly switching to the BARF programme, and secondly, having the patience to ride out the storm of [decreasing] bouts of Eclampsia over a number of generations.

Treating Eclampsia

If you have a bitch that develops Eclampsia, you must get her to a vet as soon as possible. However, you can help matters with some very simple first aid.

The most essential thing is to get some calcium and a source of simple sugars - e.g. honey - into her as rapidly as possible. Any form of calcium will do, such as milk, calcium tablets, or better still, one of the soluble forms of calcium such as Calcium Sandoz.

Many breeders will use milk and honey, or even better, milk, Calcium Sandoz and honey or glucose.

To a cup of milk add two teaspoons of Calcium Sandoz, two teaspoons of honey - a quick acting carbohydrate, a teaspoon of dolomite - as a source of calcium and magnesium which calms the nerves - half a banana - it contains complex carbohydrates and vitamin B 6 which is calming. Whisk it all up in your blender.

If using powdered milk and you do not have any other form of calcium you may make it a little stronger, e.g. one and a half times the recommended strength. If you have calcium tablets, two or three of these may be crushed up into 250 ml [one cup] of milk together with the honey, banana and dolomite.

If your bitch is reluctant or not able to drink this mixture, feed her with a syringe, making sure you syringe it very gently into the side of her mouth with her head tilted back at a comfortable angle. This is to ensure she swallows it. It is important she does not 'breathe' it in. If it ends up in her lungs, it is likely to cause aspiration pneumonia.

Get her to a vet as soon as possible for a proper assessment and for an injection of calcium and what ever other treatment he feels is necessary. This will usually include the pups being taken from her and weaned if it is a bad case. Take your vet's advice on this.

The bottom line is, if you want to beat Eclampsia, feed the BARF diet for all of a bitch's life and do not supplement with calcium before the pups are born. The only time you may have to use a calcium supplement is after the pups are born, but even this will eventually become unnecessary if you continue with the BARF diet through several generations.

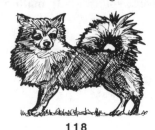

CHAPTER SEVEN

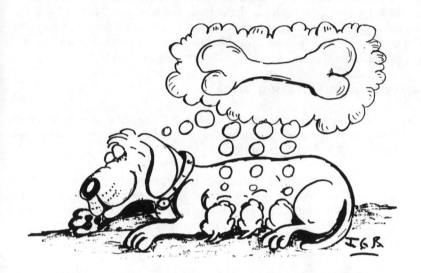

FEEDING THE LACTATING BITCH

The hardest work a bitch can do!

Being a mum feeding pups is one of the hardest jobs a bitch can do. In terms of energy expenditure, its only canine equivalent would be a sled dog dragging a sled over hundreds of kilometres of frozen wasteland for an equivalent period of time. Both these activities require a similarly huge amount of top quality food if the dog is to continue its work and not lose weight or condition or deteriorate in health.

That is why a lactating bitch, at peak lactation, with a large litter of pups ...

... can be fed as much as she wants!

A lactating bitch with a large number of pups ...

... at the height of her lactation, is the only situation [apart from the sled dog] where **it is imperative that top quality food should be continually available.** By top quality food, I mean a diet designed for growth but slanted towards the special requirements of a lactating bitch. Do note that the specific needs of the lactating bitch are quite different from the sled dog's needs. However, the sled dog's diet is another story!

The food for a lactating bitch ...

- ... must have all the nutrients necessary for the repair and functioning of her body, **plus** all the necessary ingredients for producing high quality milk - in vast quantities.

- ... must be very concentrated. Being a 'growth-type' of diet it must have high levels of energy, first class protein, first class fat, first class minerals, an over-abundant supply of vitamins, and be low in carbohydrates and unnecessary components. What I have just described is the lactation version of the BARF diet.

What about artificial calcium?

A lactating bitch with large numbers of puppies is the only situation which occasionally justifies feeding artificial calcium. Artificial calcium is usually required when a bitch has received an inadequate sort of diet all her life or has an unusually large number of pups to feed. The diet which leads to Eclampsia is usually a badly designed home made diet. For more information on Eclampsia please read Chapter Six.

Should we feed her commercial dog food?

No. Definitely not. Because lactation is a most unusual and demanding time, I want to say to you right now, if you want first class results, feed the BARF diet for lactation. In my experience as a practising veterinary surgeon for over twenty years, there is no way any artificial cooked and processed food can possibly equal the results produced by a dog's biologically appropriate diet - particularly during lactation. The BARF programme is an absolute must.

Preliminary reading

Have you turned straight to this chapter, without reading anything else in this book? If so, I would strongly suggest you read Chapters Three, Four and Five in Part One of this book, which describes the BARF [Bones And Raw Food] diet in detail.

Have you read my first book **Give Your Dog a Bone**? If not - and you have time - it would be a great idea to read it as well!

Have you done that? Great. Now read about ...

The MODIFIED BARF DIET for lactation

General principles ...

Our whole aim is to get as much milk forming food into her as possible so that she can easily care for her large litter and not lose any condition herself.

The only time you limit the AMOUNT of food fed to a lactating bitch - is when her litter is very small. That means NOT feeding her ad lib at peak lactation. Instead, during that second to fourth week , simply increase the amount she is fed on a pro-rata scale to the guidelines I outline later in this chapter. Naturally you will be feeding her the modified BARF diet for lactation.

Yes, it should be a growth type diet, which means - as we have discussed in Part One of this book - not a lot of change to the basic BARF diet, but that change will take into account her need for ...

- **an adequate intake of liquids to make milk**

- **high levels of good quality protein**

- **a calcium rich balanced source of minerals**

- **a source of concentrated energy**

- **the B vitamins to help her use that energy**

- essential fatty acids plus vitamin E to stabilise those essential fatty acids

- vitamin C to boost the immune system and to help cope with the stress

- vitamin A for the health of her immune system and the internal lining of her mammary glands

Apart from the need to supply your lactating bitch with raw meaty bones - particularly, because they supply the minerals she needs, including calcium and phosphorus - **high levels of protein are absolutely essential for the production of milk.** This means that protein supplements are an excellent idea. Eggs, cottage cheese, perhaps brewer's yeast, if she is not allergic to it, are all great sources. They can all go into the pattie mix.

The three basic foods for your lactating bitch will be ...

1] The raw meaty bones ...
2] The pattie mix ...
3] The fortified milk mix.

1] The Raw meaty bones ...

... MUST form the basis of the lactation diet

You must feed your lactating bitch with top quality raw meaty bones. This is for her greatest health, for best milk production and therefore for the pup's greatest health. I cannot emphasise this too strongly. However, I am not talking about the large beef bones or other bony off-cuts. We are not looking to keep her teeth clean and give her psychological benefits at this stage.

Nutrition is our major concern. What our lactating bitch needs are chicken wings, necks and carcases. Raw turkey necks and wings would perform the same function. These raw meaty bones will act as a source of top quality protein, all her balanced mineral requirements - particularly calcium and phosphorus; they are a brilliant source of Omega-6 essential fatty acids and a concentrated form of energy in the form of fat.

Large dogs have no problems crunching through these. However, if your large bitch refuses them for some reason, which can happen, or if she is a small bitch and weary from the task of being pregnant and giving birth, then I strongly suggest you mince these portions - bones and all - and incorporate them into the pattie mix. Do not let her refusal to eat these things prevent her from receiving what she needs.

Appetite stimulants include multi-B vitamins, a zinc supplement, and surprisingly enough - a nip of gin. In some cases I have had to administer a shot of cortisone to get things going, but this is something you would have to discuss with your vet, as such a drug can only be administered under veterinary supervision.

If your lactating bitch will not eat raw meaty bones ...

... for whatever reason - in their whole state - then those raw meaty bones must be minced and **fed as minced raw meaty bones.**

WARNING: DO NOT just feed plain mince without the bones to your lactating bitch. Eclampsia will almost certainly follow. DO NOT just give a calcium supplement in place of the bones. The bones supply a whole lot more than calcium. In other words make sure you DO FEED THE RAW MEATY BONES!

2] The Patty mix for lactation

consists of ...

1. raw crushed vegetables and/or fruit -

2. plus the mince, which in this case is made from raw meaty bones

3. plus additives.

The bulk of the patty must consist of the mince made from the raw meaty bones ....

With the basic BARF patties, the emphasis is on vegetables. **With the lactation patties, the emphasis is more on the minced raw meaty bones.**

The mince should form between 60% to 80% of the pattie mix. It must be made from raw meaty bones - chicken wings or necks etc.. This emphasis on the mince increases if the bitch is refusing to eat the raw meaty bones as such.

That means the vegetables and fruit will form between 20% and 40% of the pattie mix.

The vegetables will include such things as silver beet, spinach, celery, members of the cabbage family, root vegetables such as carrots and sugar beet. Use whatever fruit you can get hold of, including such things as tomatoes, apples, oranges, mangoes, grapes, bananas - or whatever is in season.

To a 2 kg mix of the above we add the following ...

Yoghurt - low fat and plain - one small tub
Eggs - raw and preferably free range - 3 to 5
Flax seed oil - 3 -4 dessert spoons
Raw offal such as liver, heart, brains etc. - e.g. half a lamb's liver
Garlic - 1 or 2 cloves
Kelp powder - 3 or 4 teaspoons
B vitamins and vitamin C - a mega dose of both.
Cottage cheese - 230 gm or about half a pound
Brewer's yeast - 2 tablespoons

Plus other healthy food scraps - such as small amounts of cooked vegetables, rice, cottage cheese etc., particularly where these will stimulate your bitch's appetite.

IMPORTANT
It is ESSENTIAL that your bitch eats everything you have put in the mix, so MAKE SURE THE WHOLE LOT IS MIXED INTO ONE HOMOGENEOUS MASS. THAT WAY YOUR BITCH CANNOT SEPARATE WHAT SHE WANTS FROM WHAT SHE DOESN'T WANT.

Any surplus not fed on the day - should be formed into patties, frozen, then thawed out and used as required. Add the vitamin E just before you feed the patties - e.g., for a 25 kg. [55 lb] bitch give 400 i.u. daily.

Feed your lactating bitch cod liver oil every day

E.g. for a 25 kg [55 lb] bitch, give 3 to 4 ml daily.

3] The fortified milk mix

Consists of ...

> One cup or 250 ml of milk
> One teaspoon of honey
> One or two teaspoons of flax seed oil
> One raw egg [or two egg yolks] - about 60 gm
> One or two junket tablets

Blend this in a blender [or shake it vigorously in a jar] and let it come to body temperature as you would a baby's bottle by suspending the container in hot water. Keep the mixture at body temperature for ten minutes to allow the junket tablet to work.You could also try adding some vitamin drops [multi-B and C] - so long as this did not put her off drinking it.

The lactation diet is so very simple!

Feed the raw meaty bones - either minced or whole - and the patties as alternate meals and give the modified milk drink as her sole source of fluid - if she will take her fluid in this way.

If she is not willing to tackle the bones in their whole state, they must be minced.

How much food and how often?

These two questions are really the same question. This is the one time in the life of your bitch that she must be permitted to eat as much of this high quality food as she likes. There will be absolutely no harm done by letting her eat ad lib - as much as she likes, particularly if she has a big litter to support.

A goal you have for your bitch ...

... after the pups are born **is that she should have the same weight or perhaps a bit more than she had at about the time she was mated.**

Your next aim for her is that **she should have maintained this weight or a fraction more by the time the pups are weaned.** What this means is that she should not deplete her own body reserves during the period of lactation.

If you can achieve the aim of no weight or condition loss during lactation AND produce a large litter of healthy robust pups without having to supplementary feed them, then you will know that you have been feeding her properly. Actually, you will know even better when she continues with good fertility and no weight loss over the next heat cycle and the next and the next - etc..

When to start feeding for lactation

Feeding for lactation begins before your lactating bitch is born. In other words if your bitch is to be really good at making milk which will rear strong healthy puppies, she should have chosen her parents wisely. Ideally, she should have been born of parents raised on the BARF programme and been raised on that diet herself.

Most breeding bitches today have been reared on commercial dog food. As a result they are not the magnificently healthy animals we would wish them to be. Many breeders comment that they have to have their dogs on the BARF programme for several generations before they are exhibiting freedom from breeding problems and absolutely top health, including the ability to produce adequate milk to rear a large healthy litter.

What if you are only just starting?

Maybe your dogs have not been on the BARF programme for several generations. Perhaps you are only now commencing to feed them properly. Do not panic. **You have to start somewhere, and there is no time like the present.** By making that change right now, you are ensuring that your dogs, and this includes your lactating bitch[es], will be doing the best they possibly can.

As far as your lactating bitch is concerned, even if you have only just made the switch, she will do far better than she would had she remained on her previous diet. Her puppies will do even better.

The first meal for that new mum

Let us go straight to the day your bitch gives birth. On that day it is possible your bitch did not eat at all, although that is not always true.

What most bitches do eat the day their pups are born are the afterbirths or placentas. Do not stop your bitch from eating them. Eating the afterbirths is part of a natural cycle of events that has developed for good reasons. A natural solution to a number of problems.

For a wild dog, eating the afterbirths hides the evidence that a birth has occurred which reduces the chance of attack from other predators. Of course that particular advantage does not have much applicability today, but the next one does.

By eating the afterbirths, your bitch not only cleans up her own surroundings, thus reducing the possibility of flies and disease etc., but she also receives an extremely nutritious meal to carry her through the next couple of days.

Afterbirths are a rich source of first class protein. They are a raw concentrated food, full of blood-forming and milk-forming elements. The ingestion of this meal allows a bitch to spend the next several days with her new born litter - without the need to move away from them to obtain food. This ensures she is able to give them her full attention. They receive their first milk or colostrum - a rich source of anti-bodies and nutrients including vitamin A - and also they do not become chilled because she has left them. Those first couple of days are absolutely vital.

She must reman protectively curled round them in those first few hours after birth, stimulating them and licking them dry with her warm, comforting and constantly active tongue. All of this maintains their body temperature over which they have no control. Pups at this stage are SO vulnerable. It is essential they do not become chilled. They must have her warm body constantly available to stop chilling. They must have - constantly available - a supply of rich warm milk. They need to sleep, wake, nurse and sleep.

They need her tongue to stimulate them to urinate and defaecate and remove same. If those pups are able to get off to a good start, they have a much greater chance of future good health and therefore survival. The colostrum they receive in those first twelve to twenty four hours after birth is extra protection against disease. Mum has packed that colostrum full of antibodies against all the local pathogens her body has encountered. She has also packed it full of immune-stimulating nutrients like vitamin A.

While it is true that pups do receive antibodies from their mum whilst inside her, nevertheless, the more they receive - in the colostrum - the greater the protection they have against a world full of potentially deadly enemies.

That is one of many good reasons for allowing the bitch to do her own thing at the time of birth. The less you interfere with natural processes, the better things are. Usually! Do realise that the more you do for her, the more she will expect you to do. The more she is able to be left to get on with it, the better mum she will become.

The real trick is to know when to interfere. That is, to know what she should be doing - as I have just described, for example - and if any of those features or elements of those pups' existence are missing, step in and supply it for them.

The second meal - you supply - usually

After giving birth, most bitches are tired and thirsty. Exhausted and dehydrated might be a better description in many cases. Tired or exhausted because they have just completed a mammoth task, and thirsty or dehydrated for the same reason, plus they have just lost an enormous amount of fluids and electrolytes [salts]. These fluids and electrolytes were in the pups they gave birth to and also in the fluid-filled sacs which surrounded those pups.

That is why one of the best foods you can give your pups at this time is the fortified milk mix...

... which as you remember, consists of one cup or 250 ml of milk, one teaspoon of honey, one or two teaspoons of flax seed oil, one raw egg [or two egg yolks] - about 60 gm, and one or two junket tablets plus multi-B and C vitamins.

This is blended, brought to body temperature, and kept at body temperature for ten minutes to allow the junket tablet to work.

Preferably, you will have tried this mix on her already and know that she will drink it and that it does not give her diarrhoea. Quite often a bitch who cannot tolerate straight milk can quite happily drink this mixture without it giving them diarrhoea. It is always better to try strengthening the milk up rather than watering it down when diarrhoea is a problem.

Your bitch is going to be a cannibal for a few days

NO, hopefully she will not be eating the pups, but she will be drawing on her own bodily reserves and making use of the afterbirths she ate, as well as drinking that milk drink. That is why it is most important that she be a robust sort of bitch at the time of giving birth. Not fat of course, but robust, which means having been on the BARF programme.

Your bitch may well be hard to please at this time

Newly made mothers can be difficult. There are no guarantees on what they will or will not want to eat and/or drink. I certainly cannot guarantee that every bitch will want the same thing exactly. It will depend a lot on what she is used to eating, her state of health, and in many cases she will refuse what normally she would be quite happy to eat.

Many bitches will not eat any solid food at this time at all. Some bitches want only solid food and stubbornly refuse to drink at all. You really do have to tune into your bitch, be patient and be prepared to offer alternatives if one type of food is refused. What it is important for you to understand is her needs. She needs liquids to make the milk, she needs protein food to make the milk and she needs mineral rich food to make the milk. The mineral rich food must be high in calcium of course. She needs energy. That is why the milk recipe I gave you above is so good. It fills all those needs perfectly.

Sometimes bitches in those first couple of days do not eat or drink at all, but simply draw on bodily reserves. If your bitch does not eat, and you are not sure whether she does have a problem or not, do have her checked by a vet. There could be something wrong.

129

A vet check after giving birth is important anyway

Once she appears to have finished giving birth, or if you are not sure that she is finished, or if there is a problem such as a discharge that you are unsure of, or if she is passing fresh blood - **whatever, do take your bitch to the vet for a check up.**

Even if everything appears to be normal, still have her checked. It is important to make sure she does not have any pups left inside - dead or alive, that she did get rid of all the placentas or afterbirths, and perhaps most important of all that she is not haemorrhaging [bleeding from inside her uterus or vagina]. Haemorrhage at this time can be fatal!

Your vet may or may not recommend an oxytocin shot or one of the more modern derivatives of ergotamine which do a similar job. These drugs cause her uterus to shrink down - ejecting any afterbirths and other fluids left in there - as well as helping to control haemorrhage.

Of course, every time the puppies suck on her teats they cause the release of natural oxytocin. However, I must say that I know of no controlled trials to show that this single shot by a vet under the stressful conditions of a veterinary surgery could out-do the continual release of oxytocin when the pups suckle their mum in the peace and quiet of home. **The release of oxytocin when the pups suckle is the bitch's natural way of ensuring that her uterus is cleaned right out and ceases to haemorrhage.**

It is an excellent idea to keep a record of her rectal temperature in the first week or so following whelping. You can obtain a rectal thermometer from your vet or chemist.

To take her temperature - first shake the mercury down. Now lubricate the mercury end with soap and then gently work it into the rectum to a depth of approximately two inches using a twisting motion. Once in there, make sure that you hold the thermometer with the mercury part at the end pressed firmly against her rectal wall, and is not just sitting in a lump of faeces. Hold it there for two minutes. If her temperature goes higher than 39.3 degrees Celsius, and she is not eating, and not bright, get her to the vet quickly. She may have an infection in her uterus.

Uaginal discharges

A dark red or reddish brown discharge occurring after all the puppies are born usually indicates that the uterus is completely cleaned out. A bright red discharge means she is haemorrhaging. Take her to your vet immediately.

If you see a copious brown or green discharge on the second or third day after whelping, this could mean a retained afterbirth or even a dead puppy left inside. If that is the case your bitch will be visibly unwell. No energy, a raised temperature, and usually a loss of appetite. Again, a visit to your vet is imperative at this point.

Hungry puppies ...

If your puppies cry a lot it means that they are hungry and/or cold. You must attend to this problem immediately. Such a situation is rare to non-existent when you have a healthy bitch producing plenty of milk. It is unfortunately common where bitches are fed an inadequate diet - such as one of the commercial dog food diets, or a poorly formulated home-produced diet. She may also be sick - again - not uncommon with a poor diet because her immune system and therefore her resistance to infection is so low.

If there are problems of this nature, get her to your vet to treat her specific illness, and switch her to the BARF diet, including the modified milk drink to build that resistance.

If all attempts to stimulate milk flow fail, and you do not have another bitch to foster those pups - they will have to be hand raised. See Chapter Nine which deals with orphan puppies.

An almost fool-proof method of stimulating the production of milk ...

in a bitch whose milk appears to be drying up is to feed her the modified milk mix. You will be doing this anyway.

Jacqueline Blackall, a long-time adherent to the BARF diet, and breeder of Cavalier King Charles Spaniels, swears by the use of the herb Fenugreek as a stimulator of milk production in bitches. She adds one or two teaspoons to each meal she serves her pregnant bitches.

The lactation diet proper

Once you have got your bitch over those first few days, it is usual for her appetite to return. Her attitude returns to being more bright and alert, although she is still focussed on the puppies rather than you. She has no choice. Those pups are very demanding and will become even more so.

Their demands for milk will peak at about week three and continue for one or two more weeks, by which time you will have begun to wean them.

In the meantime, the questions that begin to run through your mind include - what should she be eating right now to support herself and all these hungry puppies? How often should she be fed? How much is she allowed to eat?

Do we feed her 'ad lib' for the whole of lactation?

It will not be necessary for her to be fed ad lib during the first week [unless at this time she is severely underweight]. The pups are only small and not drinking the amount they will be during the third and fourth weeks. As a guide, for an average to large litter in that first week, you will feed about one and a half times - in weight - what she would normally have when not pregnant or lactating - and of course we are talking about feeding her the lactation modified BARF diet.

In the second week ...

The rule of thumb is to feed her twice as much as normal.

Should we 'humanise' the pups or leave them alone?

Conventional wisdom says that "So long as there are no problems with the pups it is best to leave them alone for the first two weeks, particularly discouraging visitors from handling them." The question is - "Is that good advice?" Mostly I have to disagree with it. It is during these first two weeks that these young pups are establishing their early identity. They have to come to believe that they are both humans and dogs. They have to learn to trust other dogs and to trust us. Now is the time to gently accustom them to being handled **all over** by a wide variety of people.

Typically, the places older dogs hate being handled are their mouths, their tails and their feet. Spend some time with each pup - handling them all over in a kind and gentle way - every day if possible. A major concern by some about such a thing is the passing on of disease to these pups. If they have had their colostrum, and are healthy pups with mum on the BARF diet - there are no problems. Obviously don't be silly about this. For example, you would not allow another breeder whose dogs all have Parvo handle them!

Another concern is that pups of this age should not be disturbed too much, and should get as much sleep as possible between feeds. That is true, so I suggest no more than two sessions daily, of being handled.

Do worm them at two weeks of age ...

... and then every fortnight until they are twelve weeks of age.

In the third week ...

... the pups are becoming quite large, growing rapidly, and not yet started on solid food. Now is the time she is having to produce maximum milk. As a rough guide, she will need three times her normal amount of food. Now is the time to feed her ad-lib and it is probably just as easy to feed her that way. From a practical point of view, as much as she can eat in three or four meals per day.

If your bitch has a history of Eclampsia ...

Extra calcium may be required. For more details on Eclampsia, please read Chapter Six - which deals with Eclampsia.

WARNING: Do not under any circumstances feed the calcium in place of the bones. It must be fed AS WELL as the bones.

We have found that with time and patience the Eclampsia problems disappear when bitches are fed the BARF diet from birth [where possible], before and during pregnancy, during lactation and in the periods when they are between litters - technically known as the 'inter-oestral' period.

Weaning the bitch

What we are talking about here are the problems faced by your bitch when the pups have been weaned and she is still producing a whole heap of milk which is no longer required. For information about weaning the puppies, please turn to Chapter Eight.

The time when the pups are weaned from their mum leaving her with the dilemma of excessive milk production can vary enormously, depending on the policy of the breeder and the state of the bitch's milk supply. However, all that is discussed in Chapter Eight.

If the pups have not left mum already, the pups are ready to be weaned and leave mum completely at around seven to eight weeks of age. **The question is, what do we do with mum?**

For many bitches fed processed food - there is no problem. They ran out of milk weeks ago!

However, bitches which do have milk at this stage should have their food and liquid intake severely restricted from this point.

We have to give the bitch's body the message that the milk is no longer required. Where pups have stayed with their mum for the whole seven to eight weeks, the pups would have been gradually increasing their solid food intake, and decreasing their milk intake over that period, in which case the stimulus for milk production - those pups sucking on their mother - would have been lessened, and she may be starting to produce less milk.

To help this 'drying up' process you will now do the opposite to the lactation diet. You are going to cut down on the milk-forming elements in the BARF diet she is receiving and increase the vegetable content.

- **You will reduce the total food intake. She can have her over-all food reduced to about one quarter of the weight or volume of what she has been having. She should be kept on that level for the next forty eight hours.**

- **Stop the raw meaty bones. By doing that you reduce protein, minerals and fat. Do not give her any chicken wings or necks etc. until her milk has begun to dry up.**

• Stop the milk drink altogether and let her drink water only.

• Even the water should be restricted for twenty four hours, not leaving it with her but allowing her access to the water for ten minutes every four hours or so.

• As a general guide, make the vegetable content about 75% with the mince being about 25%. The mince is now lean minced meat with no bones.

• Reduce the amount of oil and kelp and eggs similarly.

• Give her some big bones to chew on to keep her occupied and happy.

Keep in mind that those recommendations are for a well bitch with plenty of milk. If your bitch is underweight and not well, and not producing a lot of milk, you will probably not need to do any of that. She may in fact need exactly the opposite! She may need to continue with the lactation diet to build her up! At this point you must use your own judgement on how far you should reduce and restrict her food and water intake. If you are in any doubt about her state of health - do consult your veterinary surgeon.

As her milk dries up you will gradually return her to the level of feeding she was on prior to becoming pregnant - the BARF diet of course. You will adjust the amount and the quality of the BARF diet you are feeding her on the basis of her weight and condition.

She is now moving into ...

... the inter-oestral period

This is the three to seven month period between litters when your bitch does not appear to be doing very much. However, do not be fooled and do not neglect her in this period. This is a very critical time.

The inter-oestral period is the time when your bitch is getting ready to produce more puppies.

• Her uterus is undergoing repair and reconstruction in readiness for another pregnancy.

135

- Her bones are stocking up on calcium, phosphorus, zinc and other minerals in readiness for the lactation which will follow.

- It is a time when the essential fatty acid stores are replenished.

- It is a time when her muscles, which may have lost some of their lean muscle mass - their protein - to the milk, have an opportunity to repair and restore.

- All of these processes depend on proper nutrition. It is vital you do not just put her on some awful dry dog food at this time.

- She is rebuilding her immune system.

You absolutely must feed her the BARF diet during this time of restoration. Breeders who neglect their bitch when she is 'dry,' as is so common, do so at the risk of their entire breeding programme.

Let us now move on to the next chapter where we look at how to wean the pups.

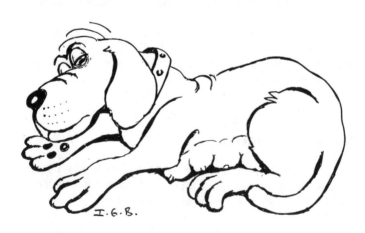

CHAPTER EIGHT

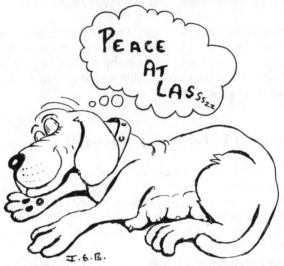

WEANING THE PUPPIES

Weaning pups - a very simple task ...

... and yet many breeders make it one of the most difficult times for both themselves and their pups. Not only that, foods fed to pups during weaning often cause colic, diarrhoea, and a lifetime of allergies and related problems.

Weaning puppies is the process ...

... where we **gradually** change the pups from their mother's milk - which should be their only source of food and liquids after they are born - to the sort of food they will be eating for the rest of their lives. This change-over should be gradual, without trauma or fuss, and should not result in digestive upsets or a set-back to the pups. If you follow the advice in this chapter, that is exactly how you will find it to be.

When do puppies get weaned?

The age when puppies need to be weaned or have to be weaned from their mum varies a lot. Like other things in life there are no hard and fast rules.

However, weaning should not be a thing you suddenly decide to do today and have completed by tomorrow. Ideally, weaning starts at about three to four weeks of age and finishes at about eight weeks of age. It is a gradual process for both mum and the pups. In this way it is entirely stress free for all concerned. Mum, pups and breeder.

That is not how it is for many breeders

In the vast majority of cases - particularly where bitches have been fed modern processed foods - the need to wean becomes an emergency situation. Mum has run out of milk! The pups need to be weaned - right NOW! The question at that point often becomes - "what on earth do we feed them?!" It gets worse. Quite often those pups are not in any way ready to be weaned. They are often too young, which means they have immature digestive systems which may not react well to solid food.

How will I know that this emergency state has arrived?

Hopefully it will not - but if it does you can't miss it because the puppies will tell you. They will be hungry, which means they will be very restless, active, and cry a lot. If the litter is past four or five weeks of age there will be other signs as well. Mum will be spending less and less time with them. She will be quite frustrated by their constant hunger and their 'attacks' on her to procure milk. She will particularly resent their teeth.

As the puppies' teeth get more numerous, and the pups become bigger, stronger, and hungrier, the pain caused by their sharp teeth will override her maternal instincts and she will begin to reject them.

If the bitch starts to regurgitate her own food for the pups, that means her instincts are saying the pups are ready to be weaned. If you have not begun the weaning process already this is a signal that perhaps it is time you did!

Weaning should be under your control

It should be a planned-for event. The best results will be obtained when the bitch is fed properly as I have already described - so that she has plenty of milk. That way you can decide how and when to introduce the pups to solid food.

The more attention you have paid to feeding mum since her birth, through growing up, becoming pregnant, giving birth and suckling those puppies, the greater chance that she will have sufficient milk to carry those puppies through to weaning. That is, to the time when their digestive systems and their immune systems are able to cope with other foods - the foods the pups need to be weaned on to - suitable foods - let me emphasise.

It is only when a pup is past the third week of age ...

... that you can begin to think about starting it on solid food in a serious way, although as you shall shortly see, you can let young pups play with raw meaty bones a little earlier than this to get them used to the idea.

However, the longer you can keep pups drinking their mother's milk, the better it is for them. They grow better, both mentally and physically, and their chances of developing food allergies is greatly diminished. The earlier you start them on foods other than mother's milk, the more digestive upsets you are likely to see, particularly if the food is something inappropriate such as commercial dog food or baby cereals etc.

Ideally puppies should be kept fully on their mother's milk ...

... until they have reached at least four weeks of age. Prior to that time, the ability of these very young puppies to digest and assimilate foods other than their mother's milk is very poor. What they particularly find hard to digest - even at this age - are the cereal-based diets many breeders attempt to feed them. This includes the human baby cereals as well as the canned and/or dry and/or semi-moist dog foods soaked in water or milk as advocated so often.

To recommend any of the artificial foods as weaning foods is BAD ADVICE!

Unfortunately, with today's commercially fed bitch ...

... keeping the pups fully satisfied past the third or fourth week may not be possible, because in many cases, milk production begins to peter out round about this time. Let me stress to you that this is a malnutrition problem. It starts out as malnutrition of the bitch and ends up as puppy malnutrition.

It gets worse. The way many people wean their pups today does little to help the situation. This is because the food fed to both mum and the pups is typically cereal-based.

Cereal-based food is something very foreign to a little carnivore's digestive system. If that cereal based food is processed dog food of some description, the situation worsens. Such products contain heat damaged proteins and heat damaged fats together with an awful chemical cocktail of colourings, preservatives and flavour enhancers etc.. A lethal mix indeed!

You will know when your bitch's milk supply is becoming inadequate ...

... because the pups will become restless, active and hungry. They will cry a lot. Their mum will be spending less and less time with them. She will be getting away from them at every opportunity. If loss of milk is combined with puppies teething, she will begin to actively discourage them. Teething pups sucking and biting on empty teats are very painful. The problem is, the less milk she produces, the more hungry they get. The more hungry they get, the more they chew on her teats. The more they chew on her teats, the more reluctant she is to feed them and the less milk she produces ... etc. etc.. A vicious cycle has been set in motion.

Mum often lets you know when it is time to start the weaning process

She will often let you know round about the fourth week of the pups' life. This is usually a mum that is coping well. A mum with plenty of milk, and still enjoying the pups. The message is simple and clear. She will begin to regurgitate or vomit partly digested food for the pups. This is how wild dogs such as wolves and dingoes begin to wean their pups onto solid food. This is a signal to you. It is time to start those pups on solid food if you have not already done so.

Many breeders adopt a policy of early weaning ...

Often as early as three weeks of age. They usually do this so they can sell the pups early. Sometimes it happens because mum develops Eclampsia. Sometimes it is done because mum has run out of milk, but it is usually done for the breeder's convenience and to reduce costs. The idea is to have the pups off their hands by five weeks of age.

Another reason for early weaning is that the breeder is concerned for the health of the bitch. They do not want to "take too much out of their bitch."

Breeders know that by weaning the pups early, their bitch will be in better condition for the next pregnancy. On modern [for modern read 'poor quality'] foods I have no doubt they are correct. However, if you are feeding your bitch properly on the BARF programme, such a move is rarely necessary. Lactating bitches that are, and have been properly fed, can cope with feeding masses of puppies for long periods with ease.

The major problem you face with early weaning ...

... is the immature digestive system of the puppies. A digestive system not yet ready to cope with things like cereals. Such foods are likely to cause colic [tummy pains] and diarrhoea, followed by bowel infections, dehydration and- worst of all - dead puppies.

Unfortunately, where early weaning is adopted as a policy, the cost in terms of future puppy health can include lifetime problems. Pups kept on their mum are more balanced individuals, both mentally and physically.

A major problem associated with early weaning is the production of allergies. By introducing too much foreign material too early to a developing but immature immune system you are setting the scene for future allergic reactions to that food. This does not happen one hundred percent of the time of course, but it happens often enough to be a major problem in the dog world today. It is a basic cause of many problems later on in life. Allergic skin and bowel problems such as eczema and inflammatory bowel disease, and a whole host of auto immune diseases which will surface at a later date. **These will be labelled as problems with "no apparent cause."**

Where a bitch is able to maintain the pups without supplementation and without the need to wean the pups early, this demonstrates that the breeder is feeding mum right and feeding the puppies right.

There are many medical reasons for early weaning ...

And if you are faced with one of these - fine - go ahead. The obvious one, apart from a lack of milk, would be milk fever or Eclampsia. Once again, let me say that Eclampsia disappears when the BARF programme is being used in a kennel. See Chapter Six for more details on Eclampsia.

If you successfully wean your puppies early ...

Well done - it is not an easy task. As I always say, I have no argument with success. However, my strong recommendation is that if mum has sufficient milk for those pups, and there is no good medical or husbandry reason to wean them early, for the sake of the future health of the pups let her keep feeding them for as long as possible.

The bottom line is that I do not recommend early weaning of pups unless it is for genuine medical reasons. The younger a pup is when it is weaned, the more problems it will have both at weaning and as its life progresses, UNLESS you feed it appropriately for its age.

If the puppies are younger than three weeks of age ...

... and mum can no longer feed them for whatever reason, they should be regarded as orphan puppies. That is, start them off on the orphan milk, and keep them on that orphan milk for as long as possible. Gradually change them onto solid food as I shall shortly describe. If the pups you have need to be regarded as orphans, please turn to Chapter Nine which deals with orphan pups in detail.

If the pups are four to five weeks of age ...

... and you have to wean them straight away for whatever reason, you will have to make a decision whether to regard them as orphan puppies - or not. Please use your common sense. If they have lots of teeth and have already started on solid food, you can continue with the solid food as their entire diet without the need for milk. If they have not been started on solid food, now is the time to begin.

Offer them the raw meaty bones as described below. If they are very immature be prepared to use the milk formulas I describe in Chapter Nine and combine the orphan method with the BARF method of weaning.

Let's get down to it!

THE BARF METHOD OF WEANING - it is so easy!

When the pups are about three weeks of age ...

... you can introduce them to raw meaty bones. I would suggest chicken wings, necks or carcases [or turkey or duck] - whatever is available. They should not be frozen. Bring them to body temperature. Do not under any circumstance cook them. Also, do not challenge young pups with old and rancid chicken pieces. Those pieces should be warm, raw, fresh, and sweet smelling.

To give the pups something to get hold of ...

... and to increase the smell and taste factor - so important for creating interest in this food - cut into these pieces with a cleaver or a knife. Make as many cuts as you wish, but do not turn them into mince. Throw these pieces of chicken in with the pups. They are there to be played with.

The pups will smell them, roll in them, growl and fight over them, suck at them, possibly chew a bit at them, maybe even eat little pieces. Mum may challenge the pups for these pieces. That is no great concern. If she wants to eat them - very good - just throw in some more. If she becomes a real problem, simply remove her from the pups for a couple of hours. When the pups have finished with these bits of bone and meat, or they become a bit smelly, and mum has not eaten them, remove them from the pups. Replace them every day - with fresh pieces.

If the pups don't have many or any teeth ...

... that is not a problem. Different breeds and strains cut their teeth at different ages. If mum is being fed properly the pups are getting all they need from her. It is not important that the pups actually eat these pieces. If mum has been and is being fed the BARF diet, there will be plenty of milk. What you are doing is getting the pups used to the presence, the sight, the smell, the texture and the taste of raw meaty bones.

On some days offer them some pieces of raw liver to play with. Like the bones, they may eat some of this and they may not. Again, it does not matter if the pups don't actually eat the liver at this stage - they will eventually.

By the time the pups are four weeks old ...

They will not only be playing with the liver and the raw meaty bones, they will actually be eating them or wanting to eat them. If this is difficult because the pups are very small or have few teeth, now is the time to present these pieces in a more broken up or possibly minced state. Use your judgement here. Large breeds such as Rottweilers and Shepherds etc. will have no problems at all with eating large pieces of both liver and the raw meaty bones. They will be crunching through them with gusto and delight. In other words only do what you have to! The less work you have to do in breaking up their food - the better it is for you and for the pups.

By the time the pups are five weeks old ...

They will be eating the chicken pieces - usually without them having to be broken up at all, especially with the larger breeds or those breeds where the teeth come early. It does not matter if your pups still cannot crunch through them or don't have many teeth. Keep breaking or mincing those pieces until such time as they have the teeth to handle them whole. Like most dietary changes you make, this change from mince to whole pieces will be a gradual change. However, it is important that by the time these puppies are weaned, they are eating these pieces whole. In fact by eight weeks, most of the bigger breeds will be swallowing them whole. That is OK, however, if they are doing this - now is the time to switch them to carcases - chicken or turkey or whatever you are able to obtain.

By the time the pups are six weeks old ...

They will be well and truly eating solid food - the raw meaty bones - as the major part of their diet. They will still be receiving some milk from mum, [provided her diet has been and continues to be adequate - e.g. the BARF diet], but she will be spending less and less time with them. Now is the time to introduce the patties. Use mince derived from necks or wings or carcases. Mince it yourself, keeping in mind that any mince you buy is suspect so far as what it contains, both in the way of basic ingredients and also in the way of chemical preservatives.

At seven weeks of age ...

... the pups will be 95% weaned. They will not actually need the milk mum is producing, although they may still be drinking some. Mum will be spending very little time with them, and she will possibly be starting to dry up a little. and then again - may be she won't because after all, she is on the BARF diet!

The six to eight week stage ...

... is vitally important nutritionally. This is the stage of extreme puppy curiosity which means it is the time to add the various components of the BARF diet to your puppies' menu. At this age puppies will try and eat everything and anything. That makes it the time to teach them to eat as wide a variety of foods as possible. Dogs that learn to eat everything as puppies will as adults eat a broad range of foods. This makes it easy to feed them when they are adults. It ensures you can easily feed them their balance of nutrients.

At eight weeks of age ...

They will be completely independent of mum and fully weaned on to the BARF diet. This means they should experience very few problems when they arrive at their new homes - so far as food acceptance and upset tummies are concerned. They simply continue with the food they are used to.

Isn't that lovely and simple!

Things you should note about this weaning programme

The major advantage of this method is its simplicity. If you are feeding mum the BARF diet, she will have plenty of milk at the third, fourth, and fifth week. During that fourth to fifth week when the pups are starting to get their teeth, instead of using those teeth to chew on mum because they are so hungry, they are using those teeth to chew the bones and to genuinely remove the hunger. As a consequence, the pups are less hungry when they suck on mum - less frantic - they do less damage to mum's teats. As a result she is happy to let them continue. She is not put off her milk by severe bites to her mammary glands.

This is a win win win situation. The pups are satisfied with biologically appropriate food, mum is comfortable and happy to continue producing milk, and the pups have as much milk as they need. This contrasts sharply with bitches and puppies fed modern foods. The bitches are unable to produce sufficient milk for their pups and the pups are fed inadequate weaning foods. The result is poorly grown pups, bitches that fail to recover properly from pregnancy and lactation and frustrated breeders .

You will also note that I am not suggesting that you start your weaning programme by feeding cereal or canned dog food or dry dog food turned into a mush. I am also not suggesting that you feed milk - except to those pups regarded as orphans - see Chapter Nine.

It is important that the pups actually begin their weaning programme with solid food, and there is no better solid food than raw meaty bones. With the BARF method of weaning, diarrhoea is never [or rarely] a problem, and it very rarely causes allergy problems, whereas grains and other foods commonly used to wean pups are a major cause of both diarrhoea in the pups, and allergies later on in life.

Pups which spend their first few months of life eating these biologically inappropriate foods lay the physiological foundation for a lifetime of ill health. The immediate problem caused by grain-based foods is an assault on an immature digestive system resulting in digestive upsets.

The long term problems caused by grain-based foods in puppyhood relate to an assault on an immature immune system, resulting in a mass of problems such as allergies [usually skin or digestive] and various auto-immune diseases.

However, the role of raw meaty bones is more than physiological – it is also physical

The very best way for young puppies to cut their teeth is by feasting on raw meaty bones. Far better than on mum's mammary glands.

However, those raw meaty bones play an even more valuable role in a young pup's development. They are vital for the proper development and growth of young puppies' bones, joints and muscles. Those pups are undergoing a valuable form of eating exercise as they rip and tear and wrestle and fight over their bones.

This exercise, along with the appropriate nutrition provided by those bones, provides the only sound foundation for bones and joints that will ultimately develop to be be free of Hip Dysplasia and other juvenile skeletal diseases.

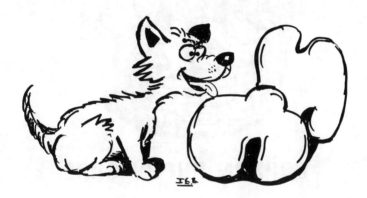

CHAPTER NINE

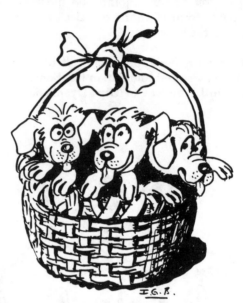

ORPHAN PUPPY CARE

Do not panic!

Perhaps the most important words the novice needs to hear when faced
with the prospect of raising orphan puppies - is - do not panic. if you are
faced with raising a litter of orphan puppies, realise it can be done. Those
pups can be raised and it is much easier than you might imagine.

What is an orphan puppy?

An orphan puppy is is one that has been separated from its mother and
possibly its litter mates before it is three weeks old. After a puppy is three to
four weeks old, you can allow it to begin eating solid food. It may then be
regarded as an early weaned pup which is basically an orphan which you
are starting on solid food.

Dealing with newborn puppies

Most of the following advice applies to any newborns - orphan or otherwise.

The importance [or otherwise] of colostrum

It is extremely beneficial but not essential that newborn pups receive adequate quantities of their mother's colostrum in the first twelve hours of life. The colostrum is the first milk their mother produces. It is rich in antibodies and also vitamins, particularly vitamin A.

The antibodies which come from the bitch are there to protect the newborn puppy from all the disease organisms the bitch has encountered in her life, including those diseases she was vaccinated against. The vitamins in the colostrum, particularly vitamin A, provide a much needed boost to the puppies' immune system

The newborn puppy's ability to absorb antibodies from the colostrum begins to decrease immediately after birth. At the same time the level of antibodies secreted in the milk begins to decline at about the same rate.

As a result, twelve hours after the puppies are born, their ability to absorb antibodies is only half as good as it was at birth, and after twenty four hours the pups are unable to absorb any worthwhile amounts. At this time, the milk has very low levels of antibodies in any case. So for maximum protection against infectious disease, all pups should receive their dose of colostrum sooner rather than later, preferably in the first six to twelve hours after whelping.

Wherever possible, make sure that pups receive colostrum as their first milk rather than any other milk

If pups drink any milk other than their mother's milk during that first twelve hours of life - for example cow's milk - they will absorb the proteins whole, and may possibly develop allergies to them later on. This is because newborn pups have the capacity to absorb proteins whole rather than digest them. In other words they absorb the antibodies - which are protein - rather than digest them.

Apart from being high in nutrients and antibodies, colostrum has a laxative effect.

This is important because newborn puppies can become constipated. That is, blocked up with the faeces [called meconium] that formed while they were inside their mum. If this is a problem, see your vet who will organise some mini-enemas.

If the pups did not receive any colostrum ...

... for whatever reason, do not panic. **Those pups DID receive antibodies from their mum across the placenta before they were born.**

Some vets will inject some of the mother's serum - or some other dog's serum - into the pups. However, the amount of extra antibodies the pups receive by this method is not worth the effort. **It proves far more valuable to inject the newborns with vitamins A, E, D, B complex, and C.**

Dealing with pups that are dehydrated, weak and chilled

If you have pups that are dehydrated, weak and chilled: before allowing them to suck on their mother, or - if they are orphans - before giving them any sort of milk replacer - you must ...

- re-hydrate them

- give them some energy

- bring their body temperatures up to about 38 degrees Celsius.

To re-hydrate them and give them some instant energy, they need glucose and warm water

This can be given with a spoon, an eye dropper, a syringe or a stomach tube or whatever. The solution is made by dissolving a tablespoon of honey or glucose in a cup [250 ml] of warm [body temperature] water. Give five mls of this solution every fifteen to thirty minutes.

Raise their temperature slowly – over several hours if you have to.

The newborn puppy is unable to control its body temperature during the first few weeks of life. In fact newborn puppies are not able to obtain full control over their body temperature until about four weeks of age. Their body temperature will therefore vary depending upon environmental temperature.

If pups have a low temperature...

... all their activities are suppressed and this includes both suckling and digestion. If you force feed [with milk] pups that have a low temperature they will continue to deteriorate. In addition, because the milk does not move out of the stomach, the pup will often vomit and inhale the milk into its lungs, causing pneumonia and death. That is why before allowing the pups access to any sort of milk, their temperature must be raised to about 38 degrees Celsius, and the pups must be rehydrated.

Healthy newborns have the ability to slow their metabolic rate

They will slow their heart to slow oxygen consumption and reduce oxygen needs and to conserve what energy reserves they have left. They can maintain the circulation of their blood at a very low blood pressure. In other words, do not give up on cold, weak newborns with a slow heart beat. They can be revived, but it has to be done slowly.

That is why it is important NOT to feed them until their body temperature is up to 38 degrees Celsius. Indeed it is not a good idea to over-stimulate their heart. Do everything slowly. Hydration is very important.

If there is severe dehydration, it needs to be treated by a vet who may elect to give subcutaneous fluids, or if the problem is extreme, fluids can be given either intravenously or intraosseously - i.e. into the bone marrow.

To warm the pup[s] slowly, use the lead light method - see page 158 - and/or hot water bottles and/or electric blankets and/or the warm - not hot - oven method. But don't cook them!

Once the pups have received a source of energy such as glucose or honey, they have been rehydrated, their temperatures have been raised to normal and they have become normally active, they can be put back with mum, or started on a milk replacer if they are orphans.

Should puppies that are older than 24 hours become chilled for any reason, it can be dangerous. When the rectal temperatures drop below 94 degrees Fahrenheit [34.5 degrees centigrade] the pups will stop nursing, or if they do nurse, it is ineffectual. These pups will cry and if not treated within a few hours will pass the point of no return, and will die some time within the next 24 hours.

Suitable milk replacers for puppies

If you do need a milk replacer to supplement a mum with a poor milk supply or to completely replace her, you do have to choose it carefully. **In Australia the product 'Biolac' for pups works beautifully.** It has been produced to closely approximate bitch's milk - unlike most of the other products currently available. It is the only one I recommend. In other countries I have no idea which ones are any good.

If you are uncertain of what to use - that is, you do not know if the products available to you work well - then I strongly suggest you use the following formula.

Home made replacement milk for orphan puppies

250 ml full cream milk - raw, pasteurised, or reconstituted milk powder
20 ml natural yoghurt
2 egg yolks from 55 gm eggs
10 ml [2 tsp] of flax seed or hemp seed oil - cold pressed of course
10 ml [2 tsp] honey
10 drops of a B vitamin supplement such as pentavite
250 mg vitamin C, e.g. Ester C, or calcium or sodium ascorbate. [Use ascorbic acid if that is all you can get.]
One crushed junket tablet

Blend the ingredients and then allow to stand in a double warmer for fifteen minutes at body temperature. Re-blend to ensure it is liquidised before feeding.

How much 'milk' and how often

Like most things associated with feeding there are no hard and fast rules. However, the following guidelines may be used as a guide or a place to start. After that, it is very much a matter of common sense and judgement.

The ounces method. During the first week, start off with about two ounces [60 ml] per lb [454 gm] of body weight per day, increasing that amount gradually to approximately three ounces [75 to 90 ml] per lb, by the end of the first week.

During the second week, gradually increase that amount so that by the end of the second week you are feeding up to four ounces [100 to 120 ml] per l lb of body weight daily, and by the end of the third week you are feeding up to six ounces [150 to 170 ml] per lb of body weight daily.

By the fifth week you will be starting to decrease the milk, because at three to four weeks you have started getting that puppy [those puppies] on to solid foods, so that by weeks six to seven you have completely weaned the puppy off the bottle or the tube - if tube feeding. The pup[s] may still be drinking milk, but they will be lapping it from a dish, not being tube fed or fed with a bottle.

Another method used to work out how much milk to feed puppies is to use the percentage method. By this method you feed about 15 % of the pup's body weight per day at birth, and gradually increase this amount to forty percent of the pup's body weight per day at four to five weeks of age.

Another more simple method or guide you may use to decide when a pup has had enough - is to look at the pup. The abdomen should be slightly enlarged but not greatly distended after each feeding. Of course if the pup is drinking from a bottle, he or she may decide that for you.

On that point, let me also say that most people use a combination of demand feeding by the pup, and schedule feeding by yourself.

The pups should be fed every two to five hours. In other words, they will be fed between five and ten times daily. If they are strong and robust puppies, feed them five times daily. That means **you feed one fifth of the calculated daily amount at each feed.**

The only time it will be necessary to feed every two to three hours is when and if the pups are very small and very weak.

Sample calculation

Supposing you have a **newborn pup that weighs 230 gm or about half a lb.**

If you are working out how much to feed **by the ounce method,** then a half lb pup needs to be fed one ounce or thirty ml per day. If it is a robust pup and you are feeding it five times daily - then you will feed it approximately **six ml at each feed.**

If you are working out how much to feed **by the percentage method,** 15% of 230 gm is 34 ml per day, and so this would work out at **seven ml at each feed.**

I suggest you use the figures I am giving you as a check to see if the amount that bottle fed pups are drinking is about right. On the other hand, if you are tube feeding, you will be more reliant on these figures as a guide when deciding how much to give.

On that note **please let me stress the dangers of overfeeding:** it is much safer to underfeed slightly than to overfeed. There is a high risk of regurgitation or vomiting followed by pneumonia when feeding large quantities of milk frequently. This is very much a matter for judgement. **It is certainly best to underfeed during the first several days when you and the pup[s] are getting used to the idea.**

Be sure and warm the formula to body temperature. The simplest method I know of is to sit the bottle of formula in a pan of hot water. **Test it on your wrist to make sure it is not too hot before feeding it.**

Make sure all your equipment is kept clean and sterile. Sterilise all equipment with one of the proprietary lines used for babies.

Keep unused formula in the refrigerator. Try and only make up enough for each day. If you want to make more than that ahead of time, then you must freeze the formula in daily amounts.

Methods of feeding

There are two basic methods. **Bottle feeding and tube feeding.**

Bottle feeding orphan pups

When using a nipple bottle, make sure the formula does not run out too quickly. When you invert the bottle it should ooze out slowly - but you should not have to squeeze it to get it out. If you need to enlarge the hole to get it to run more freely, use a hot needle.

When using the nipple bottle, first squeeze a drop of milk onto the nipple and then insert it in the puppy's mouth. Never squeeze milk out of the bottle into the puppy's mouth. If you do, the pup may aspirate the milk into its lungs resulting in pneumonia and death. **Let the pup suck it out of the bottle.**

Tube Feeding

This is an excellent method when you have lots of pups [or one] and not a lot of time. It is fast, easy, safe, clean and anyone can learn to do it.

Ask your vet to get you a 15 inch or 35 cm feeding tube. Have it ready - ahead of time - just in case. It must be the type of feeding tube that can take a syringe.

On the tube, mark the distance from the tip of the puppy's nose to the end of the last rib. That is slightly in excess of the amount you will need to pass to get the tip of the tube into the stomach.

When you go to pass the tube, if it will not go that far, it probably means you are in the trachea or wind-pipe. Pull it out and start again!

Do not pass the tube past that marked point. If you push the tube in too far, it may double, which means when you pull it out, it may come out doubled which is traumatic for the pup. Re-mark the tube at least once a week.

Before passing the tube, put the tube on the syringe, suck up the formula into the syringe, and then expel all the air bubbles.

Sit in a chair. Have a towel on your lap. Have the puppy cradled in a semi-upright position, head slightly flexed and comfortable and firmly held. Now pass the tube gently over the tongue. The puppy will swallow it.

If you are not sure of your technique initially, and you have no one to guide you, practice with a small amount of warmed water in the syringe rather than milk. A small amount of water will cause the pup to cough if the tube is in the wrong hole, but it will not do any real harm. However, it is almost impossible to get the tube in the wrong hole - the trachea - with a healthy pup. Also, if the pup is able to squeal or cry etc. when the tube has been inserted fully, then you are in the correct hole.

Once you are satisfied that you have the tube in the correct hole - the oesophagus - go ahead and administer the formula over a period of thirty to sixty seconds. Do not just squirt it in over a couple of seconds. The puppy needs the extra time in order to allow expansion of its stomach. Regurgitation is rare if you are gentle and relatively slow.

If regurgitation does occur, withdraw the tube and do not give any more until next feeding time.

Following feeding you should always 'burp' the puppy - just the same way you would a baby by sitting the pup up and gently tapping its back.

You should also stimulate urination and defaecation - both before and after feeding. The mother does this by licking the genital area. You do not have to go that far! Use a cotton ball moistened with warm water.

For a pup's correct mental development, it should be kept with other pups. Please note that orphan puppies will develop tremendous behavioural problems if they are raised without the companionship of others of their species.

The only potential problem with raising them all together - all of the time - can be the incessant sucking and bullying that sometimes occurs with orphan pups. If this happens, a degree of separation may be necessary, with individual areas for each pup. Once again, this is a matter for your ingenuity, common sense and patience. However, no matter what, those pups must spend some time together for their normal healthy mental development.

You must have a set of scales

It is vital that the pups are weighed frequently and that a record of those weights is kept. The weight gain you see with the pups should follow roughly what is expected for the breed. Your breed society should have some figures to give you an idea of this.

When you weigh the pup[s], keep things consistent. For example, you might weigh them every morning, before the first feed of the day, after they have urinated and defaecated.

Bedding for the orphan puppy

Blankets or rags work nicely, as does dust free, deodorised wood shavings. For more information on the value of wood shavings, see Chapter Five - The Whelping Box.

The surrounding temperature for orphan puppies during the first week of life should be kept at around 80 to 95 degrees Fahrenheit [30 degrees Celsius], during the second to third week around 80 degrees Fahrenheit [27 degrees Celsius] and the third to fifth week around 75 degrees Fahrenheit or 23 degrees Celsius.

Housing for the orphan puppy ...

... can be a simple cardboard box, a wooden box - whatever. This can be heated in a variety of ways. That includes a thermostatically controlled heating pad, a hot water bottle [which is the least reliable] or the lead light system.

I prefer the lead light system. Please note that the lead light could be an actual heat lamp. However, many people suddenly faced with an orphan puppy or an orphan litter may not have a heat lamp, but most people can get hold of a lead light.

The lead light system is based on the same principle as the chicken brooder.

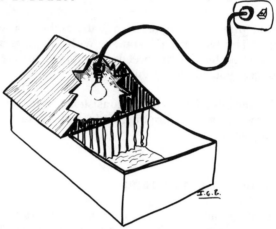

You may make this system as elaborate or as simple as you like. The part of the box warmed by the lead light should be covered - either with a properly made roof as in the diagram, or else use some wire or wood over which is draped some blankets or towels to keep the heat in. Use a one hundred watt globe, not a forty watt globe like a friend of mine, who lost the orphans he was trying to raise as a result of trying to save a few cents on his electricity bill!

Note that one end of the box is not heated. This end is there to enable pups that are becoming over-heated to crawl into a cooler area. In other words they regulate their own temperature.

Of course if you have another animal that wants to act as a foster mother, that is great; use it. You will probably have to supply the nutritional requirements, but the foster mum will provide body warmth and animal companionship, together with the all important tongue for stimulation of urination and defaecation.

Weaning the orphan puppy

To wean the orphan puppy follow exactly the same procedure you would follow for any other puppy raised by its mother. See **Chapter Eight**.

PART THREE

BONES BUILD BONES

INTRODUCTION

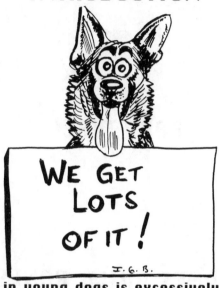

Bone disease in young dogs is excessively common ...

... and becoming more so. It has reached epidemic proportions despite enormous efforts to get rid of it. At least 90% of the dogs that develop Hip Dysplasia, Elbow Dysplasia, or any of the other skeletal diseases should not have done so. The reason they have these problems is because they have not been raised correctly. They have been mismanaged.

Over the last 40 years it has become an article of faith in the dog world that **bad genes cause skeletal problems in pups.** An almost religious faith in this doctrine has underpinned the massive but ineffectual eradication campaigns we have been using to fight these problems. The reason for these poor results is that while genes play a basic role in producing these problems, the removal of those genes may well be impossible and in many cases undesirable.

There is a simpler solution to the bone and joint problems which are plaguing our modern dog population. That solution does not involve mass radiography and mass culling. **It involves a few simple changes in puppy management.**

Management of the growing puppy is vital

It decides what sort of framework will support that pup for the rest of its life. For **an individual puppy,** knowing its genetic background is of little value. The only important factor is how it is raised. **If you can raise the puppy correctly from the start using the BARF programme - of biologically appropriate diet and exercise - there is little chance of skeletal disease.**

Sound management builds sound bones.

There are three forms of puppy MISMANAGEMENT

- Modern puppy mismanagement

- Old fashioned puppy mismanagement

- A combination of the two

Modern puppy mismanagement ...

... which is now so common - **uses processed food, excessive food, excessive calories, excessive protein and excessive calcium together with inappropriate or excessive exercise** to produce the whole range of modern bone diseases such as Hip or Elbow Dysplasia. These are usually seen when the puppy is young. However, it does not end there. Modern mismanagement will almost certainly produce degenerative joint disease in some form or another when the dog is older. In other words, with modern mismanagement, these problems can almost be guaranteed. Sooner or later!

Old fashioned puppy mismanagement ...

... on the other hand is uncommon these days and **involves severely deficient diets which lack calcium, vitamin D, phosphorus, or other nutrients.** These are the diets which produce the rickets type diseases of weak, bendable, easily broken bones. Problems which are relatively rare these days. Fortunately, should you mismanage only slightly, or you catch the problem sufficiently early - before permanent damage is done - you can usually save the situation.

The remedy for modern mismanagement ...

... the mismanagement of excess, involves stringent dietary and exercise regimes. If these fix the problem, the outlook is great. If the problem requires surgery, you probably have a pup which may have lifelong problems or may even require euthanasia.

The remedy for old fashioned mismanagement ...

... the mismanagement of deficiency, involves a return to a normal diet. If caught early enough, a return to healthy normality is highly likely. If not, a crippled pup or euthanasia is the likely outcome.

Modern Puppy Mismanagement - a Costly error

Millions of dollars are wasted attempting to produce pups with healthy bones. This includes the high cost of purebred pups, the food bills, the calcium supplements, and the inevitable vet bills associated with hip scoring, elbow scoring and the treatment of deformed pups. However, the costs involve more than money.

There is also the pain. Millions of dogs suffer painful lives because of the way they were raised. Many owners have no idea of the pain their dogs are suffering.

Then there is the terrible waste of excellent puppies. Puppies that should have given their human family love, companionship, and pleasure are being euthanased.

There is also a huge loss of genetic potential. Every pup which is desexed or put to sleep because of skeletal problems is a loss of irreplaceable genetic material. This does not have to be.

Finally, do realise that most of the arthritis seen in older dogs has its basis in mistakes made during the rearing of that dog.

The simple way to prevent skeletal problems in pups ....

.... Is to raise them on a diet based on Raw Meaty Bones, the BARF diet. This has been the basis of canine bone and joint health for millions of years, and it continued to be that way until the mid thirties in the USA and England, and till the mid sixties in Australia.

The switch to modern foods, calcium supplements, and a modern approach to exercise most certainly eliminated the reasonably uncommon skeletal diseases of deficiency, the rickety type problems. Unfortunately it replaced these simple and relatively uncommon old fashioned problems with an epidemic of problems such as Hip and Elbow Dysplasia and a host of related skeletal diseases in our modern over fed and over exercised dogs.

Can you ask your vet to confirm this?

Unfortunately the role of management in producing either skeletal health or disease is not part of our training. Instead we rely on getting rid of the genes which cause these problems. We kill and cull.

On top of that we are trained to do lots of things which promote skeletal problems.

- Many of us recommend and even sell commercial pet food.

- We are not trained in the use of a dog's natural diet. Raw meaty bones and other raw whole foods.

- So many of us sell or recommend calcium supplements.

- We appear to be ignorant of the damage excess calcium causes.

- We are often guilty of offering poor or no advice regarding the exercising of growing pups.

The end product of a veterinary profession trained to be salespeople for the pet food companies ...

... together with very little experience in common sense management of growing puppies, and an almost total reliance on killing and culling to remove skeletal problems, is an increase in bone disease in dogs. From the miniature breeds to the giant breeds. Especially the giant breeds.

I am fortunate. My background in Agricultural Science which emphasised the role of management in animal health and disease has shown me why our continuing emphasis on kill and cull is not working. There are much better, more creative, and happier solutions. Eliminating genes is not the be all and end all to these problems.

I have a vital and urgent message for all dog lovers

Juvenile bone and joint disease in dogs can be prevented and therefore eliminated by simple, inexpensive, easily learnt and highly effective management techniques.

So what is SOUND MANAGEMENT?

Sound management involves **feeding and exercise.** Get these right and skeletal problems disappear. The basis of bone health for dogs is

- to limit all exercise to play only

- to feed a properly formulated BARF diet in limited amounts

- to grow the pup slowly.

Warning: even the BARF diet fed to excess can produce juvenile skeletal disease. You must do it properly.

It is absolutely vital that puppies be grown slowly, without artificial calcium supplements on a low fat diet, and that their exercise is both appropriate and adequate, neither too much nor too little.

These are the simple but powerful tools available to you. No money to spend, no special equipment required, and nobody to consult. You can use these ideas straight away, confident that Juvenile Bone Disease can be a thing of the past, no matter what the breed, the circumstances or the food available, and no matter what 'nasty' genes your dog[s] may have inherited for juvenile bone and joint disease.

It is also vital that you understand - where you have employed these techniques and have still produced one of the so called heritable diseases such as Hip or Elbow Dysplasia - NOW is the time to kill or cull. You may do so with confidence. This pup has bad genes that absolutely must go!

Who Should Read this?

If you have anything to do with puppies - keep reading. This section is written principally for puppy owners, but also for dog breeders, veterinary surgeons, puppy pre-school teachers, obedience trainers, pet shop owners and show judges. It is written for anybody who needs to know how to raise pups with healthy disease-free bones and joints.

If you are a breeder whose pups have bone or joint problems, read on, and learn how to eliminate such problems in one generation.

If you own a pup which has problems with its bones and joints, read on and learn why they happened and what to do about them.

If you are about to buy a pup, keep reading - you need this information.

If you raise pups with no problems, keep doing what you are doing. I have no argument with success. However, think about the long term health of your pups. Do your pups live longer than the average for their breed, free of Degenerative Joint Disease, other forms of arthritis and other degenerative diseases such as liver failure, skin disease, cancer, diabetes, kidney failure, heart disease and so on? Do they die suddenly at an advanced age with little or no suffering? If not, then you have not yet got it right. Keep reading.

Can we eliminate all skeletal problems?

I would love the answer to be an unequivocal YES! - but of course that is not possible. The answer is - YES - MOSTLY, but not completely.

There will always be exceptions, and when these appear - that is the time to kill or cull.

The diseases which should mostly disappear when the BARF programme of feeding and exercise is used include ...

... all the old fashioned rickety type problems together with the modern diseases starting with Osteochondrosis, Osteochondritis, Hip Dysplasia, Elbow Dysplasia, Wobbler Syndrome, Dropped Hocks, Splayed feet, Bone Cysts, Carpal Instability/Flexion Syndrome, Patellar Luxation, Aseptic Necrosis of the Femoral Head [Legg-Perthes Disease], Rickets, Nutritional Hyperparathyroidism, Hypertrophic Osteodystrophy, Panosteitis, Septic Arthritis and all forms of arthritis or degenerative joint disease in the older dog.

Don't let all those complicated names phase you!

Just realise that nearly every problem they represent can be prevented by adhering to sound management principles.

One more thing

Sound management will produce immediate results and more complete results than trying to breed these problems out. However, there is one drawback. You must never let your management slip, because when you do - the problems will return.

As you read on, note that I place special emphasis on Hip and Elbow Dysplasia. These two problems are vexing the dog world and the veterinary profession in a way that no other problem ever has. However - they don't have to. They can both disappear tomorrow by simple but sound scientific management techniques. That is the central message of this book.

At this point you have lots of questions.
Keep reading.

The rest of this book is designed to answer them.

CHAPTER ONE

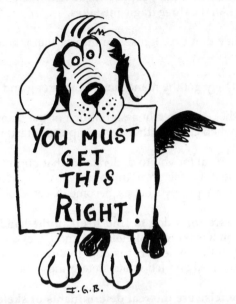

I.G.B.

CORRECT MANAGEMENT
OF PUPS –
– AN OVERVIEW

Faulty management lies behind practically every case of canine bone disease in puppies. This includes all the old fashioned ricketty type diseases **and** the modern ones including Hip Dysplasia, Elbow Dysplasia, The Wobbler Syndrome, Dropped Hocks, Splayed feet, Bone Cysts, Osteochondritis Dissecans, Legg-Perthes Disease, Slipping Patellas and any other problems involving altered, abnormal or diseased bone growth.

What is more, it also includes much of the arthritis seen in older dogs.

The reason why bone problems are increasing is that many breeders, most new puppy owners and the people who advise them such as vets and dog food companies, make three tragic mistakes.

- Firstly, they don't recognise the impact that management has on the problem,

- Secondly, they get the management bit wrong and ...

- Thirdly, they incorrectly assign much of the blame to bad genes or genetics, when clearly other more important factors are involved.

It is absolutely crucial for you to understand that puppy management is the fundamental, the only factor of any practical value which may be used to determine whether a puppy's bones become diseased or healthy.

It is extremely rare for a dog to find itself in the hands of a nasty set of genes hell bent on wrecking its skeleton. Although every dog's genes play a major role in deciding whether it is able to develop skeletal disease, it is how a dog is exercised and fed which determines whether it actually will.

Feeding and exercise are the real determinants of skeletal health. For all practical purposes, when building a dog's skeleton, all we need to be concerned about are the materials we use to build those bones together with the stresses and insults, placed on or suffered by those growing bones.

It is essential we do our best to match the requirements of a pup's body to its long time heritage of natural food and the sort of exercise and rate of growth experienced by its ancestors. For success we need to be as true to nature as possible.

The more we depart from a dog's biological background and attempt to impose our own ideas of how it should be managed, the more we test its ability to grow and function normally. Commercial dog food, badly designed home produced food, excessive food, artificial calcium supplements, and inappropriate exercise, are the methods people use to produce skeletal disease.

Breeders and puppy owners who adopt these faulty management techniques stress their pups' bodies well beyond their biological capacity to adapt. The consequence is bone disease, amongst other problems.

A properly balanced raw meaty bone and crushed vegetable based diet, fed in limited amounts and teamed with an appropriate exercise regime comes very close to an iron clad guarantee that you will produce normal healthy bones and joints in your puppies every time. No matter what the breed and no matter how many 'bad genes' those pups have supposedly inherited. Such a programme makes it almost impossible to fail. It is easy.

If we eliminated management errors, the incidence of Juvenile Bone Disease should drop from its present level of around 60% to 80% in some breeds, to a more acceptable 5% to 10%.

Most of the juvenile bone diseases arise as a result of the following mistakes made during the rearing of pups.

1] Deficient diets which are lacking in one or more essential nutrients

2] Excessive artificial calcium

3] Excessive food, particularly excess proteins and fats

4] Pups that grow too fast - because of [3]

5] Pups that become obese - because of [3]

6] The use of processed food with its heat damaged nutrients

7] The failure to feed pups raw meaty bones and crushed raw vegetables

8] The failure to limit exercise to play only until the pups' bones are mature

Faulty management either allows bone problems to surface, or it directly produces those problems. That is, it allows a genetic problem to surface, or it actually produces the problem by itself. Most of the time, it is a combination of both these methods, each to varying degrees, depending on the individual dog, the genes it has inherited and the way in which the pup is fed and exercised.

Once you understand the impact of faulty nutrition and inappropriate exercise you will realise what powerful tools you have available to you to almost totally eliminate bone problems from your individual dog, your clients' dogs or your kennel. And what is more ...

It is all so Incredibly Easy

Raw meaty bones and raw crushed vegetables. These are truly magic foods. They have been magic foods for puppies and adult dogs for hundreds of thousands of years. These are the foods dogs have evolved to eat over countless generations. These are the foods their whole physiology is designed to handle, actually craves, and definitely requires in order to grow and function normally.

Raw meaty bones and raw crushed vegetables are cheap, they are available, and it is beyond me why people would want to make life difficult for themselves and their pups by basing their diet on anything else.

Many people, when they discover the simplicity of the BARF diet refuse to believe such a simple programme could make such an incredible difference. On that basis they refuse to follow it.

I have been feeding my own dogs this way for decades, as have thousands of my clients and people who have read my writings, together with countless numbers of other dog owners and breeders who have simply figured this simple truth out for themselves, or have continued to feed their dogs as their fathers and mothers and many many generations before them have done.

Not only is the BARF diet well balanced, if fed properly, your puppy has the best chance of growing lean and healthy. Not the sort of pup that grows fat and fast.

However, let me warn you, even a natural diet fed to excess or incorrectly balanced, can result in both an excessive growth rate and obesity.

If you do choose to follow the whole BARF programme, then do follow it. Make sure for example that when your pup[s] are fed meat on the bone, they eat the bone as well as the meat. If they eat the meat only - disaster will follow.

Do not over feed them and make sure that their diet IS balanced - over time. If you do not follow the whole programme, but go off on some tangent of your own - you may be faced with problems. For instance, a meat only diet which contains a lot of fat, will be a diet which is low in calcium, high in calories and high in protein. Such a diet can be equally as disastrous for the growth of a puppy as starvation.

I will even go so far as to say you will produce far healthier puppies using a good commercial dog food in limited amounts and no supplements, than using fresh products badly.

However, if you do choose to feed your pups properly following the BARF programme fully, you will be rewarded with lifetime health for them.

Feeding raw meaty bones ensures that your Maltese Terrier, or your Papillon, or your Bull Terrier or your Saint, or your Rotty, or your Great Dane, or your German Shepherd dog **receives every mineral required in perfect balance for healthy bones.**

So far as calcium is concerned, Raw Meaty Bones should be the only form of calcium which you should need to feed to your pup.

Those raw meaty bones help prevent all other dietary imbalances, they help control speed of growth, they help prevent obesity, and they ensure plenty of healthy chewing exercise. Isometric exercise which can exercise the whole body.

Most important of all you must be convinced of the absolute necessity of keeping your pup lean and hungry and growing slowly. You must limit its growth rate to between 60 and 70 percent of what it is capable of doing. This simply cannot be stressed too strongly. A slow rate of growth becomes more and more important as the size of the breed increases.

All of this is as true for the Giant breeds as any other breed. If you don't realise it already, you will quickly discover how susceptible these breeds are to any problems with their diet. When raised on processed foods, or home produced diets badly done, they walk a tight rope in terms of nutrition until they are over 12 to 18 months of age. Any slip up and they will pitch over into a yawning abyss of skeletal problems.

However, that life path changes dramatically if the diet you choose for your giant breed is a biologically appropriate diet based on raw meaty bones and raw crushed vegetables. The BARF diet. Suddenly that tight rope becomes as broad as a footpath. Much more tolerant, much kinder.

Raw meaty bones and crushed raw vegetables make your large dog much less sensitive to the effects of its genes. Those genes which predispose it to bone disease. They even make it much less sensitive to the effects of the wrong sort of exercise, or even to the occasional poor choice in the rest of its diet. They act as a buffer against all the other factors which help produce bone problems.

The right sort of exercise is vital!

- **The only reliable and healthy form of exercise** a pup should have until its bones are mature, is eating exercise together with short walks, free running and play.

- A pup must never be exercised or walked or run until exhaustion. A pup must always stop when it wants to. Before it becomes excessively tired. Before it becomes sore.

- It must never have any jarring sort of exercise where it is constantly jumping down on things.

- It should not be encouraged to dance around on its hind legs. If a dog must perform that trick, wait until its bones are mature.

- And do not allow it to become fat.

If you only learn one thing about exercising pups, learn how important it is for them to eat raw meaty bones as a form of exercise, and that the only other permissible form of exercise for a pup is play.

Realise that young bones are soft and easily moulded.. We want the forces that work on those bones to mould them into the correct shape. Excessive and jarring exercise will damage and/or force those bones to become the wrong shape. The beginning of either Juvenile bone disease, or Osteoarthritis later on. **"As the twig is bent..."**

People tell me what I recommend is too simple. What do you think? Does it sound too easy? Let me encourage you to put aside your scepticism, particularly you vets and long time breeders, and 'give the BARF programme a go.' The chapters which follow are designed to help you to make that decision in favour of the BARF programme.

In the next chapter, I take you through the origins of skeletal problems in pups, from their obscure beginnings in the 1930's to their current position of prominence today.

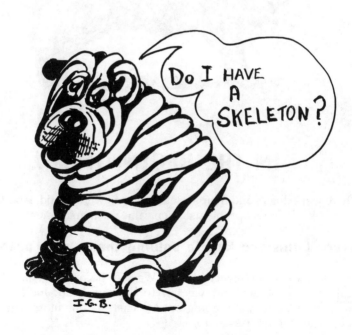

CHAPTER TWO

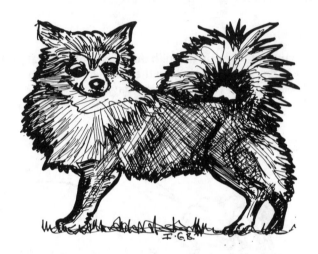

IN THE BEGINNING ...

... there were dogs - and their skeletal systems were sound. And there were very few problems. Then came mismanagement...

History holds the key to solving these bone problems

It pays to look at the bigger picture. We can become so enmeshed in the details of a problem that we fail to lift our head, look around and appreciate what is really going on. Nowhere is this more true than with modern skeletal diseases in dogs.

As scientists, the way we look at the bigger picture of a disease is to look at the history of that disease. This is called epidemiology.

Epidemiology is literally the study of epidemics

That is, how epidemics or outbreaks of disease change over time. If we can relate these changes to changes in the animals' environment, we can find vital clues as to what is causing the problem.

Let us now examine the historical or epidemiological evidence which shows us what those conditions were and are, that allowed bone problems in young pups to first appear, and then over a period of twenty years become an epidemic which has continued non-stop, growing in size and complexity, for a further forty or fifty years, despite our best efforts to eliminate it.

The story of skeletal problems in our dogs ...

... begins with the sudden appearance of Hip Dysplasia in the 1930's, and continues to the present day where skeletal disease in pups is found to consist of a vast array of problems, is widespread and common place.

Dog owners today assume that this is how it has always been. Very few of them realise that at the beginning of the twentieth century, the modern skeletal diseases which we take for granted today, were all relatively rare conditions.

Hip Dysplasia was the first Juvenile Bone Disease recognised in dogs. An Australian vet,   Tom Hungerford, in his internationally renowned text "Diseases of Livestock", tells us that **Hip Dysplasia "first attracted attention in 1935."**

By 1965, a mere 30 years later ...

... Hip Dysplasia had been identified in 55 breeds of dogs world-wide, and was found to be widespread throughout each of these breeds. Unfortunately, the skeletal problems did not stop with Hip Dysplasia. Sometime between the 1930's and the 1960's a multitude of other problems such as Shoulder, Elbow, Hock and Stifle Dysplasia appeared.

There are a heap of questions that nobody is asking!

- How is it that Hip Dysplasia and later on other skeletal problems such as Elbow Dysplasia could suddenly appear and then apparently spread rapidly through many different breeds?

- Did Hip and Elbow Dysplasia exist before 1935? If they did, were they rare or common?

- If they were common, why weren't they recognised earlier?

- If they were non-existent before 1935, where did they come from?

- Why do these skeletal problem appear mostly in the larger breeds?

- Why do they continue to increase in frequency?

- Why can't we eliminate these problems despite mass radiography and mass culling?

- What does all this mean in the light of the theory that these are inherited diseases which can be eliminated by genetic means?

Do we have answers?

Hip Dysplasia was considered a rare disease when it was first described. This is important. Hip Dysplasia and other skeletal diseases are not rare today. Their presence in most breeds of dogs is accepted as normal today.

If Hip Dysplasia and the other skeletal diseases had been common, the vets of the day could hardly have missed them.

Hip Dysplasia is not a disease to be ignored! A disease seen in all the large and giant breeds where affected dogs waggle their bottoms as they walk, like old cows with flattened and grossly widened hips. A disease which results in extreme difficulty when rising from a sitting position, and difficulty in turning. A disease which can be crippling and where every movement is filled with pain.   A disease which in its mildest form shows a markedly shortened stride and painful back problems, often proceeding to severe lameness. Sometimes the   hind limbs can become almost totally useless.

Could all those other skeletal diseases have been missed?

Elbow Dysplasia, deviated legs, the Wobbler Syndrome, dropped hocks, splayed feet - if diseases such as these had been common diseases as they are today - could all these have been missed prior to the 1930's? That seems hard to believe.

Then came the view that genes are to blame!

The view that Hip Dysplasia is an inherited disease ......

..... Was born in 1945. At first Hip Dysplasia was thought to be caused by a single gene. If that had been true Hip Dysplasia would have been very easy to remove by breeding. However, breeding did not solve the problem. For that reason it was decided that Hip Dysplasia was caused by many genes.

The gene theory itself was not questioned

Since that time, the dog world has taken the gene theory for granted and spent much time, effort and money, using it as the basis for the eradication of both Hip and Elbow Dysplasia, via a number of massive and on-going world-wide breeding schemes. The validity of the gene theory as the basis for eliminating these problems has never been questioned.

This is despite the fact that the incidence of all forms of juvenile bone and joint disease has continued to increase dramatically.

It seems difficult to believe, in fact highly unlikely, that a mass of nasty genes hell bent on wrecking our dogs' bones should suddenly appear in the dog population some 60 to 70 years ago and from that time spread like wild fire throughout all breeds of dogs. That sort of thing happens with infectious disease agents such as bacteria or viruses, but not with genes. It is much more likely that the genetic structure of our dogs has remained unchanged.

In other words, if Hip Dysplasia and Elbow Dysplasia are genetic problems, it must be that the genes which cause them have always been present in our dogs. If that is the case, **there must be other factors which are causing these skeletal diseases in our pups .**

There must be something else going on?!

There is little doubt that if these skeletal problems suddenly appeared during the 1930's, and were subsequently found to be widespread and rapidly becoming more common, that factors other than heredity were and are responsible for causing them to occur.

There is strong evidence to show that these problems appeared suddenly as a direct result of a radical change in the way we raise our dogs. That these problems are not due to to any change in our dogs' genetic structure.

If that is so we have to examine very closely what HAS changed to produce these problems

If those genes were always present but unable to express themselves, we must doggedly pursue that factor or factors or 'right conditions' which occurred in the mid-thirties and which allowed those genes to express themselves. There is little doubt that those 'right conditions' are continuing to allow these genes to express themselves today - in many cases - even more so!

The conclusion we must draw from this is that to get rid of these diseases, there is very little point in trying to **change** the dogs' genetic structure, as we have been trying to for the last forty to fifty years. Without success.

Instead we need to eliminate the changes which produced these problems

Much simpler, much quicker, much cheaper, less heartbreaking and above all - much more successful.

This approach is true for both the common skeletal diseases such as Hip and Elbow Dysplasia and the less common 'mystery' diseases such as Panosteitis and Hypertrophic Osteodystrophy.

Will we vets re-think our position?

In science, when a theory is proposed, it is tested to see if predictions made on the basis of that theory come true. If they do not, the theory is supposed to be modified or abandoned and a new theory sought to explain the observed phenomena.

Back in the 1940's a theory about Hip Dysplasia was put forward. It said something along the lines of - **'Because Hip and Elbow Dysplasia are due to bad genes, the best way to eliminate them from our dogs is to breed them out.'**

We have been attempting to breed these problems out for the last fifty years. The attempt has failed! The problems remain. In fact they are probably increasing!

That means we should be looking for a new theory to explain what we are seeing.

We vets need to rethink our position entirely. All we need do is open our eyes to see the problem as it is, the courage to abandon a few cherished beliefs, and the common sense to make a few management changes.

- We need to understand that these diseases were rare in the thirties.

- We need to identify the environmental changes which allowed them to appear.

- We must eliminate those changes rather than attempt to remove genes which have not lived happily with those changes.

This should reduce the incidence of these problems to the pre 1930's level.

Let us go back to the mid-twenties

This was the time in both America and England that commercial dog food was becoming more popular as the staple diet of domestic dogs. Particularly the larger breeds and particularly those dogs in a kennel situation.

The Juvenile Orthopedic diseases began to appear en masse when dogs were, for the first time in their evolutionary history, fed largely on commercial dog food. Dogs had stopped eating bones for the first time ever. This failure to eat bones and the widespread use of commercial dog food was combined with heavy artificial calcium supplementation. Something that dogs had never had to cope with during their entire evolutionary history.

This scenario which occurred in America and Britain in a big way from 1935 onwards, was duplicated much later in Australia during the 1960's. In Australia, the change to commercial dog food was hardly noticed. It was welcomed by the vets of the time who together with most pet owners viewed it as a step forward. However, there is always a price to pay for 'progress.'

Australia loses its dog-feeding innocence

It is a human trait to think and act as if the current situation is the way things have always been. When it comes to feeding our pets we are no different. Pet owners think and act as if processed pet foods have always been there for us. As if this is how we have always fed pets. "Is there any other way?" But of course processed pet foods haven't always been available. **Pet food is a modern phenomenon.**

Prior to 1966, there was very little pet food for sale in Australia. 1966 was the year that pet food hit the Australian market in a big way. People have forgotten this of course. If you mention to pet owners that thirty years ago in Australia there was very little pet food and that most people fed their pets on human food scraps including raw meaty bones, they look at you in wonderment and disbelief. Pet foods in Australia have certainly made a rapid take over of both the eating habits of our pets and the minds of pet owners.

It seemed great at the time

Owners and vets alike welcomed processed pet foods. The owners enjoyed the convenience. Not only that, they could rest easy knowing that they were feeding their pets the 'best possible food' - according to both the ads used by the pet food companies and their local vet. The vets welcomed the 'pet food era' with open arms. It made their life a lot easier. It eliminated the need to explain the principles of sound nutrition to their pet owning clients. Or so they thought. The pet food companies had done all the work for them as far as they were concerned. Another reason we vets continue to welcome these products, particularly in hindsight, is that processed pet foods have completely eliminated a number of classical nutritional diseases.

Our pets' problems used to be simple!

Our pets used to have simple problems. Simple to diagnose and easily remedied if they had not gone too far. If they had gone too far, euthanasia was the sad but obvious and necessary solution in most cases.

Prior to the widespread use of processed pet foods in Australia ...

... there were a number of diet related disease problems seen in our pet population. These involved simple nutrient deficiencies and occasionally excesses. Usually a deficiency or excess of a single nutrient.

An all cereal diet caused [mostly] a protein deficiency.

An all meat diet, which was relatively common, produced a calcium deficiency.

An all liver diet produced a vitamin A excess.

An all fresh fish diet produced a vitamin B1 deficiency.

An all egg white diet produced [among other things] a Biotin deficiency.

A high fat diet produced a vitamin E deficiency.

Fortunately, these problems were not all that common with the possible exception of the calcium deficient diet caused by an all meat diet. However, there is little doubt that the modern processed foods have eliminated such problems almost entirely.

From a veterinary perspective, the existence of scientifically formulated, complete and balanced processed pet foods has completely eliminated the need to explain nutritional principles to the pet owning public.

Sounds great! Sure does. But everything has its price. Has the elimination of a few simple deficiency diseases - together with the convenience that processed pet foods bring us - been worth it? What are the costs here?

Unfortunately not all changes are for the best

Progress is not always what it seems to be. When the Australian pet population changed from a predominantly fresh food diet to a cooked and processed food diet, the diseases our pets suffered shifted in character as well. This change occurred in Australia in the mid-sixties. In America it changed dramatically in the twenties to thirties, and in England it may have changed even earlier.

While it is true that a number of classical deficiency diseases have disappeared with the widespread consumption of processed pet foods, the need for vets to understand nutrition, to explain correct nutrition and to offer clients an alternative to cooked and processed pet foods has never been more important.

Why is this? It is because we have jumped from the frying pan into the fire, to use a very old but apt expression.

Now our pets have complex problems

These changes in our pets' eating habits, as wonderful as they have seemed to both the veterinary profession and the public at large, have not only eliminated a number of simple deficiency diseases, **they have also produced an enormous increase in the type and frequency of degenerative diseases.**

This wholesale switch of the nation's pets to processed pet foods has resulted in a dramatic increase in such problems as arthritis, cancer, skin conditions, heart and kidney disease.

More pertinent to this chapter is that the widespread use of these foods has also resulted in an enormous increase in skeletal diseases such as Hip Dysplasia.

With the advent of the scientifically produced complete diets in Australia in the mid-sixties, [much earlier in other countries, such as the UK and the US], most of the classical diseases of deficiency and excess disappeared. This has been hailed as a great step forward by the veterinary profession. HOW WRONG CAN YOU BE?

By switching our pets from a predominantly raw whole food diet based on raw meaty bones, to the biologically inappropriate cereal based pet foods, we have exchanged a few simple easily fixed and relatively uncommon problems for a virtual epidemic of - very common but complex, expensive to diagnose and treat - degenerative diseases.

These degenerative diseases, like the simple nutritionally based diseases seen in the pre-pet-food era, are all caused by excesses and deficiencies. However, they are not simple diseases caused by simple nutritional problems.

Our new set of nutritional problems are much more complex, subtle and insidious. They are caused by multiple deficiencies and excesses all working together. The diseases caused by these artificial foods are rarely linked to those artificial foods.

While it is true that every single one of these degenerative disease conditions have always existed, it was never to the marked degree we now see in our modern pet population. In the case of Juvenile Bone Disease in our dogs, that problem has risen from relative obscurity or rarity in the 1930's to become one of the most vexing and costly problems facing the pet owning public today.

The question we must ask ourselves is this ...

... has the elimination of those few simple problems of nutritional deficiency been worth the enormous increase in the degenerative disease problems that have taken their place, not the least of which is the Juvenile Bone Diseases in our dogs?

Do vets know of these changes in disease patterns?

While a wealth of knowledge exists in research journals and academic circles concerning the relationship between modern processed foods and degenerative disease, very little has filtered out into the world of clinical practice. While some of this information is beginning to be taught in medical schools, it is not so for the vets.

The average veterinary practitioner appears to be totally ignorant of the role of nutrition in either causing or preventing these degenerative disease processes.

Of course it does not take a genius to figure out why the veterinary profession has no idea of the origin of the degenerative diseases

Our veterinary undergraduates are taught their pet nutrition either by representatives of the pet food companies, or teachers who push the pet food programme to the exclusion of all other feeding methods.

Therefore it comes as no surprise that these highly impressionable undergraduates develop an unshakeable faith in these nutritionally inadequate foods.

They have no idea that the very diseases they spend so much of their undergraduate time learning about could easily be prevented by switching their clients' dogs to a more suitable diet.

The unfortunate bottom line to all of this is that today's vet will tell you that a highly expensive brand of pet food, often imported from overseas, and sitting on their shelves just waiting for you to buy it, is the absolutely best way to feed your young, growing dog.

No questions are to be asked - no argument is to be entertained. The facts are however, that even if you do manage to raise a sound puppy using these foods - and yes that DOES happen, eventually one or more of the degenerative diseases will emerge as a direct result of this food being fed.

Distinct patterns of change have been noted in the orthopaedic diseases seen in our teaching Hospitals.

But their significance has been ignored

The veterinary clinic at Sydney University sees more difficult bone and joint problems than the average practice. These cases are referred by private practitioners who lack either the expertise, the equipment or the will to handle them.

In the 1960's and 70's we used to see lots of Rickets

When I was a veterinary student at Sydney University in the mid 1970's, the principle type of bone problem referred at that time were the ones caused by nutrient deficiencies. The most common deficiency was a lack of calcium. **Calcium deficiencies occurred when pet owners fed their pups an all meat diet.** Although we did see problems caused by nutritional excesses, that is, problems such as Hip, Shoulder, and Elbow Dysplasia, they were less common.

Over the next fifteen years that whole situation was reversed

By the mid to late 1980's referral cases involving bones and joints at Sydney University had become principally problems of excess. These were problems of poor bone and joint formation due to overfeeding in general and an oversupply of calcium in particular. The problems of deficiency, such as those caused by insufficient calcium due to an all meat diet, so common 15 years previously, had all but disappeared.

In that very short period of time, the pendulum had swung from one extreme to the other. Problems of excess including Hip, Shoulder and Elbow Dysplasia had largely replaced the deficiency problems.

Why the change in the type of bone problems seen?

The simple answer is that there had been a dramatic change in the eating habits of the nation's dogs. We Australians had stopped feeding our dogs on raw meaty bones and food scraps. We had switched them to a diet of mostly cooked and processed foods. We began to do this in the mid-sixties, with the changeover pretty well complete by the mid-eighties. [Note that we were some thirty years behind the USA and UK in making this change.]

As a result, the disease patterns in our dogs had changed from simple single nutrient deficiencies and excesses which were relatively uncommon, but when they occurred were easy to fix, to complex and - unfortunately - exceedingly common diseases of degeneration and permanent damage.

Included amongst those degenerative diseases were the Juvenile Orthopedic diseases. These modern bone problems, the direct result of this new 'excessive' style of feeding and management, have proved difficult to prevent, difficult to treat, and have produced lifetime problems in the multitudes of animals that have succumbed to them.

Let us try and put all this together

You will recall that a little earlier in this chapter I asked the question "what HAS changed to produce these problems? What is that factor or factors, what are those 'right conditions' which occurred in the mid thirties which allowed the genes responsible for the modern Bone Diseases to express themselves and which continue to allow them to express themselves today?"

At least part of the answer to that you now know. It is very simple. Those right conditions or factors which allowed the increase in Juvenile Bone disease which began in the thirties and continues today were the decrease in raw food and raw meaty bone eating combined with the increased use of commercial dog food and calcium supplements.

There is little doubt that the increase in what was once a rare group of diseases is a direct result of a world wide change in the way pups are reared, particularly their eating habits and growth rates.

The skeletal diseases in growing dogs have become so common that today the elimination of Hip and Elbow Dysplasia is the main focus of breeding programmes in breeds such as the German Shepherd, Great Dane, St. Bernard etc.

It is tragic that the major thrust of our breeding programmes is the elimination of a group of diseases. An entirely negative set of aims!

So what happened to cause these problems?

On the basis of the available evidence it was the abandoning of a BARF type diet and replacing it with cooked and processed foods together with calcium supplements, which triggered these problems of degeneration, including the skeletal diseases in our puppies.

Also heavily involved is another factor which this chapter has not as yet touched upon.

This is the excessive and inappropriate exercise regimes which have accompanied the increasing urbanisation of our dogs.

This important aspect of our dogs' changing environment will be dealt with more fully in the chapters which follow.

What I want you to realise is that ...

... These dramatic change in our dogs' environment ...

... have allowed genes which in the past caused very few problems, to suddenly be able to wreak havoc on our pups' skeletal systems. **Genes which under these modern conditions of diet and exercise will most definitely produce Juvenile Orthopaedic Disease in our young dogs.**

If that is true - and the evidence to support that proposition is overwhelming - we may conclude that until we rethink our management practices - particularly the way we rear our puppies - we will continue to fail in our endeavours to eliminate skeletal disease in our pups.

To put the whole question of managing puppy growth in perspective, we will now look at how young dogs have been fed down through the Ages, starting with our dogs' ancestor - the wolf and other wild canids.

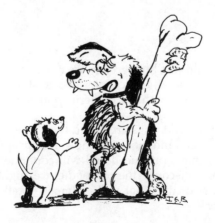

CHAPTER THREE

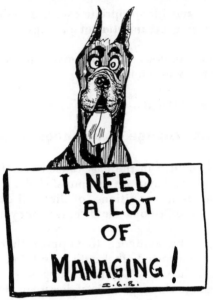

PUPPY MANAGEMENT – THEN AND NOW

To help you understand just how greatly we have changed the conditions under which pups are reared, this chapter looks at the rearing of pups in the wild and compares this with our modern approach to raising pups.

By understanding how wild dogs are raised to be free of orthopaedic bone disease, we will understand not only how inappropriate exercise and inappropriate foods have produced and will continue to produce these problems, we will also discover the sort of diet we ought to be feeding our dogs today. The sort of diet that will [almost] totally prevent skeletal problems in our pups.

We will also look briefly at the way pups were raised in the pre-pet-food era. Prior to pet foods, most pups were raised in a similar fashion to wild dogs. That is, in such a way that problems such as Hip and Elbow Dysplasia were relatively rare conditions.

We pay dearly for modern puppy management

The price we pay is the bone disease we generate. We have produced perfect conditions for its production. This is because modern foods and a modern approach to exercise are biologically inappropriate. On the other hand it is rare for wild pups to develop bone disease, and that includes Hip and Elbow Dysplasia. Why? Because a wolf or a dingo or an African wild dog's diet and exercise as a pup prevents the creation of these problems.

There is a vast gulf separating these two approaches to rearing pups.

An important question ....

Can [or should] modern dogs be raised like wild dogs?

It is now generally agreed that the ancestor of the modern dog is the wolf. What is not clear is how long that domestication process has been going on. It may have been as short as 10 000 years or as long as 50 000 years, or possibly more. No matter how long it has been, that process of domestication where our ancestors removed the 'wildness' from the wolf, involved thousands of years of selective breeding. They took an animal that could well have seen them as food, and by selective breeding, produced an animal that became their best friend.

In this process, our ancestors produced hundreds of 'different looking wolves.' These various "breeds" - as we now know them - were and are, all different shapes and sizes. Each breed was developed in a local area for a particular task or tasks. Whether it was hunting for large prey, exterminating vermin, guarding, herding, being a companion, a foot warmer, whatever, each breed fulfilled a set of needs in the society in which it was developed.

189

The result is that each breed is not only different to look at, but also has a unique mind set which relates very much to the task[s] it was bred to perform.However, our dogs also retain many of their wolf-like characters, including their pack mentality. This includes the need to either lead or be led.

Today, as we train our dogs, we need to be aware of both the unique mind set of our particular breed and the basic pack mentality, the wolf-like traits, which still dominate our dogs' thinking.

The point I am making in regard to this discussion on bone disease in pups, is that to produce the dog, our ancestors made only two basic changes to the wolf.

They changed the wolf's appearance and they changed its mind. What they did not change, was the basic internal workings or physiology of the wolf. There was no need to.

As a result, the basic workings or physiology of modern dogs is no different or very little different to their ancestor the wolf. Modern dogs grow and function [and malfunction] in very much the same way as the wolf. **That is why the food and exercise requirements of today's growing pup are the same as those of a young growing wolf.**

To produce a fully functioning adult dog, our modern pup needs to grow in exactly the same way as the wolf pup. If we vary the food and the exercise too drastically, we will alter the finished product. We will produce damaged goods. To be more specific ...

The basic environment which the modern dog requires for healthy bone growth in terms of food and exercise is exactly the same as it was [and still is] for the wolf.

So although we have carried out selective breeding to alter our dog's outward appearance and mind, we have not asked it to cope with, nor have we selectively bred it to deal with any dramatic change in feeding or exercising. UNTIL NOW.

A modern experiment

One of the large National Parks in the USA has recently become home to a group of wolves. Wolves had not lived there for something like fifty or sixty years. Approximately half a dozen wolves were returned to the park several years ago [time of writing 1997], and over a period of six or seven years those few wolves had multiplied to a healthy 100 plus.

QUESTION: What is important to dog owners and breeders about this little happening? ANSWER: This little happening, and the fact that it has been so simple and so successful has enormous implications for what modern dog owners are trying to do in their attempts to raise sound stock, particularly as regards skeletal health.

Think about how these wolves have survived

They have had no vets to radiograph their hips and select sound breeding stock. There have been no progesterone tests prior to breeding, no ultrasound to detect pregnancy, no blood tests to ensure that health is perfect, no caesareans, no injections after giving birth, no worming, no extra calcium, no vaccinations or puppy checking, or treatment of problems.

There are no dog food companies out there supplying them with super premium foods. There is no one to make sure that their every meal is complete and balanced. There is no one to make sure they never eat egg whites. No one to protect them from eating bones. No one to cook their food and to make sure they do not contact dangerous bacteria such as E. coli or Salmonella, and most especially no one to ensure they receive the correct ratio of calcium to phosphorus so they will have perfect bone growth.

All those wolves had was themselves. They were on their own as they have always been and doing just fine. The only individuals who have not been doing fine have been the local farmers. Losing stock, and becoming [rightly or wrongly] afraid to venture into the forest once again because of the age old fear of wolves.

We have much to learn from this experiment

Wolves rely on their stamina and strength to survive. Any animal unable to hunt or compete with the others for food because of skeletal problems would certainly not survive. The free moving healthy looking wolves I observed, appeared to have perfect bone and joint health.

Why are these wolves - without the 'benefits' of modern veterinary technology, without truckloads of super premium dog food, and without calcium supplements - doing so well?

The answer is very simple. They are living in a biologically appropriate environment in terms of food and exercise. They are getting what they need. They have no need of modern technology.

By contrast our dogs are not receiving what they need in terms of diet and exercise. That's why they can't grow healthy skeletons. Despite our technology. ..... **our dogs are doing badly!**

Let us go on and examine the lifestyle of this experimental group of wolves. The lifestyle of any group of wild dogs. That lifestyle will show us the basic principles which we should use to determine how pups should be fed and exercised today, for maximum present and future health. Particularly the health of their bones and joints. You will discover that such a diet is simple, straightforward, and uncomplicated. Just like the lives of those wolves.

How wolf pups eat and exercise

After it has been weaned, a wolf pup's only responsibility is to play, do as it is told, learn, sleep, keep an eye out for danger and eat. Not much different to how it is - or should be - for juvenile humans or modern pups today. A relatively simple life. A relatively tough life. This is a time when young wolves discover in relative safety how life is for a wolf. A time when the weaklings are weeded out. These are the foundations which build a smart, tough, lean and healthy adult.

First, the eating ...

Wild dogs do not eat regular meals. Nobody plans their meals. Nor do they have   an all meat diet. On the other hand, not one single meal is complete and balanced. Raw bones with meat are a major part of their diet. Lots and lots of it! In the winter they dig up and eat frozen food. They eat offal such as liver and heart. They eat raw eggs. They eat decaying material. Food that is slightly off.

They may eat once a day or five or six times a day, depending on the season and what sort of food is available. They have days when they go hungry. They have days when they pile food into themselves almost beyond capacity. They eat when food is available, and as the urge takes them. They eat a wide variety of foodstuffs. Insects, bark, soil, birds - complete with their tiny bones and feathers - whatever. Every meal they eat is totally raw. Not one skerrick of it is cooked. Ever.

They eat vegetables including herbs, from the gut of their prey. This vegetable material is raw, totally crushed and partly digested. They eat faeces.

A wolf's diet contains almost no grains.

Wolves never eat cooked grain

In eating the intestinal contents of their prey they will eat some grain which is usually immature and green. Most certainly they do not eat a totally grain based diet like the modern dog, subjected to a lifetime of dried dog food.

Even if their prey had been eating mature seed heads, by the time the wolf pup or adult gets to eat this grain, it has been ground to a paste and soaked in the juices of the herbivores intestines. A totally different product to the masses of cooked and processed grains fed to dogs today. Not only that, these few grains are mixed in with a mass of other grassy and herbaceous material.

For a wolf - not one single meal consists of dry dog food. They don't eat canned dog food either.

Feeding for Weaning

As tiny pups, still with their mother, the wolf pups are well looked after. After weaning things change dramatically. However, before we tackle that, let's look at the weaning process itself. This deserves our attention as it has important lessons for how we wean our pups today.

Wolf pups are not weaned using cereals or bowls of milk or mushed up dried or canned dog food, or bread soaked in milk. From the moment the weaning process begins, the wild pup begins a diet which is based on the carcases of other animals - mostly herbivores.

Mum begins the process by vomiting. She vomits up food for the pups, starting when they are three to four weeks of age. These young pups crunch their way through and eat any tiny or soft bones, they rip and tear at the meat attached to larger bones, and they suck and chew at the organ meats swimming in a sea of fermenting totally crushed vegetable material. All totally raw. They also eat whatever they can scavenge from left over carcases left lying around their immediate vicinity. This includes - once again - raw meaty bones and bits of liver and raw partly digested totally crushed and sometimes fermenting vegetable material.

The young pups are not protected from faeces ...

... with its E. coli or Salmonella or Campylobacter or a myriad of other bacteria or protozoa. Instead, they eat it and develop healthy immune systems, well able to deal with the normal bacteria and other micro-organisms in their environment. In addition, they are able to - and of course have to - build a resistance to intestinal worms.

When weaning time comes around, do your pups enjoy similar 'advantages'? The question is, how far should we adapt these principles as we rear our pups today?

Certainly I am not suggesting we should allow our pups to be wormy or to be needlessly exposed to high levels of pathogenic bacteria by feeding them meat that is rotten or anything like it. They should not however be totally protected from such things. Their food must be raw. I am strongly suggesting that what young wolves or dingoes or foxes eat, deserves our very close attention. This is what we need to duplicate.

Once wild pups are weaned ...

They don't join in the serious hunting, but of course they do a lot of "play-hunting". Insects, lizards, rodents, whatever moves is fair game. They may even catch and eat some of these. This is important. Not for what they are eating so much, but more for how they are being exercised. **Those few lines contain the vital information on which to base the exercising of modern pups.**

Wolf pups mainly eat at the family dinner table. That is, they share in whatever the older wolves have dug up, hunted or scavenged. However, even this food is not easily won.

When mum looked after them the young wolves had a degree of protection. After weaning it is a different story. They are no longer pampered or cosseted. No more favourable treatment. The pups have now plummeted to the bottom of the social heap. Instead of being number one when meal time comes, when the hunt is over, when that old or **frozen** carcase is dug up or discovered, the young weanlings as the lowest members in the social order are last in to the feast. **They have to fight for every morsel and scrap of food they get.** 'Manners' for a wolf pup consists of not eating until the older wolves 'allow' them. That is, when all the others have had their fill. The pups then have to fight amongst themselves, until they too have established an order of dominance.

Because the wolf pups only get to eat the leftovers, most of the choice bits have gone. So what is left for them? There will be bones with scraps of meat, little bits of organs such as liver, heart spleen etc., that the adults in their ravenous haste missed. Lots and lots of gut contents, consisting of masses of plant material, raw, crushed and fermenting.

Because wolves and other wild dogs follow the herds of deer, bison, antelope etc., pulling down the young, the old, the injured and the sick, one of the foods always available for them is the faeces of the animals they follow. This is an important part of their diet. They actually require those healthy bowel bacteria. That is why modern dogs seek out and eat faeces. Their own, other dogs', cats' faeces - whatever they can obtain.

The habit of eating faeces supplies a young pup with first class protein, essential fatty acids, masses of vitamins and plenty of healthy fibre.

Research tells us that faeces eating by the young of many species plays an important role in bowel and brain health.

The bacteria in faeces help in the development of the immune system of the bowel and undoubtedly assist in the prevention of such problems as inflammatory bowel disease.

The essential fatty acids present in faeces have been shown to play a vital role in the full development of the central nervous system, particularly the higher functions of the brain. This is something we have to take very seriously.

Poor brain development could well be one of the factors behind much of the unprovoked aggression we are seeing in modern dogs fed processed food. Another brain problem which could be related to this is epilepsy.

I am not suggesting that our pups should necessarily eat faeces - although in the Australian country-side, young teenage and adult dogs certainly do eat plenty of nutritious and healthy cow, sheep, rabbit, horse and other herbivorous faeces. What I am saying is that we must find suitable substitutes for our dogs today.

This is the basis on which we may confidently supplement our young pups' diet with yoghurt and other sources of probiotics; vitamins; healthy clays; essential fatty acids from fresh, cold extracted oils and first class protein such as egg yolks - all combined with raw crushed vegetable material.

It is important to note that young wolves, like adult wolves, **never have a meal that is complete and balanced.** Instead, they are raised on a wide variety of foods. Those young wolf pups are most certainly not raised on a meat only diet and they are not raised on cereals. They receive no calcium supplements.

Their diet is balanced - eventually - over many many meals - both large and small. In a strict scientific sense, that is what their bodies are designed to cope with.

Wolf pups do not eat at regular times

The food supply is not regular.They are not spoon fed. They have to battle for their food. Obviously the food needs to be adequate for survival and healthy growth. However, it is very rare that their hunger is ever fully satisfied. These pups are lean and hungry most of the time. There are periods when they may go for twelve or more hours without food. As a result, they are not fat and roly poly. They never grow at anything like their maximum growth rate. As a result they grow SLOWLY.

Let me repeat. THE WOLF PUP GROWS SLOWLY. It is not biologically appropriate for a wolf pup to grow at its maximum pace. There is at least one very simple reason for this. A wolf pup raised at top speed will develop skeletal problems!!

The pups do not get to eat a lot of fat. Wild game is always very lean. The relatively small amount of fat which is present is not saturated, but full of essential fatty acids. Quite different to the fat found in modern farm fed livestock; saturated and lacking in essential fatty acids.The pups mostly miss out on the fat because the adult hunters will preferentially eat it first. The pups get most of their essential fatty acids from their habit of eating faeces and gut contents - chewed up vegetation.

One thing you should be realising by now, is that crushed up vegetable material is a vital ingredient in a puppy's diet. If it is to be a healthy pup!

The older wolves will always eat until they are absolutely jammed full of food, go back to camp, vomit, and then eat their vomit at a more leisurely pace. Naturally, little bits of this mixed up mess of food are left and the pups can dart in and grab bits and pieces of it. In the process they also eat bits of dirt and leaves and sticks etc. Soil, grass and other fresh plant material are also eaten by these hungry wolf pups quite deliberately.

That in essence is how the weaned wolf pup eats and grows

- Its diet is based on raw meaty bones.

- It is a totally raw diet.

- A diet rich in plant material, but totally devoid of cooked grain.

- No processed food.

- No masses of steaming white rice.

- Some meat - never minced, but always raw.

- Some organ meat -always raw.

- Not a lot of fat. Almost no saturated fat. No cooked fat, but plenty of essential fatty acids.

- A diet rich in vitamins.

- A diet full of bacteria including masses of E. coli, Salmonella, Campylobacter and many many more so called pathogenic bacteria, all of which play a role in immune competence, including most particularly bowel health.

- A wolf pup's diet is constantly varying, both in quantity and quality of food. As a result, there are no regular meal times or meal sizes, and not one single meal is complete and balanced.

- The wild pup let me repeat is always lean, always hungry. It is never fat and roly poly. As a consequence it is highly unusual for it to develop juvenile orthopaedic bone disease.

There is so much to learn about rearing pups from the above story. Go back and read it carefully. Note simple things like ...

- Pups do not need supplementary calcium

- Pups do not need processed food

- Pups do not need cooked grain meals

- Pups do not need a feeding routine

- Pups do not need their meals to be complete and balanced

- A pup's food should not be cooked

- Frozen food [thawed] is fine for pups

- Pups require their whole feeding routine to be complete and balanced

- Pups need to be fed a diet based on raw meaty bones

- A major part of a pup's diet should be raw crushed vegetable material

- Offal is a normal part of a dog's diet

- The healthy equivalent of faeces is a normal part of a dog's diet

- Healthy soil or clay is part of a dog's diet

- Dogs should grow up lean and hungry

- An occasional short fast will not be harmful and may be of benefit

- Pups should be exposed in a controlled manner to bacteria

- Pups should be weaned using raw meaty bones

- Pups should not be weaned with cereal foods or processed foods

- Pups should never be grown at their maximum growth rate

- Pups should be kept lean - not fat and roly poly

- Pups require to be supplemented with foods which replace faeces. This is important for brain and bowel health.

If you can use the above as a check list and say yes - that is how my pups are raised - there is very little chance your dogs will develop skeletal problems.

The exercise regime of the wild pup

From the moment it is born, the wild pup is not only eating the right food to build sound healthy bones and joints, it is also involved in the sort of exercise regime which has precisely the same aim.

A pup's struggling/walking exercise begins in a saucer shaped whelping circle that mum creates in the earth. This simple depression enables maximum conservation of warmth, and maximum puppy safety. As exploring newborns, the pups are able to tumble safely back into mum's protectively curled body. That soil formed depression also provides optimum traction or grip for young paws. This is vital. Young pups that slip and slide around on slippery surfaces are destined for bone and joint problems. Wild dogs never have this problem.

From those first struggling moments to find a teat and begin sucking, through the many encounters it has with that teat and with its brothers and sisters as it struggles to find that teat again or that 'just-right-spot' to sleep or stretch, through its first walking steps, the young wild pup is constantly moving and stressing all its bones and joints.

By the second week following birth, there is much definite wrestling and struggling. This play fighting can look pretty serious at times, and it has a serious purpose. It is preparing those pups for a lifetime of struggle, and part of that preparation is the building of strong healthy bones and joints. Once again, a soil base is essential - providing good traction for those growing and developing legs.

As a wild pup grows and attempts to walk, the soil base on which it lives provides the perfect grip it requires. This ensures optimum use and therefore development and strength of those little legs and their bones and joints. You will never see puppies raised in the wild developing into 'swimmers.'

The next major addition to a wild pup's exercise regime, is when mum begins to vomit up food to begin its weaning programme. Now those pups have something to fight over. Ever watched three week old pups fight over raw meaty bones? Ever heard them?! Now they are really working. Pulling, tugging, chewing, the whole body braced, to win possession of that precious morsel. Exercising jaws, necks, shoulders, back and legs. This is the beginning of a lifetime of essential bone eating exercise.

A pup that eats and rips and tears at bones from its earliest days develops a strong, lean muscular body with healthy bones and joints. This is in stark contrast to a modern pup raised without bones. Both the muscles and the bones are thinner and weaker and the joints are looser. This lack of eating exercise ensures such pups are much more prone to skeletal problems such as Hip and Elbow Dysplasia.

At five weeks the young pup has added a very juvenile form of 'play-hunting' to its exercise regime. Insects, rodents, lizards - whatever. Notice I said 'play-hunting.' Apart from eating, everything the pup does is a form of play. Play is the key word for the rest of that juvenile puppy's puppyhood. Play hunting, play fighting and just plain playing. Only the adults hunt. There is no serious hunting, or even fighting, till a pup reaches adulthood.

On that important point let us come back to the present for a moment. When it comes to modern dogs, the rule of thumb is that the smaller and lighter the breed, the sooner it can begin to stress those bones. Maybe as young as eight months. With the Giant breeds however, they must wait until fifteen to eighteen months.

This is important. **Pups do not, should not, indeed must not undergo any long periods of running or walking or jarring exercise until their bones have ceased to grow and have begun to harden.Playing pups stop when they are tired.** No long boring walks on a lead for wild pups. They wrestle and fight with each other instead. The importance of play as the major form of exercise is that a young pup can stop as soon as it starts to hurt or become tired. In that way, no excessive strain is placed on young growing bones. If pups had to seriously hunt before their bones were ready, the stress placed on those young bones would be sufficient to permanently damage the bones.

From our observations of young wolves growing and developing in the wild, we may draw some very important principles of exercise which should be applied to all growing pups today. Particularly the members of the larger and Giant breeds.

Pups should only receive two forms of exercise ...

- Play

- Eating exercise

Pups should not

- be given long hard runs as seen when hunting.

- be subjected to long boring walks.

- have their bones and joints 'jarred' - by constant jumping - for example.

What about dogs in the 'Pre-Pet-Food' era?

How were they raised? The answer to that is - not too differently to wild dogs. Of course they did not have to hunt for their food. For most domestic dogs in the 'pre-pet-food era', much of their diet was still composed of raw meaty bones together with other food scraps. Most importantly, the bulk of that food was raw. This diet definitely included plenty of vegetable material. Not always raw however.

Traditionally the dog was fed the food scraps of the humans who raised it. Certainly some of its food was cooked, including some leftovers consisting of cooked grain. However, the bulk of its diet reflected very much the sort of food on which wild dogs were and are raised.

What about exercise? In this respect, most dogs were raised in much the same way as wild dogs. Not too many fancy whelping boxes, more soil and straw than slick newspapers. Like the wild dogs, dogs in the pre-pet-food era spent most of their youth playing. Mostly they had large expanses to play in, so nobody felt inclined to take young pups for long boring walks in order to exercise them.

These dogs were not over-fed. This is because everybody was very relaxed about feeding dogs. It was simple and straightforward. Everybody knew how to do it and trusted their instincts. THEY KNEW THAT DOGS ATE BONES. There was no drama if they forgot to feed the pups. They would have scavenged something for themselves anyway. Nobody was racing to produce the 'biggest, roundest, fattest, most calcified, biggest-boned, 'bestest', largest, beautest- dog - ever, in the shortest possible space of time.'

The bottom line for these dogs raised in the pre-pet-food era is that the degree to which they experienced ill health reflected the degree to which their owners departed from that biologically appropriate method of feeding and exercising that nature developed over the hundreds of thousands of years of the wolf's evolution.

Feeding the modern pup

When we consider how wolves/dogs were raised in the 'pre-pet-food' era and compare that to our modern methods of husbandry, we can only conclude that the changes we have made to feeding and exercising have indeed been dramatic, and that their effects on puppy growth have been traumatic and catastrophic. In the light of this let me rephrase a paragraph you have just read:

The degree to which modern dogs experience ill health reflects the degree to which they are subjected to biologically inappropriate methods of feeding and exercising. Let us now look at those biologically inappropriate forms of puppy management so rife today.

1] All the food a modern pup eats is cooked ...

For the first time in its evolutionary history we are asking our dogs to eat nothing but cooked food. This is biologically unacceptable. A very dramatic change. Not too much of this is even home cooked food. Mostly it is commercially produced processed food. Usually either canned or dry food. Cooking is a process which destroys many of the life enhancing factors found only in raw foods. These include enzymes and many natural anti-oxidants and other anti-degeneration factors.

2] All the food a modern pup eats is based on cooked grain ...

The vast majority of the food eaten by the modern dog is composed of cooked grain as the most fundamental and major component of the diet. Another dramatic and biologically unacceptable change. Dogs have never in their evolutionary history - until now - eaten cooked grain. The results on health are devastating.

3] Meat meal and rendered fat come next ...

The cooked grain is teamed up with meat meal [with its damaged protein] and rendered [read highly damaged and damaging] fat.

In both the US and the UK it is not illegal to use rendered fat from domestic animals in pet foods - and there are reports that this is happening - together with flea collars and other dangerous chemicals such as the euthanasia solution in some of these deceased and rendered pets.

Aside from the dangerous chemicals it contains, that rendered fat contrasts strongly with the healthy fat so full of essential fatty acids that our dog's ancestors ate. These heat destroyed components are biologically unacceptable. They do not support healthy growth. They do not support a healthy life or contribute to a healthy old age.

The meat meal bears very little relationship to the healthy raw meat eaten by a wild dog.

4] Now add the chemical cocktail ...

Add loads of refined sugar, loads of salt, chemical colourings - dyes, to make the product look like something it is not. Add artificial chemical flavourings to make it taste like something it is not. Add flavour enhancers to make sure the animal eats something it ought not to. Add chemical antioxidants [known carcinogens] to ensure the product does not become obviously rancid.

What a lethal cocktail!

5] Now add the legally required nutrients ...

These are the currently known to be essential vitamins and minerals. The legal constraints on commercial pet foods do not require them to include vitally important biologically essential anti-oxidants and anti-degeneration factors present only in whole raw foods.

As a result, these products do not contain many of the essential factors we **do** know about such as enzymes, nor do they contain many of the essential factors we don't yet know about, the ones yet to be discovered and only present in whole raw natural foods.

6] Now add the complete and balanced myth/disaster ...

Every meal for the modern pup is complete and balanced. This necessity to have all the food fed to a dog in a "complete and balanced" form makes that food a slowly lethal cocktail. The combination of minerals and vitamins all cooked together makes many essential nutrients totally unavailable for our dogs. For more details on this particular problem see chapter 6 in **Give Your Dog a Bone**.

7] The modern puppy diet omits bones ...

This omission is another nail in the coffin for the modern dog. **The omission of raw meaty bones from the diet of the modern dog is central to the formation of bone disease in pups.**

Because the modern pup does not eat bones it misses out on all the essential nutrients bones supply including its calcium in perfect balance and form, together with all the other minerals required for healthy bone formation in perfect balance and form.

The result is that the modern pup obtains its minerals in a totally inappropriate form. The modern pup also misses out on its eating exercise. This eating exercise is a vital component of the exercise regime designed to grow healthy disease free bones and joints.

8] The modern pup does not eat vegetables or fruit ...

Instead it eats dry or tinned processed grains. Another complete disaster. The lack of crushed vegetables makes a monumental contribution to the production of degenerative disease in dogs, including problems such as Hip and Elbow Dysplasia. The modern pup does not eat the gut contents of a herbivore or anything like it. It does not eat faeces or anything like it. As a result it fails to receive a mass of essential nutrients as described in previous paragraphs, including probiotics - so essential for its bowel and over-all health.

Do you like what you are reading about modern dog feeding?

It gets worse!

The dry dog foods lack water which can help produce such problems as bladder stones, cystitis, and even bloat.

The canned dog food contains too much water which also can produce its own set of problems - for example, if it is used in lactation, the food is too 'dilute' to support the needs of the bitch.

The modern puppy does not have to exercise to obtain its food. That is, it does not have to expend any effort other than chewing, to eat its food. This lack of eating exercise does nothing for the teeth and gums. Instead it encourages periodontal disease and thin wasted looking limbs.

These are diets which have not withstood the test of time like the dog's biologically appropriate diet - the BARF diet. They are low in vitamins, particularly B, C, E, and quite often A.

For a pup particularly, they often contain dangerously high nutrient excesses - including calcium, fat, and protein. This combination is a disaster in its effects on bone health.

These products are often deficient in minerals such as zinc and copper because of their high calcium content.

For these products we pay enormous prices and live in expectation of them producing sound animals. The advertising that prompts us to buy such products is a monstrous misrepresentation of the facts. A very sad joke.

In summary we have to conclude this modern processed food diet is just so ... Poor ...

It often contains too much poor quality protein, lots of unnecessary and highly dangerous to health sugar, very low levels of essential fatty acids, too much calcium, too much salt [sodium] and too much phosphorus. It is a diet high in added chemicals such as colourings, flavourings, preservatives including artificial antioxidants. It is food devoid of the anti-ageing factors present in whole raw natural foods. No natural antioxidants, no enzymes. It is full of biologically inappropriate essential fatty acids, and biologically inappropriate complexes between cooked proteins and carbohydrates ... etc., etc..

Exercising the modern pup

For most modern pups, their home after weaning consists of a very tiny space compared to what wolves, dingoes and our dogs of yesteryear enjoyed. Most are forced to spend their time in small yards, or even smaller houses. This situation is occasionally relieved with trips to the streets and pavements on a leash for a long and very often boring walk.

What most of them are NOT able to do, is spend their growing days - between weaning and adulthood - in free running exercise and play with fellow pups.

The cramped conditions, the lack of freedom to run and play, together with the necessity to take long boring walks wreaks havoc on a young pup's bones. When that pup is tired out on that long boring walk - it cannot stop - it has to walk home. This causes irreparable and irreversible damage to soft and relatively vulnerable bones and joints.

These problems become worse:

- the bigger the breed,

- the heavier the breed,

- the fatter the breed,

- the more fast growing the breed,

- the more poorly engineered the breed,

- the less well muscled the breed,

- if the pup is being fed incorrectly.

- It is further compounded when breeds such as the St Bernard and the Labrador Retriever are involved. These are breeds which have been bred to spend much of their time as puppies being supported by snow and water respectively. Unfortunately, they no longer enjoy such an environment.

We are asking the dog to cope with enormous change

Over a very short period of time, approximately fifty or sixty years, and in many cases much less time than that, we have drastically altered the way our dogs are fed and exercised. They no longer eat raw meaty bones as the basis of their diet. They no longer eat raw food of any kind. For the first time in their evolutionary history they are eating a basically cooked diet. Not only that, it is a diet based on cooked grains and filled with poisons.

Their exercise regime as pups has gone from free running play which stopped when the puppy wanted it to, to forced route marches. Long boring walks or running which goes on well past the point where the puppy wants it to stop. There is no eating exercise and very little playing exercise.

These enormous changes to our dogs' diet and exercise have been sudden. There has been no chance to adapt. One of the results has been dramatic changes in our pups' bone and joint health.

What has been our response? To fix the diet and the exercise? Not at all. We have not diagnosed that to be the problem.

We have in fact made an inappropriate diagnosis.

Our diagnosis is not exactly correct

We have labelled the problem as genetic. The result of that diagnosis has been to attempt to alter the genetic make-up of our dogs so they can cope with this dramatic upheaval in their lives.

Having made a not necessarily incorrect but certainly a useless diagnosis, the inevitable outcome has been and will continue to be failure.

This is such an important point and is crucial to our understanding of why these bone diseases are occurring. When we observe skeletal diseases in our pups, we are looking at the response of the modern dog to a drastically altered feeding and exercise regime.

Our response to this situation is to attempt to select those individuals which will not develop orthopaedic bone disease in the face of this dramatic change. **We are attempting to alter our dogs' genes so they can cope with this modern way of feeding and exercising.**

To put that another way, our schemes to eliminate problems such as Hip and Elbow Dysplasia, or any of the other skeletal diseases seen in Juvenile canines are attempts to eliminate those individuals which cannot cope with modern foods and our apparent need to over-exercise and inappropriately exercise young pups.

We are attempting to eliminate those individuals which do not have proper bone growth in the face of these massive insults.

This results in enormous numbers of dogs being culled from our breeding programmes. Mostly to no avail. How futile. What a waste.

The problem is, not a single dog has the genetic capacity to deal satisfactorily with these changes. We do not have any dogs with the genetic capacity to fully cope with modern food or exercise regimes.

It is highly unlikely that there ever will be in the foreseeable future, dogs which have the genetic capacity to live long healthy lives when fed and exercised as pups are today.

We are walking down a path which will either come to a dead end or end in disaster.

Please read the chapters in **'Give Your Dog a Bone'** which deal with raising puppies, with eating bones, with eating vegetables, fruit, cereals and offal.

Re-read the BARF diet. Then compare and contrast what you do when you raise pups. If you are a newcomer to the dog world, compare all of this with what you would have done before having read this.

Think carefully. Which environment of diet and exercise do you want your pup to grow up in?

The modern environment of biologically inappropriate dog food, excessive protein, excessive calories, fast growth rates, calcium supplements, excessive exercise and bone disease, or the time honoured way of puppy rearing which produces healthy longevity, abundant reproduction and sound bones, free of Hip and Elbow Dysplasia etc., etc., etc..

To further our understanding of this problem of skeletal disease in our pups, the next chapter deals with how bones should grow - NORMALLY!

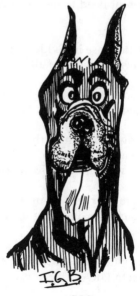

CHAPTER FOUR

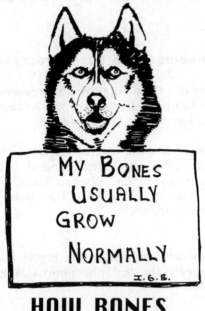

MY BONES
USUALLY
GROW
NORMALLY

I.G.B.

HOW BONES SHOULD GROW – – NORMALLY!

The aim of this chapter is to help you understand bone growth. Once you understand the BASIC MECHANISMS of bone growth, you will understand how modern mismanagement can so easily upset that process.

In this chapter you will be introduced to the technical term

- ENDOCHONDRAL OSSIFICATION -

211

Endochondral Ossification is a fancy name which describes how bones grow. This term is important because it is ALTERATIONS or changes in the process of Endochondral ossification which are the start of all of the bone diseases.

Bone growth involves two basic processes

Firstly the formation of a matrix or template or ground substance which is made from cartilage in the shape of the bone. Cartilage is a pliable firmish material composed of protein and carbohydrate.

The second process is when this preformed cartilaginous template turns into bone as minerals, principally calcium and phosphorus are deposited into it. This process is called mineralisation. Vitamin D plays a number of vital roles in this process along with hormones, and also calcium, phosphorus and other nutrients.

The combination of cartilage production together with its subsequent mineralisation by calcium and phosphorus is given the name of Endochondral Ossification.

For our purposes we may think of Endochondral Ossification as being normal bone growth - where ENDO means inside, CHONDRAL refers to the cartilage, and OSSIFICATION means turning into bone. Literally the process where minerals are deposited into cartilage, turning it into bone. When this process of cartilage **formation** and **mineralisation** goes wrong, either separately or together - we have **ALTERATIONS in Endochondral ossification.** That is, we have bone growth gone wrong which is skeletal disease of one kind or another.

The mineralisation of a puppy's bones ...

... starts in the last two to four weeks before a pup is born. Minerals - principally calcium and phosphorus - start to infiltrate the cartilage. The cartilage is being calcified or ossified or mineralised. Let me say again that this apparently simple, but very vital process where cartilage grows and is transformed into bone is called 'Endochondral Ossification.'

As the long bones in the limbs grow ...

... they become both thicker and longer. That growth occurs because cartilage cells multiply in number and grow in size and produce cartilage material around themselves. Eventually all of that new cartilage becomes mineralised and turns into hardened bone, except for the cartilage in the joint, which stays as 'joint cartilage.'

This process of bone growth – [this Endochondral ossification] occurs in three distinct areas within the bone. [See diagram on page 214.]

1] The growth plate is where bones grow in length. The growth plate is found near each end of the bone. The cartilage cells of the growth plate continue to reproduce and produce new bone until the bones have reached their mature length. Then they change into bone cells, at which time they no longer produce cartilage. The growth plate has changed from cartilage to bone. Growth in length has ceased. This usually occurs around the time of sexual maturity.

2] The growth of the joint occurs by an increase in the number of cartilage cells in the joint itself. The bit of cartilage which covers the end of the bone never becomes calcified, but remains as cartilage for the remainder of the dog's life. And so it is known as the joint cartilage.

3] The growth in thickness of the long bones occurs all along its length. A membrane of cells which covers the shaft of the bone produces new cells in layers round the outside of the bone. These new cells lay down the new bone material directly. They do not bother with the step of forming cartilage. The ground substance is mineralised as soon as it is formed.

Please note that these cells which produce the new bone of the shaft have the capability of being either cartilage cells or bone cells. For example, if the bone is broken at any stage, these cells multiply as cartilage cells to carry out the repair process.

That is why we can regard the growth of a bone in width as being the same process of Endochondral ossification that we see in the growth plate and the joint.

That means it will go wrong in much the same way.

As the bone grows in width, older bone is dissolved away from the inside of the bone and so the walls do not become too thick, and the width of the marrow cavity gradually increases.

How Bones Grow - Normally

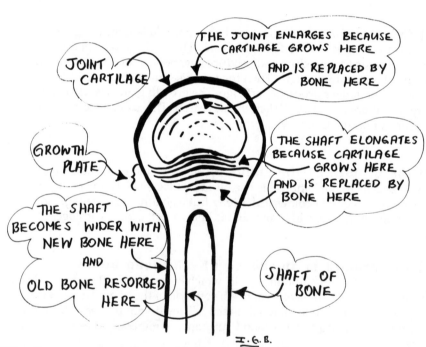

What I want you to understand is that bone growth occurs ONLY in those three places - the growth plate, the joint and the shaft of the bone.

That means that it is only in those three places that things can go wrong. These are the three places where skeletal disease occurs if the conditions for bone growth are not right.

Of those three growth areas ...

... the **growth plate is probably the weakest point.** It is highly sensitive to any problems the puppy may have with nutrition, or trauma. For example, all of the angular limb deformities are associated with damage to the growth plate.

The joint is almost as sensitive. The diseases we see when poor nutrition and trauma affect bone growth in the joint include Hip Dysplasia, Elbow Dysplasia and Osteochondritis Dissecans. Such problems can affect the shape and health of that joint for the rest of a pup's life.

The shaft of the long bone is the least sensitive to problems with nutrition and trauma. This is because preformed cartilage is not involved in the growth of the shaft. The cells that are produced go straight into bone cells without becoming cartilage cells first. They secrete a ground substance that is immediately mineralised, rather than starting out as soft and easily damaged cartilage. Nevertheless, there are at least two bone diseases of pups which involve this process. One is Panosteitis, and the other is Hypertrophic Osteodystrophy. The growth process in the shaft is in principle no different to the growth in the growth plate or the joint. It is affected by poor nutrition and trauma in much the same way.

The role of hormones in bone growth

There are a number of hormones involved in bone growth. Some examples include thyroxine from the thyroid gland, growth hormone, parathyroid hormone and one of the forms of vitamin D which is actually a hormone.

Sounds complicated doesn't it!? Don't worry. What I want you to realise is that **hormone production and function - except in very rare instances - is totally dependent upon nutrition.** In other words, if the nutrition goes wrong - so does hormone production and function.

So for all practical purposes we can forget hormone production and function as a cause of bone and joint problems. We can concentrate on nutrition when we discuss those factors in a puppy's life which are involved in skeletal disease or health.

Bone growth is a dynamic explosive process ...

... with numerous simultaneous processes - all dependent upon one another - including the formation of new cells, the production of cartilage and its mineralisation with calcium and phosphorus.

This requires a mountain of new protein, plus other nutrients such as copper, vitamin C, vitamins, minerals, and essential fatty acids. In addition, all of the hormones involved in bone growth, including iodine dependent thyroxine, must be functioning normally. Also, for bone growth to occur normally, there must be placed on those bones the normal stresses that a puppy encounters in its day to day activities. Those stresses must be present, but they must not be too excessive. **They must not become trauma.**

This process of bone growth ...

... will continue for at least two years after birth and possibly several more years, before a dog has mature hardened fully functional adult bone.

- That is why careful management of growing puppies must continue until such time as the bones are fully hardened and mature. The food and the exercise must be just right if a puppy's bones are to grow in a normal healthy way.

What I want you to remember from this chapter ...

... is that the **growth plate**, the **shaft** of the bone and the **ends** of the bone - the joints - are **three active areas of growth** in the bones of a puppy. They are three areas of **'Endochondral ossification.'**

If those three growth areas within the bones are not given the conditions they need for normal growth - right up until the time they have become mature hardened adult bone - their growth will be abnormal. There will **'alterations in Endochondral ossification.'** That is, there will be bone disease.

Let me conclude this chapter by saying that when we begin to discuss bone disease in young dogs, particularly pups of the giant breeds, just remember ...

1] **Skeletal disease in the bones of young dogs only occurs in the three active areas of growth.** The joints, the growth plates and the shaft of the bone.

2] Skeletal disease only involves one basic process - **alterations in Endochondral Ossification.** That is, mineralisation of cartilage gone wrong.

3] Those alterations in Endochondral Ossification in the growth areas of the bone are caused by faulty management.

All very simple!

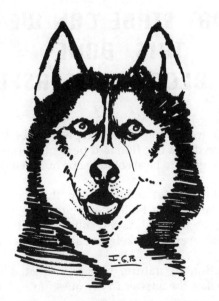

CHAPTER FIVE

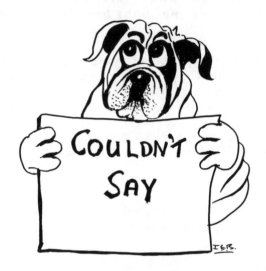

AT WHAT STAGE CAN WE SAY
THIS BONE
HAS BECOME DISEASED?

I have a question you need to consider. "Is it possible for bone formation in our puppies to proceed in a one hundred percent normal fashion so that their bones and joints grow to be absolutely one hundred percent perfect?"

Before you answer that, let me just say that bone growth, or Endochondral Ossification, has built in safeguards to ensure - as far as is possible - nothing goes wrong. As a result, wild dogs rarely develop skeletal problems. **However, their skeletons are never perfect.**

There is no perfection in nature. Nature is just a broad range of possibilities. That makes the answer to my question - NO ... Every bone and joint system ever formed is to some degree imperfect. That is why ...

218

... there are no definite boundaries between normality and disease.

Skeletal disease or health is not an 'either or' situation. It can be difficult to decide whether a given bone or joint is healthy or not. Every bone and joint has genetic, nutritional, immunological, hormonal, physical, infectious and physical factors which decide how it will grow. It is not possible for all those processes or the bones they form to be one hundred percent perfect. This lack of precision means that there are no definite boundaries between normal bones and joints and diseased bones and joints.

In other words there will always be **alterations in Endochondral Ossification.** Every bone ever formed will either be essentially but not completely normal, or progressively more to the abnormal side of average, and be diseased.

The three growing points in bones are totally dependent upon correct nutrition and correct levels and types of exercise and other stresses to ensure both they and the bones they are producing are made strong enough to support the weight and activity of a growing pup.

Any nutritional deficiencies or excesses and any physical insults that upset the normal patterns of growth will very quickly be reflected in some alteration of the growth of these young bones. That is - **alterations in Endochondral Ossification.**

It is easy to miss the first signs of bone disease

At what stage do we decide that the bones or joints have become diseased? When do we know that a given dog has a skeletal system that has passed across a broad and hazy boundary to enter an area we call disease?

The decision is arbitrary. Is is based on the **DEGREE** to which there are problems or imperfections in a given bone and joint system. Take a hip joint for example: the more a hip joint grows to the abnormal side of average - the more likely we will say there have been alterations in Endochondral ossification. That is, we will label it diseased.

Because the transition from normality to disease is a very gradual process ...

... we often miss the first signs. If we ignore a dog enough, we may allow the destructive process to continue to a point where PERMANENT DAMAGE will occur.

That is why, when skeletal growth starts to go wrong, early detection is absolutely vital. If a problem can be detected early enough, it can be halted before any damage is done. All that is required to halt the disease process in most instances are some simple changes in nutrition and exercise.

This is management at work. The fact that such processes can be halted by changes in nutrition or exercise also tells us that it was faults in this management process which caused the problem in the first place.

Suppose you are the owner of a young Great Dane.

In your enthusiasm to get things exactly right, let us suppose you get the nutrition bit pretty well correct, with just some minor imperfections. For example, you may allow a slight excess of calcium to appear in the diet. You add a little bit each day - just to be sure, not realising that the diet you are feeding actually has just the right amount. This may cause no problem. Cartilage formation and mineralisation may proceed reasonably normally.

However, suppose you go to a dog show and discover that most of the other Dane pups of similar age are well ahead of your pup in size and weight. This observation together with the criticisms made about your pup, causes you to re-think your feeding regime.

You change the diet. Suddenly your young Dane's growth rate is made to increase dramatically. You have changed the diet to a more protein and calorie rich food. The pup now begins to put on weight. At first this seems fine. However, bit by bit, that increasing weight is placing more and more stress on those highly vulnerable young bones.

During this growth spurt, which is so easy to produce in puppies of the giant breeds, the mineralisation of the cartilage quietly and subtly begins to proceed in a less than optimal fashion. Before you can realise it, that skeletal system is heading closer to and may even begin to cross that boundary between normality and disease.

A return to the show ring brings applause for this improved appearance together with more free advice. That advice sees an increase in the exercise regime of that young pup.

The owner has been persuaded to indulge his pup in lots more walking and running and jumping. 'To build up its muscles.' Sadly, those bones and joints, weakened by incorrect nutrition, are now being subjected to the twin evils of excessive weight and excessive exercise.

It is not very long before that pup's skeleton has been pushed across that broad boundary between health and disease.

Within a week or two of these changes, the pup begins to feel sore in its bones and starts to limp. Once the pup begins to limp, we detect that change from normality. We can see clinical disease. The problem is we may be too late. We may be now be seeing alterations in Endochondral Ossification that have already resulted in permanent damage.

These problems do not happen overnight

The more we subject a pup to these faulty conditions of nutrition and exercise, the closer we push it to disease. Mostly, people have no idea this is happening until it is too late. This is because we see disease as a cut and dried issue. An 'either/or' situation. With skeletal disease, we are often not aware of critical changes in weight, growth rate, and the way a pup moves. Changes which herald the onset of problems, and which if rectified early enough could totally prevent skeletal problems from occurring.

However, not only do we often fail to detect these problems well before permanent damage occurs, but when these problems are detected ...

... we say - "Oh, it has bad genes."

Our faulty diagnosis means we fail to replace those faulty conditions with more appropriate growing conditions.

And so the problem continues!

This short little chapter is here to emphasise the following points ...

- most modern bone diseases are caused by a multitude of factors, not just one single cause - bad genes.

- The factors which influence and control normal skeletal growth are the very same factors which cause disease.

- The line between normal and abnormal bone growth is hazy and ill defined. There is no definite cut off point. No point where you can say "this bone is perfectly healthy while this bone is diseased."

- That is why - if we can catch a problem early enough - we can get rid of the factors which are working against skeletal health and boost those that are promoting skeletal health. In fact we can often stop the problem dead in its tracks.

We may therefore conclude that skeletal problems are

1. Totally preventable - if we manage our pups correctly

2. Totally 'producible' by mismanaging our pups.

3. Totally treatable if we catch them early enough!

.... Ignore the early tell tale signs of problems when something can be done - and you will see skeletal disease develop.

I now want to introduce you to the disease process in growing bones that is first seen when bones begin to cross that hazy boundary between normality and disease. That MOST BASIC disease process, the one we see first in all these conditions is a process called OSTEOCHONDROSIS, and the next chapter is devoted to it.

CHAPTER SIX

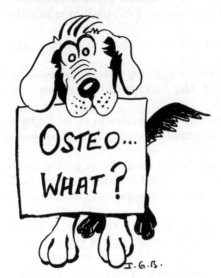

OSTEOCHONDROSIS –
– THE BASIC CAUSE
OF SKELETAL DISEASE

It has been difficult to find a consensus as to what **Osteochondrosis** actually means. One definition says that it is "... any of a group of disorders of one or more ossification centres in young dogs characterised by degeneration or aseptic necrosis followed by re-calcification. Epiphyseal aseptic necrosis." If that means nothing to you - don't worry!

Yet other definitions indicate that Osteochondrosis simply refers to pathological alterations in Endochondral Ossification. It is this wider definition that I am adopting.

I am saying that Osteochondrosis is ...

... an alteration to the normal process of mineralisation of the growing bone. Usually that means a FAILURE to mineralise.

I am going further however and also saying that ...

... With very few exceptions, Osteochondrosis is the basic disease which underlies **all of the skeletal diseases** we see in pups.

Osteochondrosis means alterations in Endochondral Ossification or disordered bone growth. Bone growth gone wrong.

Osteochondrosis is the name I am giving to those alterations in bone growth which are caused by either excesses or deficiencies of nutrition, and by excesses [or possibly deficiencies] of exercise or trauma.

- The OSTEO bit means bones, the CHONDR bit refers to cartilage and the OSIS bit means sick or not well or disordered. That is, Osteochondrosis or OCD is a sickness in the way that cartilage grows and turns into bone.

Let's just call it OCD

What I am presenting here is a unified approach to understanding skeletal disease. I am broadening the definition of OCD and saying that most of the Juvenile Bone Diseases, are the result of one basic disease process - **Osteochondrosis or OCD.** In other words, all these different diseases have occurred due to alterations in the way in which cartilage is turned into bone during growth. This includes both the relatively uncommon old fashioned skeletal diseases caused by nutritional deficiencies - the ones we call Rickets - and the modern types caused by excesses, including Hip and Elbow Dysplasia.

If we can halt the disease process in the early stages of Osteochondrosis, we can usually prevent permanent damage.

There are two types of OCD

One is caused by deficiencies, and the other is caused by excesses. It was the OCD of deficiency that we used in the past to wreck our puppy's bones.

Today we use OCD of excess as the modern way to wreck pups' bones. In this chapter, I am going to concentrate on the OCD of excess.

Modern OCD, or OCD of excess, is the basic skeletal disease which results from **over nutrition** and **trauma** to the growing points in the bone. It has replaced old fashioned OCD, or OCD of deficiency as the most popular way to wreck pups' bones.

OCD and modern skeletal diseases

All the modern skeletal diseases start with OCD. Where they end - the final disease state - whether it be Hip Dysplasia or Elbow Dysplasia or whatever, depends on a pup's genes and what type of insults, both nutritional and traumatic that pup's bones and joints receive as it grows.

Most of the skeletal diseases we see today are diseases of excess. Excesses of nutrition and exercise. The diseases resulting from modern OCD have LARGELY replaced old fashioned OCD diseases, which were mostly due to single and simple causes of deficiency.

They all start out slowly and subtly. It is difficult to tell when the disease process begins. Because the boundaries between disease and normality are indistinct, it can be difficult to decide whether a bone or joint is diseased or not.

They all have many causes. Because so many factors control this process, it is our management - good or bad - which can push an animal across that broad and hazy boundary into disease, or retain it safely on the healthy side.

Veterinary textbooks tell us that the cause of OCD is not known. I am here to tell you that ......

The factors responsible for Modern Osteochondrosis are

1] Nutritional imbalances including excessive calcium. If any of the nutritional factors necessary for normal bone growth are incorrect or missing - there MAY be a disturbance to Endochondral ossification. If that happens - there will be OCD - abnormal bone growth. BONE DISEASE.

2] **Rapid Growth rate** --- Which is the result of interaction between Nutrition and Genes

3] **Trauma to the growing points of bones. If there is a physical disturbance** to these growing points - some form of trauma - there MAY be a disturbance to Endochondral ossification. If that happens - there will be OCD - abnormal bone growth. BONE DISEASE.

4] **Genetic predisposition. If hostile genes are present** - and they always are - to some extent - Osteochondrosis WILL NOT USUALLY OCCUR UNLESS one or more of the above factors are present. If that happens - there may be a disturbance to Endochondral ossification. That is - there will be OCD - abnormal bone growth. BONE DISEASE.

Our pups cannot cope with modern living

Modern dog owners and their vets expect a   puppy's bones to grow, repair and function   normally, because we assume that the inbuilt safeguards which are supposed to protect a bone against problems as it grows are in place and doing their job.

However, those safeguards were designed for a totally different environment. Those safeguards were not designed to protect against modern living. Puppies have not inherited the ability to deal with excessive foods, and foods too rich in calories, protein and calcium. Nor have they evolved to cope with the excessive and incorrect exercise we throw at modern pups. Exercise regimes which traumatise bones and joints already damaged by incorrect nutrition.

Modern puppy owners are pushing young puppies' bones well beyond their biological limits and producing - Modern Osteochondrosis - OCD.

The bad news out of all this is .....

- Firstly, when a pup is found to have developed OCD in one bone or joint, that does not happen in isolation. It will have many other bones and joints affected as well. When a dog develops Elbow Dysplasia for example, it will usually be found to have Hip Dysplasia and a host of other skeletal problems as well.

- Secondly, if we don't call a halt to OCD by changing the nutrition and the exercise which caused it, the OCD will rapidly develop into named skeletal diseases such as Hip and Elbow Dysplasia.

The good news out of all this is .....

- Firstly, because we know what causes OCD, we know what causes skeletal disease. This means if we can recognise OCD early enough - AND do something about it - we should be able to prevent most skeletal disease in our dogs.

- Secondly, if we start treating these skeletal problems early enough with the BARF programme, all those potential skeletal problems will either disappear or have their damaging impact on the pup much reduced.

Where does OCD occur?

Remember the three growing points in a bone? Both modern and old fashioned OCD is a disease of the growing points of the bone. It is a disruption of the normal process of bone growth. **It is a disturbance to the mineralisation** of any of the three growing points of the bone. That is - in the **joint**, at the **growth plate**, or along the **shaft**.

These are the points at which all the modern skeletal diseases occur.

Let us first look at Modern OCD in the cartilage of the joint

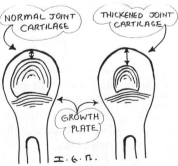

NORMAL JOINT CARTILAGE   THICKENED JOINT CARTILAGE

GROWTH PLATE

I. 6. N.

When joint cartilage develops modern OCD we see **softening and thickening of the cartilage in the joints.** It may also become painful. This problem may be seen in any joint in the body. We commonly recognise it in the shoulders, elbows, knees and ankles of growing pups.

Please note we also see disordered cartilage growth in the **hip joint**. It contributes to the syndrome we call **Hip Dysplasia**. Disordered joint growth is the very essence of Hip Dysplasia!

Hip Dysplasia is in part, an abnormal development or growth of the articular part of the bones which form the hip joint. The two bones which form the joints become abnormally flattened. Therefore by definition, Hip Dysplasia is a form of modern OCD. It has common beginnings with every other skeletal disease we see in pups.

Next we look at Modern OCD of the growth plate

1] Enlargement and weakening of the growth plate area.

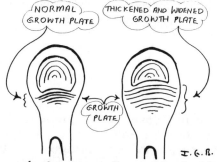

The growth plate is where growth in bone length occurs. With modern OCD this is seen as excessively enlarged wrist or carpal joints - which may be painful - in the larger breeds of dogs. For disease to occur, this enlargement and weakening of the growth plate is usually combined with **trauma.** That trauma, it should be noted can be either the normal movement of the pup, or excessive exercise or the effects of the pup being overweight.

2] Uneven growth of growth plate ...

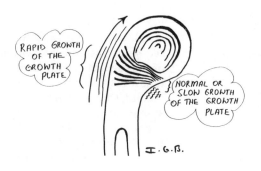

... with one side of the growth plate growing relatively normally and the other developing OCD. The end result is that one side grows faster than the other and so the limb bends. We have an angular limb deformity.

3] One bone grows faster than it should

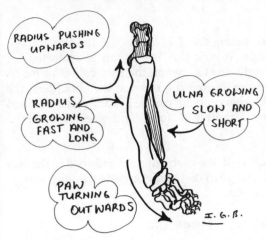

This happens in the elbow joint. We now know that this problem of mismatched bone growth between the radius and the ulna is one of THE BASIC CAUSES of Elbow Dysplasia.

It is also one of the causes of angular deformity of the wrist or carpus.

Modern OCD of the shaft of the bone

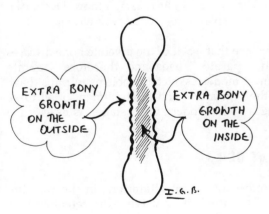

The shaft of the bone is where the bone grows in diameter. There are two well known diseases which occur when there is disordered growth in the cells which surround the shaft of the bone. One is **Panosteitis**. The other is **Hypertrophic Osteodystrophy**.

You must be vigilant for the signs of OCD!

In the pup with OCD, the very first sign seen is pain which results in lameness. This is what so many people fail to notice in their young growing pup, or, if they notice it - they ignore it - hoping it will go away.

The message is - DO NOT ignore pain and lameness in growing dogs.

There is every chance you are seeing OCD. Now is the time to act! An experienced vet should be able to pick this up. It can be detected - sometimes as early as six to eight weeks - when the pup comes in for its first vaccinations. By palpating or feeling the elbows, the shoulders, the wrists, the knees and the hocks, this problem can be instantly detected and remedial action in the form of altered food and exercise started immediately.

- Now is the time to stop OCD. If the problem can be nipped in the bud at this stage by a radical change in diet and exercise - this pup will go on to develop a sound skeleton.

If OCD is not stopped at this stage .....

...... That pup will go on to develop one or more of the skeletal problems which afflict modern pups. That is, Hip Dysplasia, Elbow Dysplasia, Wobbler Syndrome, dropped hocks, splayed feet, bone cysts etc. etc..

Be warned. Some vets still believe that each of the juvenile bone diseases are separate entities with separate causes and therefore separate treatments. In fact, because most modern skeletal problems in pups have the same basic cause, both the prevention and the treatment of all these problems - in the initial stages - the modern OCD stage - is exactly the same.

The microscopic view of OCD

What you see under the microscope is an alteration in the way the cartilage changes into bone. The problem involves the retention and thickening of the cartilage in some spots and a thinning or lysis of the cartilage in other areas.

Important facts about Modern OCD

- Modern OCD does not only occur in the long bones of the front and hind limbs of your dog. It has been discovered in practically every bone in the dog's body, and this includes the ribs and the vertebrae. That is why we see so much arthritis in our older dogs.

• Modern OCD is most common during the period of maximum growth rate in the dog - that is - around 4 to 7 months of age. It is a problem most commonly seen in medium to large breeds of dogs. It is far more common in males. This is because males grow faster than females.

• Modern OCD is known to occur in most other domestic species including horses, pigs, turkeys and chickens, and probably many others. It is only seen when these animals are forced to grow quickly. It is a modern disease, rare prior to our interference in the life of these creatures. It is also seen in humans that are grown too quickly.

• The degree of damage to bones and joints, and just which bones and joints develop modern OCD depends upon the degree of mismanagement and the genetic makeup of the pup involved.

• It is these differences in faulty husbandry and genetic backgrounds of the pups which determines where OCD develops and which particular type of OCD develops. If the OCD is not stopped at this early stage it will proceed to produce one - or more - of the various skeletal diseases.

The role of genes in producing OCD ....

...... and therefore skeletal disease is covered in more detail in Chapter Seven. However, to give you an idea of the true role of genes in producing these problems - consider the following .....

As the weight of the breed increases .... which is a genetic factor, together with rapid growth rate - another genetic factor - we see a greater chance of damage to the growing points and therefore OCD. This can happen to the growth plate, to the the joint cartilage, or to the membrane surrounding the shaft of the bone. This is particularly so in big breeds with small muscles and lots of fat such as the St. Bernard.

Conformation will increase the problem. For example an upright stance will result in more trauma than an angulated stance.

Where a large breed is also being given excess calcium and other nutritional and physical insults, the potential for damage to the growing points is even greater.

Note also the following ...

- **The presence of hostile genes cannot be changed in an individual pup** because the genes are fixed and unchangeable once you have the pup. It is nutrition and exercise - over which the puppy owner has total control - that can be changed.

- In other words, when you look to control bone disease in your pup[s], all you have to concern yourself with is diet and exercise.

- **ALL pups have a genetic tendency to develop OCD** - to a greater or lesser degree. However, understand and know that if they are raised correctly, with sound nutrition and the right exercise programme, the vast majority of such pups - no matter what their genetic inheritance - will never develop bone problems - as they currently do. This whole question of genetics and skeletal disease in pups is discussed in detail in the next chapter.

- **These factors are not independent.** The action of genes, diet and exercise is modified - accelerated, diminished or changed by each of the others. Without at least two damaging factors being present, the occurrence of the problem is much less likely. However, having said that, it is important to realise that any one of these factors occurring by themselves may also cause the condition.

- As a general rule **if more than one of the above factors is present** - it is much more likely that there will be a disturbance to Endochondral ossification. That is - it is much more likely that there will be modern OCD - abnormal bone growth. DISEASE. Commit nutritional and physical errors and combine this with bad genes - and escape is impossible. You will see faulty bone growth or modern OCD.

I know that all sounds a bit complicated. Do not be concerned. Just be aware that it is these factors which either alone, or by interacting, produce modern OCD. That is, bone disease in our dogs. The more of these predisposing factors we have operating, the more likely it is that skeletal disease will occur.

My final word about OCD is that ...

MODERN OCD is a basic underlying cause of

1] Hip Dysplasia,
2] Osteochondritis Dissecans of the
    - Shoulder
    - Elbow [known as Elbow Dysplasia] - consisting of four syndromes
        - Ununited [or fragmented] Anconeal process [UAP],
        - Fragmented Medial Coronoid Process of the Ulna [FCP],
        - Osteochondritis [OCD] of the Medial Humeral Condyle
        - Elbow Joint Incongruity or "Bad Elbow Joint"
    - Knee [stifle] Dysplasia
    - Ankle [Hock] Dysplasia
    - also joints such as wrist, hip and possibly the vertebrae and ribs.
3] The Wobbler Syndrome,
4] Dropped Hocks,
5] Splayed feet,
6] Bone Cysts
7] Carpal Instability/Flexion Syndrome
8] All forms of arthritis or degenerative joint disease in the older dog.
9] Hypertrophic Osteodystrophy
10] Panosteitis, and possibly ....
11] Septic arthritis

OLD FASHIONED OCD is a basic underlying cause of

1] Patellar Luxation,
2] Aseptic Necrosis of the Femoral Head [Legg-Perthes Disease]
3] All forms of Rickets including Nutritional Hyperparathyroidism

Please do not let all those complicated names phase you. If you grow your pup[s] using the BARF programme of diet and exercise for pups, they will not become part of your life. If you are in the midst of some sort of 'bony crisis' you will probably be familiar with some of those words. The message I offer to anyone in that situation is, keep reading and find what can be done about your particular problem.

In the following chapters we are going to explore how each of these different causes of OCD, the genes, the nutrition and the exercise impacts on the growth of a puppy's bones.

CHAPTER SEVEN

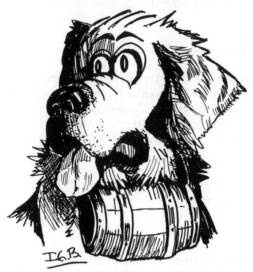

THE ROLE OF GENES IN PRODUCING SKELETAL DISEASE IN PUPPIES

In this chapter I am going to talk about the genetic basis of skeletal disease - concentrating particularly on Hip and Elbow Dysplasia. In fact where I mention Hip Dysplasia please take it as also referring to Elbow Dysplasia - or any of the other problems based on Modern Osteochondrosis or OCD.

There are two basic factors which control a puppy's bone growth. One is its genes and the other is its environment of nutrition and exercise. Which is more important?

The most basic control over bone growth in your puppy is its genes. They decide how your pup's bones ought to grow. They are the blue prints for your pup's bone growth.

Does that mean genes are the most important factor in deciding whether a dog will develop bone problems?

Not at all. Genes do not work in isolation. They always work together with the environment. That means, although your dog may inherit a mass of genes for skeletal disease, its environment may promote sound bones and joints. This may stop those genes acting. On the other hand, a dog may have inherited only a small number of genes for skeletal disease, but if the environment is unfavourable, skeletal disease may rear its ugly head! So what I am telling you is that ......

.... A puppy's genes determine if it is ABLE TO DEVELOP skeletal problems - NOT that it WILL develop them.

This brings us to a basic genetic concept which seems to be ignored by professional breeders and vets in their endeavours to produce sound skeletons. That concept is that ....

Genotype does not equal phenotype

"What on earth do those two words mean," I hear you ask. The answer is very simple - so keep reading.

A dog's GENOTYPE is the sum total of all its genes.

A dog's PHENOTYPE is what it looks like or how it is or how it works. What it has actually grown to be.

The difference between these two words or ideas is very important. The genotype of a dog is the plans or blueprints for that dog. If you could look at those 'gene plans', they would give you an idea of what that dog should or might look like. However, no living creature looks exactly like its genotype. That is what is meant by the statement that GENOTYPE does not equal PHENOTYPE.

The phenotype is how how the dog actually is or looks - which let me repeat - in many cases is quite different to what the genotype says it ought to look like. The phenotype depends on how that dog's environment has shaped its growth.

With reference to skeletal disease, most large dogs have a genotype which might be best described as Dysplastic.

That is, they have genes which will under certain conditions produce poor skeletal growth including the possibility of Hip and Elbow Dysplasia.

However, the phenotype of a dog - how it actually is - might be non Dysplastic.

It may not have any skeletal disease. It may have been grown slowly without calcium supplementation and may never have been over-exercised as a pup. For those reasons the genes for skeletal diseases such as Hip Dysplasia have not acted to produce problems in this particular dog. The skeletal disease genes have not expressed themselves.

If we radiographed that dog and found its skeleton to be normal - we would probably declare that dog to be free of the genes for Hip Dysplasia and Elbow Dysplasia. **We would say - "this dog does not have genes for skeletal problems. It may be safely used for breeding."**

Let's suppose that particular dog had an identical twin. And that identical twin was raised on as much super premium dog food as it could eat, plus added calcium supplements, plus plenty of long hard walks and running every day. Suppose that twin developed Hip Dysplasia. **We would say - "this twin has genes which cause Hip Dysplasia. We must not breed with this dog. It has a hereditary condition which it will pass to its offspring."**

Of course the truth is that our conclusions about both of these dogs are wrong.

The first dog without skeletal problems is no more free of genes for such problems than the second dog. The second dog has no more genes for skeletal problems than the first dog. **The chances of either of them producing pups with skeletal problems are precisely the same on the basis of genetics, but vastly different on the basis of how the pups are raised.**

The point I am making is that a dog's phenotype - how it looks - may tell us very little about its genotype or what sort of genes it has.

In other words, **when we take radiographs of a dog's hips or its elbows in the hope that this will tell us about its genotype - or what it might pass on to its offspring - we are totally fooling ourselves if we do not take into account how that dog was raised!**

Our radiographing is not telling us anything reliable with respect to that dog's breeding potential!

That makes our programme of keeping, culling or killing on the basis of those radiographs an exercise in self delusion. An absolute waste of time, money and resources.

But that is not what we tell puppy owners!

Puppy owners today have been led to believe that a breeder can breed pups with genes for perfect bone growth.

- Both Vets and breeders know this is not possible but they act and speak as if they believe it is.

- Breeders want puppy buyers to believe that their stock is free of all hereditary bone disease. They will do anything to promote this belief.

The idea that we can produce pups that are free of genes for skeletal disease is absolute nonsense. It is not scientific. It is at best - a statement born of ignorance - and at worst a blatant lie.

Not only is it impossible for a breeder to make such guarantees, but it must be realised that every pup ever born has a host of genes for a wide variety of defects including skeletal problems. If the effects of those genes do not show up in this individual, they will show up at some stage in a future generation.

The Genetic Myth and Our Fight Against Skeletal Disease

According to current veterinary knowledge, the genetic factor causes between 20% to 40% of most juvenile bone disease including Hip and Elbow Dysplasia. This leaves other factors responsible for a whopping great 60% to 80%. Those factors include what a pup is fed and how it is exercised.

On that basis we may conclude that nutrition and exercise must be at least 60% - 80% of the solution.

Despite the enormous contribution [60% - 80%] of what a pup is fed and how it is exercised in determining the health of our dogs' skeletons, those factors **appear to be totally ignored by breeders, dog owners and vets when it comes to eliminating skeletal problems. Instead we rely on the 20% - 40% contribution of the genetic factor.**

That would be fine if it were possible to eliminate that 20% - 40% genetic factor. **Unfortunately as you shall very shortly see, we cannot eliminate that 20% - 40% genetic factor without making VERY DRASTIC ALTERATIONS to those breeds which have skeletal problems!**

In the meantime, because the role of nutrition and exercise is ignored by, or unknown to the veterinary profession, a fundamental error has become part of canine 'truth.'

This error or myth is that ...

"... the only factor we need concern ourselves with in our attempt to eradicate Juvenile Bone Disease in dogs is the genetic factor."

As a profession we may not actually tell dog owners this myth, however we rarely tell them anything different. We allow them to continue believing that breeding is the only way to rid our dogs of such problems as Hip and Elbow Dysplasia.

Why do we vets promote this genetic myth?

- Maybe it lets us off the hook? Makes our life easier? No need to search for other explanations for these skeletal problems in young dogs.

- Does it relieve us of the need to explain how to raise pups using sound management techniques?

- Is it because we lack training in this area?

- Is it because we hope this myth and the schemes that evolve from it may do some good?

- Is it because of the profit that can be derived from veterinary work based on this genetic assumption? Certainly there is not much profit in showing people how to raise pups to be free of disease. It is definitely much easier to be lazy and concentrate on the genes.

- Is it because when you tell others an untruth for long enough, you start to believe it yourself?

- It is probably little bits of all of the above!

No matter what the reasons, millions of dollars have been spent in a vain attempt to eliminate just one Juvenile Bone Disease. Hip Dysplasia. The method used sounds simple and logical. It involves the removal of a nasty set of genes which suddenly appeared in our dogs about 50 years ago. They spread like wildfire through our dogs, particularly targeting our larger dogs - I suppose they were a bigger target - and have been hell-bent on wrecking the bones and joints of the modern dog ever since.

The theory is simple. Identify the dogs that have these nasty genes using radiographs - then remove those dogs from the breeding programme. We are trying to do the same thing with Elbow Dysplasia.

There has been only one problem with this approach

It has not worked. It is not working! The skeletal diseases, including Hip and Elbow Dysplasia continue unabated. They are not going away, and are probably increasing.

The difficulty is, it is unlikely that we shall make any great progress using genetics to reduce the incidence of skeletal problems in our dogs.

To help you understand why the genetic solution must inevitably fail...

... I want to show you which genes cause skeletal problems, and how they do it. Once you realise which genes we are seeking to remove and which genes we are seeking to keep, you will realise the impossible task we have set ourselves. You will begin to see that management is actually a lot more than 60% - 80% of the solution. It is much closer to 100%.

As a start to understanding why this is so, we have to examine the genes which cause skeletal problems.

Genes for skeletal disease fall into two categories

The most important genes are the ones which INDIRECTLY cause skeletal disease

Every dog ever born has these INDIRECT genes for skeletal problems. It is just that some breeds have more of those genes than others. **In general it is the larger breeds which carry more of these genes.** However, the presence of these genes for skeletal disease is not an automatic guarantee that skeletal disease will develop. These genes only act when a puppy is fed and exercised incorrectly.

The second category of genes acts directly.

The genes which DIRECTLY cause skeletal disease are relatively rare

In fact we are not one hundred percent sure that they exist. This group - if it exists - is responsible for only a tiny proportion of the skeletal problems we see and we can only guess at what these genes might do.

Direct genes may be responsible for causing such things as loose joints; poor quality, weak, leaky joint capsules; poor quality cartilage in the joints; unfavourable remodelling of the bones in the joints; slow muscle growth; poorly developed muscles round the joints, faster than normal growth of certain bones, and finally genes that do something else - something not yet known - but which somehow contributes to Osteochondrosis and therefore skeletal problems.

If these genes exist, then it is clear that these are the genes that we want to get rid of, because if they are present, these genes will produce poor skeletal systems whether management is sound or not. Come good or bad nutrition, inappropriate or ideal exercise.

That means, if we practice sound management and skeletal problems occur, we know that the dog in question has these direct genes and we may cull that dog with confidence.

However, let us forget these rare direct genes for the moment and examine the much more common and much more important indirect genes.

The indirect genes which cause Skeletal problems are the genes for ......

Large size,
Heavy weight,
Fast Growth,
Obesity,
Poor Muscling,
Bad engineering.

Let us examine how we might deal with or control the effects of these genes by looking at the breeds which have them

1] It is the Large Heavy Breeds which are more likely to develop Skeletal Disease

Skeletal disease occurs in the larger heavier breeds of dogs such as the German Shepherd, the Great Dane, the Rottweiler, the Saint Bernard, the Newfoundland, the Old English Sheepdog, the Labrador, or any other large heavy breed. Officially, the most well known of these diseases, Hip Dysplasia, is considered extremely rare in breeds with a mature weight of less than 11 kg.

This shows us that the first group of INDIRECT genes which cause skeletal disease includes the genes for large size and heaviness.

What can we do about these genes? THE GENETIC SOLUTION is to get rid of them by breeding our larger heavier dogs to be smaller and lighter.

The NON-GENETIC solution involving these genes is to control skeletal disease, by carefully controlling the feeding and exercising of our larger heavier dogs.

2] It is the Rapidly Growing Breeds which are more likely to develop Skeletal Disease

Skeletal disease occurs more commonly in those breeds which are capable of very fast growth. As a general rule, the larger the breed, the faster it is capable of growing, particularly the giant breeds. When pups of the larger breeds are grown at their maximum rate of growth, the incidence of Hip Dysplasia and other bone problems increases sharply.

It is possible to ruin any dog by growing it too rapidly, but the larger the breed, the more prone it is to bone problems when grown at maximum growth rate.

This shows us that the second group of INDIRECT genes which cause skeletal disease, includes all the genes for rapid growth.

What can we do about these genes? THE GENETIC SOLUTION is to get rid of them by breeding our fast growing dogs to have genes for a slower rate of growth - which means breeding smaller dogs.

The NON-GENETIC solution involving these genes is to control skeletal disease, by carefully controlling the feeding of our larger heavier dogs. Growing them slowly!

3] It is the breeds Prone To Obesity which are more likely to develop Skeletal Disease

Of the large heavy breeds, it is the breeds which tend towards obesity which have the greatest incidence of bone problems. The incidence is incredibly high in those two roly poly breeds - the Labrador and the Old English Sheep Dog. The same is true of the Saint Bernard and the Newfoundland. The Rottweiler, which can be made obese quite easily also has a high incidence of Hip Dysplasia and other skeletal diseases, as does the German Shepherd. All of these breeds are capable of putting on a lot of fat when young.

Even the Beagle or the Cocker Spaniel or the Bull Terrier or Corgi, although not great huge dogs can easily become obese as puppies.

All of these breeds will develop bone problems as a result, including Hip Dysplasia.

This shows us that this third group of INDIRECT genes which cause skeletal disease, includes all the genes for obesity.

What can we do about these genes? The GENETIC SOLUTION is to breed our dogs to have very few fat cells. Labradors, Beagles and Saint Bernards etc. to be as slim as Greyhounds.

The NON-GENETIC solution involving these genes is to control obesity by taking whatever steps are necessary to keep our pups slim whilst growing.

There is another reason for keeping pups slim. It is while they are growing that pups develop their fat cells. No more are produced once a pup reaches maturity. To keep a dog slim and healthy into older age, it is much easier if he or she has fewer fat cells to fill with fat.

4] It is the breeds which have poor muscle development which are more likely to develop Skeletal Disease

Look at the muscling of such breeds as the Labrador, the Golden Retriever, the Saint Bernard and so on. These are all poorly muscled dogs with a high fat to muscle ratio. Feel those muscles and compare them to the muscles of a Greyhound or a Doberman. By comparison they are soft weak and flabby. Every one of these dogs is highly predisposed to Skeletal disease.

This shows us that this fourth group of INDIRECT genes which cause skeletal disease, includes all the genes for poor muscle development.

What can we do about these genes? The GENETIC SOLUTION is to breed our dogs to have harder muscles and a greater muscle mass.

The NON-GENETIC solution is to carefully control the feeding and exercising of such breeds during their growing months/years, making sure they are indulged in 'eating exercise' from their earliest days, grown slowly and never allowed to become fat and lazy.

5] It is the badly engineered dogs which are more likely to develop Skeletal Disease

Engineers design and build bridges and buildings to be strong enough to take their own weight plus the weight of whatever is going to use them plus a large safety margin. The safety margin is called "over engineering".

Over time, evolution has engineered the basic structure of wild dogs to be strong enough to function normally, particularly whilst growing. They, like our bridges and buildings are "over engineered" in order to cope with the normal stresses and strains of life.

When we humans interfere with the evolutionary process by breeding our dogs to be different shapes and sizes, we violate many of the engineering principles or safeguards that evolution [God? Nature?] has put in place.

Many of our larger breeds are so dangerously 'under engineered' - for example the Saint Bernard - that when their young, soft, easily moulded, and rapidly growing bones are subjected to abnormal stresses, things can go disastrously wrong. Hip Dysplasia or Elbow Dysplasia may develop for example. The growing bones of these breeds are highly sensitive to any traumas put upon them and any faults made in nutrition.

On the other hand, breeds such as the Greyhound are very well engineered for the role we wish them to play and well able to cope with nutritional and physical traumas. Such dogs rarely develop skeletal problems.

What I want you to realise is that poor engineering is a major genetic factor which predisposes many of our larger breeds to Osteochondrosis or skeletal disease.

The engineering principles or problems - depending on how you want to look at this - involve such things as:- the shapes, thicknesses, and sizes of bones, the large size and weight of many of these breeds, the ability to store lots of fat, the presence of smaller weaker muscles and most particularly the angles of the joints of the limbs of any particular breed.

One example of poor engineering is the Chow. This breed - in common with breeds such as the Saint Bernard and the Newfoundland - has very straight legs. These result in a jarring effect on both the growth plates and the joint cartilage of the legs.

Until the advent of 'modern management practices' - poorly engineered dogs survived and grew without too many problems. However, 'modern management practices' have tipped the scales in the wrong direction.

This shows us that this fifth group of INDIRECT genes which cause skeletal disease, includes all the genes responsible for bad engineering. What can we do about those genes?

The GENETIC SOLUTION is to get get rid of these INDIRECT genes by spending a lot of time and effort breeding for better engineering in all those breeds which require it - if we can figure out which breeds need it and what changes have to be made to their structure[s].

The NON-GENETIC solution to poor engineering is to carefully control the feeding and exercising of the poorly engineered breeds as they are growing.

6] There are large breeds in which skeletal disease is rarely seen

Skeletal disease is rarely seen in the Hound breeds. These are large breeds but they are not heavy breeds. They are not fast growing breeds and they are not obese breeds. They are exceptionally well muscled breeds with a very high muscle to bone ratio. They are also brilliantly engineered dogs. They are not raised on diets which promote rapid growth or obesity. Furthermore they have undergone a long history of selection and breeding. These breeds did not appear over-night. These breeds have taken thousands of years of selective breeding to bring them to where they are today.

These dogs have very few INDIRECT or DIRECT genes for skeletal disease. They can tolerate a wide range of environmental insults and still develop a sound skeletal system. It has taken thousands of years of controlled breeding to get them to this point of 'perfection!'

Should we be using these breeds in our breeding programmes to develop sound skeletons in our other breeds? That would work, and it would be the quickest way I know of to breed skeletal problems out of those breeds prone to skeletal problems.

The only problem with that idea is that we would end up owning a lot of 'greyhound-like' breeds.

As you can see, the more of these indirect genes a dog inherits, the greater chance it has of developing skeletal problems. To put that another way, Hip Dysplasia and other skeletal diseases are usually seen in .....

... Large breeds - but such problems are worse in large, Heavy breeds - but worse in Large, Heavy, Fast Growing breeds - but worse in Large, Heavy, Fast Growing, Obese breeds - but worse in Large, Heavy, Fast Growing, Obese, Poorly Muscled breeds - but worse in Large, Heavy, Fast Growing, Obese, Poorly Muscled, Badly Engineered breeds!

The question is, what are we going to do about these indirect genes? We have two choices. We can either ......

1] Change our management practices, or ....

2] Eliminate the genes that cause the problems

It is highly unlikely that we will want to eliminate all of these INDIRECT genes

Even though they are having the biggest impact on the problem, these genes are the genes which make a breed what it is. They are responsible for the major characteristics of the dog in which they are found. They cannot be eliminated without a drastic change in the breed.

We would need to change the size and shape of these breeds and convert them to a smaller, lighter, slower growing, less obese, more heavily muscled, far better engineered breed. That would take a long time. It could be done - if we had enough time, knowledge, skill, resources and the will to do it - but the price would be unacceptably high.

We cannot eliminate these genes without eliminating the breeds in which they are found!

We may conclude ...

... that our current approach to the elimination of skeletal disease by culling affected dogs will take centuries to complete.

If it is successful, the end result will be to turn all our breeds into greyhounds or something similar.

In that event we might as well shortcut the whole procedure and begin our crossbreeding programme with greyhounds straight away!

Are you beginning to understand why the genetic solution must inevitably fail?

Can you see that the genes we are trying to remove are also the genes we are seeking to keep We have set ourselves an impossible task. That is why management is actually a lot more than 60% - 80% of the solution. It is much closer to 100%.

Instead of trying to change these indirect genes all we need do is change our management practices. We can easily produce sound pups in our existing breeds without radically changing their genetic structure. **They can be very simply produced using sound management techniques.**

There is another question that needs an answer

With respect to the indirect genes, it is highly probable that some individuals are more sensitive to these genes than others. The more sensitive individuals will more easily develop skeletal problems when exposed to only small deviations from ideal conditions of nutrition and exercise. Other less sensitive individuals will tolerate wider variations in management.

If that were the case, any small deviations from sound management would result in skeletal problems for the more sensitive individuals. This is to be expected because nobody's management will ever be one hundred percent perfect, even when following the BARF programme.

In an ideal world, such cases would be picked out early, and appropriate adjustments would be made to their nutrition and exercise regimes to call a halt to any skeletal problems that were developing. What do you do with those individuals which fail to respond satisfactorily to those improved conditions? Easy. They are culled. These dogs also have genes which absolutely MUST go.

The bottom line for genetics and practical dog management becomes ....

Although genes play a major role in the production of most of the Juvenile Bone Diseases, if we follow the BARF programme, the genes can largely be ignored because the extent to which genetic manipulation can be used to eliminate skeletal disease is **MINIMAL** compared to what can be achieved with sound nutrition and sensible exercise regimes.

By growing our dogs under ideal conditions of diet and exercise, most will develop sound skeletal systems. The very few that develop skeletal problems do have a genuine genetic problem and may be culled with confidence.

While ever the veterinary profession seeks only genetic solutions for what is essentially a problem involving exercise and diet, skeletal problems will continue.

The genes responsible for causing Juvenile Bone Disease have been present since our breeds were developed. When we started to mismanage our dogs in the mid thirties - as described in Chapter Two - these genes began to exert their effects. They began to produce the Juvenile Orthopaedic problems we are now seeing in ever increasing numbers.

Restore appropriate diet and exercise and the genes will in the large majority of cases cease to exert those effects.

While it will take untold generations to alter the genetic structure of our dogs, it will only take one generation to alter the management.

The point to take away from this discussion on genes and skeletal disease is that no matter what genes your dog inherits, it will in the vast majority of cases develop either a sound skeleton or a poor skeleton because of what it is fed and how it is exercised as a puppy.

If you get the feeding and exercise part right, the genes become relatively unimportant in the vast majority of cases.

Let us now move on and look at the vital role that calcium plays in both creating healthy bones in normal bone growth, and producing OCD and therefore skeletal disease, when it is over supplied - as is so very common in today's world.

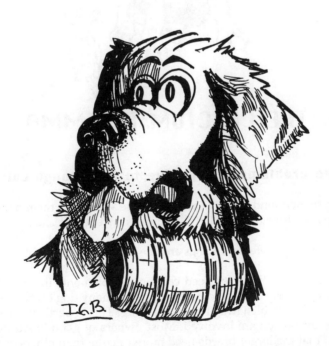

CHAPTER EIGHT

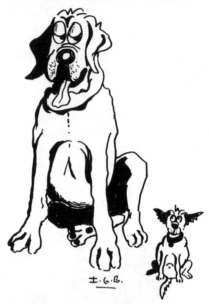

THE CALCIUM DILEMMA

Are bone problems in pups due to not enough calcium?

Most dog owners and the myriads of people who offer them advice [free and otherwise] love the wonderfully simple concept that ....

"bone problems" in dogs are due to not enough calcium.

The concept that "Puppies need calcium supplements in order to grow their bones properly" has become enshrined in many dog owners' minds as one of the unbreakable laws of puppy rearing. This is particularly so when large or giant breeds are involved. Most owners of giant breed pups are convinced that the larger breeds need more calcium than others but are not sure how that works out in practice.

Puppy owners SHOULD be concerned about calcium

Puppies do require relatively high levels of calcium for their bones compared to the needs of an adult dog. What they do not need is excessive calcium. The questions that need to be answered are:

- How much calcium is "just right", and what sort of calcium is required?

- What do we feed and what do we supplement to solve that problem?"

New puppy owners are usually the ones asking such questions. As they seek answers they speak to breeders, more experienced owners, vets, pet shop owners - anybody who, in their opinion, ought to know about these things.

What they expect is straightforward, consistent, and authoritative advice about calcium supplements. What they receive are answers that are as varied as the questions and the people they ask.

The sorts of questions people ask about calcium include ....

- What are the basic rules of supplementing with calcium?"

- Which is the best calcium supplement for my pup?

- Should I choose bone meal or dolomite or calcium carbonate or dicalcium phosphate or calcium lactate or calcium gluconate or ossol or one of the chelated calcium compounds or what?

- What about the calcium supplements with added vitamins and other minerals?

- Is milk a good source of calcium for a pup? What about bones - or are they too dangerous?

- How much of these supplements should I give?

- How much calcium do giant breeds such as Great Danes and St. Bernards need compared to say a Papillon or a Chihuahua?"

- Should the large and giant breeds be fed a different brand of food that has extra calcium?

- Should giant breeds be fed extra calcium added to the same sort of food fed to the smaller breeds?

- Do the giant breeds need the same sort of food as the little dogs - only more of it.

The people who are really keen ask their vet about the percentage of calcium present in each different form of calcium supplement. They want to know how digestible and how readily absorbed by the puppy's body each of those different types of calcium are. They are keen to buy the product with the highest percentage and most readily absorbed calcium available.

Is there a simple rational answer to these questions?

Even your vet can become confused when faced with this calcium conundrum. Advising people about calcium can be a major headache. For many puppy owners who have become aware of the questions about calcium, the calcium dilemma is a nightmare.

When new puppy owners talk to an experienced breeder

.....They will usually be given some strong adamant and apparently authoritative advice. "The only calcium supplement to use is Brand A, and feed your pup this much!" The reason these breeders appear to "know" about calcium with such assuredness is because after many difficulties and disasters, they have hit upon a system that works for them. It ties in with the way they feed. Well, most of the time anyway.

Confusion arises when those new puppy owners talk to another breeder. They soon find that every breeder has a different approach to the problem. That every one of those breeders swears blind that their way is the only way. Every other way, as far as they are concerned, will only end in failure.

This is because each breeder feeds their dogs in their own unique way ...

... and has "discovered" a unique "best" calcium supplement and unique "best" dose rate. This way of feeding and supplementing has been hard won over many years of trial and error, of disaster, tears and eventual - maybe - triumph. There is no rational explanation for what they do. They simply know from trial and error that it works - most of the time.

The bottom line for the novice breeder seeking sound advice is a dozen conflicting opinions about diets and calcium supplements. The more people they ask, the more feeding systems, opinions and horror stories they will hear regarding calcium and skeletal problems in growing pups.

To further complicate matters, the never ending search for information on calcium reveals a mountain of ever changing products. There are supplements which are - "brand new, you beaut, never been better, bound to produce the best bones ever." There are the "best ever, cannot be surpassed complete puppy foods." These promise to "solve **all** puppy growing problems forever!" Then they produce a better one which leaves you wondering about their claims for the last one!

The solution of desperation

In the face of all this - many people conclude - "better to be sure than sorry - better give those pups heaps of - some form - any form - of calcium. After all - you have to use it don't you - and it cannot do any harm - can it - ?"

Owners of the large or giant breeds often conclude that if a little calcium is good, then six times as much must be six times as good. Imagine having a puppy with legs that strong ..... fantastic!
It is commonly believed that the St. Bernard cannot get too much calcium! That bit of advice usually comes from that greatest of all authorities - "my breeder."

Unfortunately, what has evolved out of this superstition, confusion, ignorance, lies, and misinformation, is a situation where an appallingly high percentage of modern puppy owners give their puppies massive over doses of calcium.

Excessive Calcium is a major Cause of Bone Problems in Puppies

The practice of drowning puppies in calcium rich foods and calcium supplements has become one of the most popular ways of wrecking a puppy's bones in affluent societies today. Puppies raised with a diet containing excessive calcium can develop the whole range of bone problems.

The mechanism by which excess calcium causes these bone problems is by a change in the modelling process and growth rate of the bones. This is modern OCD at work. It is precisely what we know and understand regarding some of the fundamental bony changes in the modern skeletal diseases, including **Hip and Elbow Dysplasia, Osteochondritis Dissecans, dropped hocks, splayed feet etc., etc., right through to degenerative joint disease in the older dog.**

Unfortunately , in their early stages, many bone problems caused by excessive calcium , look almost exactly the same as those caused by not enough. By examining the dog, you cannot pick between a puppy suffering from an excess or a deficiency of calcium. That requires a close examination of the whole feeding programme.

As a result, when bone problems are observed in pups being fed too much calcium, the common reaction is to add even more. As you might expect, the bone problem worsens.This results in more and more calcium being fed in a hopeless attempt to correct the problem.

After a lot of money is spent on radiographs, trips to specialists, operations and all sorts of marvellous dietary manipulations and supplements, that poor deformed puppy is neutered and spends a grotesquely unhappy arthritic life, or is mercifully put to sleep.

Many a breeder's reputation has gone down the drain because of the production of defective pups. Sometimes bitter litigation is the end result with the breeder being taken to court for selling "genetically defective" stock.

Meanwhile such breeders are left scratching their heads in wonderment, still not at all sure where they went wrong.

This scenario I have seen played out on numerous occasions - so beware! In one particular case - a breeder started out following the BARF programme and produced brilliantly sound pups. For reasons best known to herself, considering the results she had achieved, she switched her dogs to a diet based partly on the BARF programme and partly on dry dog food and calcium supplements. She may have been warned by her vet and fellow breeders not to feed anything but imported dry dog food and that if she supplemented with meat, she absolutely must add some calcium to the diet. She, like many others was pressured into following the current "conventional wisdom". In this case she decided to have a bet each way. The half and half approach.

Sometimes this half and half approach works and often it does not, depending exactly on which half of the "conventional wisdom" is adopted, and which half of the BARF programme is adopted. In this particular case her choice must have been poor because disaster quickly followed.

The warning here is, the benefits to be derived from the programme I suggest are directly proportional to the degree to which you follow that programme. The more you depart from the programme, the more problems you can expect.

How Has This Calcium Problem Come About?

The "need" to drown pups in calcium with its subsequent disasters came about because of the equally horrifying effects of calcium deficient diets.

In Australia during the 1970's, there was a backlash against processed pet food. The stuff had become prominent during the 1960's. However, many people were - not surprisingly - dissatisfied with the results these products produced, and wished to return to what they believed was a natural diet.

This scenario has occurred at earlier times in both the UK and the US.

However, in the intervening period, pet owners had forgotten how to produce a natural diet. They now believed a natural diet was an "all meat" diet. Disaster. Such a diet is totally lacking in calcium. It also lacks other nutrients, but we shall concentrate on the lack of calcium for the moment.

Those weak easily broken bones seen in puppies fed mostly meat, demonstrated to vets, breeders, puppy owners and any other interested parties that "puppies - all puppies - need extra calcium". That is why the drug companies, strongly supported by vets, breeders, pet shop owners, and any one else who could make a dollar [or two] out of selling calcium supplements, were able to push so effectively the idea that growing puppies' diets must be supplemented with calcium.

This need to supplement puppies' diets with calcium became part of doggy lore or myth. "Supplement with calcium or ruin your dog" became the catch cry.

Pet food manufacturers' knee jerk reaction – add more calcium!

With all the talk of calcium deficiency and the need to supplement with calcium, the pet food manufacturers reacted by increasing the calcium content of their products .... just to be sure. To achieve this, all they had to do was add a cheap calcium supplement. That was simple. Throw in heaps more bone meal. Cost effective too. Bone meal is one of the cheapest ingredients in pet foods. They were certainly happy to do that . It actually reduced their manufacturing costs.

As a result, dog foods, particularly many of the cheaper dry varieties can contain up to 10 times more calcium than growing pups need.

At the same time as owners were being encouraged to feed extra calcium, they were also being encouraged to feed only commercial dog foods. Vets knew only too well the ill health of puppies raised on the all meat diet. They came to believe - and rightly so in many instances - that dog owners did not have the ability to properly formulate home made diets for dogs.

"Feed processed pet foods only" is now standard veterinary advice - "No more home made diets. Particularly when feeding pups!"

Unfortunately, when pups are fed these processed pet foods already containing an excess of calcium and zealous owners, anxious not to have a calcium deficiency add even more calcium, problems of calcium excess quickly follow. The pendulum has swung in the opposite direction. Owners have gone from feeding a calcium deficient all meat diet to a diet which contains a dangerous excess of calcium.

Unfortunately, many vets, breeders and puppy owners do not realise what a disastrous effect an excess of calcium can have on a growing puppy's bones.

How Does Excessive Calcium Cause Bone Problems?

There are at least two mechanisms. Firstly, excessive calcium makes other nutrients - essential for normal bone growth - unavailable, by binding chemically with them. Excessive calcium also interferes with a number of the hormones which control normal bone growth.

I suspect there are other problems not yet discovered. However, those two mechanisms are by themselves quite capable of altering bone growth. That is, causing Modern OCD. The end result can be all the bone diseases we are currently seeing in growing pups. And this includes the dreaded Hip Dysplasia.

We will now take a closer look at those two problems caused by excessive calcium.

Excessive calcium makes other nutrients unavailable

If a puppy receives too much calcium in its food, the calcium which is not needed will pass out harmlessly in the faeces. This statement is totally true of calcium supplied as raw meaty bones or in other natural forms such as in raw vegetables.

However that statement is not true of excessive calcium fed either in a commercially produced dog food, or where too much supplementary artificial calcium has been added to either a commercial diet or a home made diet.

Excessive calcium given either as a calcium supplement or as part of a cooked commercial or home made diet will attach to other essential nutrients in the diet, **forming new compounds which your pup cannot absorb.**

257

The minerals which may be lost to your pup because of excessive calcium include ...

... phosphorus, iron, copper, zinc, iodine, magnesium, manganese, chromium, molybdenum, boron, selenium and probably others.

Our knowledge in this area of nutrition like many others is incomplete. The important point is that loads of essential nutrients become bound to artificial calcium and pass out of your puppy's body as faeces. This means they are no longer available to be used by your pup.

As a a result your pup can become deficient in a whole range of minerals which were actually present in the food your pup ate! Let me stress that this is common common common.

Without those minerals present in its body, your puppy's bones are not able to grow normally. A puppy fed this way has the potential to develop abnormalities of bone growth - modern OCD - and this can develop into such problems as Hip Dysplasia, Elbow Dysplasia, Wobbler Syndrome, Dropped Hocks, Splayed Feet, etc. etc.. Let me repeat. This situation is very, very common.

Excessive calcium interferes with your puppy's hormones

The hormones which are involved in bone growth include Growth Hormone, Insulin, Thyroid hormones, the various Sex hormones, Parathyroid Hormone, Calcitonin, and probably many others. Sounds really complicated doesn't it! Well, do not worry, even the most eminent scientists in this field do not yet know how they all work.

So forget all those names and what all those hormones do. There is a much simpler way of looking at this.

Hormone production and Hormone activity are at the mercy of what you decide to feed your puppy. Nutrition is the major factor which decides how each and every one of those hormones behave themselves. It decides whether they will act normally, producing normal bones, or misbehave and produce abnormal bones.

If we use the BARF diet to feed our pups, those hormones will all function normally. The more we depart from the diet a pup evolved over countless generations to require, the greater chance there will be for error. For Osteochondrosis.

Excessive calcium interferes with at least two hormone systems involved in bone growth. Thyroxine and Calcitonin.There are doubtless other hormones involved, however, the effects of these disturbances are disastrous enough to explain most of what we see in the way of altered bone growth or Osteochondrosis in young pups.

The effect of Excessiue Calcium on Thyroid Function

Excessive calcium depresses the function of the thyroid gland. This is partly because the calcium has made the iodine unavailable, but it may also be via a direct affect on the gland itself.

However it is caused, the lack of a properly functioning thyroid gland, which is essential for normal growth, will dramatically alter the growth patterns of a puppy. This results in both a substantially reduced growth rate and abnormal bone growth.

This alteration in thyroid gland activity will affect the pup for the rest of its life. It will affect much more than bone growth. It will alter normal reproductive patterns. It may even result in infertility. However, what I want you to realise is that the effect of excessive calcium on the thyroid gland of a puppy contributes in a major way to skeletal problems in pups.

The effects of excessiue Calcium on Calcitonin Production

You recall that when excessive artificial calcium is fed, **most** of it passes out of your pup's body in the faeces. However, **some of the excess is absorbed, raising the blood calcium levels -** and this is what causes problems.

To get rid of the excess calcium constantly circulating in the bloodstream, the body secretes an increased amount of the hormone Calcitonin. Calcitonin works by decreasing the number and functioning of the reabsorptive cells in the bone.

The increased levels of Calcitonin do a great job in reducing the blood calcium levels. However, that is not the only effect.

That excess calcitonin also retards bone maturation and remodelling. It interferes with normal Endochondral ossification. It helps to produce modern OCD, which as you recall is the basic process underlying modern skeletal disease. It is the basic cause of - most of the juvenile bone disease, and yes, that does include Hip and Elbow Dysplasia, etc., etc., etc..

How much excess calcium is required to cause abnormal bone growth?

The answer to this question is - "not much!" **When feeding artificial foods,** 1.1% to 1.5% calcium in the diet is required for normal healthy bone growth. Research with Great Danes has shown that levels as low as 3% will cause abnormal or diseased bone growth. These levels are easily achieved by feeding many types of dry dog food with or without calcium supplementation.

In other words **it only takes a small excess of calcium** to disrupt the normal growth processes of a puppy's bones.

Can we solve the Calcium Problem With modern foods?

Earlier in this chapter I posed a number of questions about feeding calcium to puppies. I now want to run through a few of those questions to see if we can solve the calcium dilemma using commercial dog food and calcium supplements.

How much calcium do growing puppies need?

If you are attempting to feed a complete and balanced diet at every meal - such as a commercial product, or one that you devise with home cooking - it should contain calcium at a level of 1.1% to 1.5%, and definitely no more than 2.0%. You must also make sure both calcium and phosphorus are present in approximately equal amounts, with the amount of calcium slightly exceeding the amount of phosphorus. [That ratio for the scientifically minded is 1.1 : 1]. Is that simple or is it confusing? Do not be concerned. For the moment, please accept what I am saying and read on.

If the product you feed has that ratio between calcium and phosphorus, and an approximation will do, and the percentage of calcium in the diet is between one and two percent, things should be reasonably OK with your puppy's bones.

What do you think of these ratios and percentages? Do you find them a practical help when it comes to feeding dogs? After all, they are the correct answer.

The truth is, such an answer is of no practical value to the vast majority of dog owners unless they are feeding a commercial product which they know has calcium at those levels.

However, if you are preparing your own pet foods, how would you know that you were achieving that ratio and that percentage of calcium and phosphorus? On the other hand if you are buying any old dog food off the shelf at the supermarket or wherever, how would you know that it contained that ratio and that percentage of calcium and phosphorus? You might also ask - is this really essential knowledge?

In fact, if this is essential knowledge, you have to wonder how dog owners in centuries past right up until 30 or 40 years ago managed to produce healthy dogs, or indeed how the wild dogs have survived without people with such knowledge to help them?

Most reputable dog food producers do get the ratio bit right, but not the amount. Most dog foods contain way too much of both calcium and phosphorus. Recent analyses of a whole range of commercially produced dog foods in both America and Australia, including some of the popular and best selling supermarket brands, showed that they contained excessive levels of calcium. Some of them contained up to 10 times more calcium than is required by a growing puppy. Most of them had at least twice as much as was necessary.

The only thing you can be really confident about is that most of these commercial foods contain excessive calcium. The problem is there is no way you can know how much calcium is present in the product you are using.

The bottom line with this question is that it is all very well finding out how much calcium a puppy needs. You may find the correct answer, but when it comes to feeding your puppy, that knowledge is of no practical value. However, that is precisely what the dog food companies want you to conclude. It makes their job of persuading you to buy their product that much easier.

Let us go to the next common question.

Does my puppy need extra calcium?

Another simple question with a simple answer. ..... "If there is not enough calcium in the diet, you must add more until the correct level is reached."

Once again I have given the correct answer, but have been of no practical use because neither you nor anyone else has the slightest idea of how much calcium is present in your puppy's food. However, by answering the question in the only logical way it can be answered, I have produced another reason for pet food manufacturers to persuade you to buy their product.

Let us move to the next question.

Which calcium supplement is best?

This question too has a very simple answer. If the product your pup is eating is deficient in calcium, add any calcium supplement you want to. It does not matter which one you add. Your pup's body will absorb what calcium it requires from the supplement you give it.

If there is already heaps of calcium in the diet, very little calcium will be absorbed from the supplement that you add, no matter which one you choose.

In other words, the availability of calcium from a supplement is almost totally dependent upon your puppy's needs, and has very little to do with the form in which it is supplied. The other factor which must be present is vitamin D.

Let me remind you of something we have already covered. That is, if you add too much of that artificial calcium, bone disease will rear its ugly head.

You see, the body still absorbs too much of the artificial stuff, whereas with the natural form - raw meaty bones - this simply does not happen!

However, despite all of the above there is still the problem of having no idea how much calcium is in the diet you are feeding. You do not know whether your dog even needs a calcium supplement, let alone which one!

Also let me point out, that if you are feeding a so-called good quality commercial dog food, no supplementary calcium is needed. In fact adding calcium to these diets is downright dangerous to your puppy's bone - and general - health. Recall that most commercial dog foods have way too much calcium already. There have even been reports of some of the high priced premium brands of puppy foods having too much calcium.

Finally, let me say that when it does become necessary to supplement a young dog with calcium, the one I usually choose is dolomite. This is a combined calcium and magnesium supplement. Of all the supplementary forms of calcium it is usually the safest in terms of not causing skeletal problems.

Let me now move to the most common question vets are asked with regard to calcium supplements.

"How much calcium should I give my puppy, doc?"

What they mean is "How much extra artificial calcium should I be adding to my puppy's diet?" That also is impossible to answer. The answer required depends on how much calcium is in the diet already. As we have seen, without access to an analytical laboratory, that is impossible to know.

Another common question people ask is .....

Can milk be used as a calcium supplement?

The simple answer is that milk - whether it be cow's milk, goat's milk or even dog's milk - will not balance up an unbalanced diet.

Milk itself is a complete and balanced food for young animals. It has the correct ratio of calcium to phosphorus, and sufficient calcium for the needs of a growing pup.

If you add milk to an all meat diet in an attempt to balance the meat with respect to calcium, the only thing you will achieve will be to unbalance the milk. In short, no, you cannot use milk as a calcium supplement.

However, there is nothing wrong with adding milk to a diet which is already balanced for calcium and phosphorus. Feeding milk will not unbalance an already balanced diet.

Are calcium supplements with phosphorus of any use?

These are supplements such as dicalcium phosphate or bone meal, or any of the so called complete mineral mixes for dogs which claim to contain Calcium and Phosphorus in perfect balance for pups.

As a general rule, you add one of these types of supplements to a diet which is very low in both calcium and phosphorus, whereas you add pure calcium with no phosphorus to diets which are high in phosphorus and low in calcium, such as an all meat diet.

However, let me stress once again, it is very difficult to get this juggling act "just right" because you have no idea of the levels of calcium and phosphorus present in the diet you are attempting to 'fix up.' That is why most attempts end in failure.

The folk who do succeed, do so because they have found a system that works through a long period of trial and error. If they happen to fluke it right the first time, it is more by incredibly good luck than good judgment. Once again, we have produced another argument for feeding dog food.

Do giant breeds need more calcium than the smaller breeds?

This is perhaps the most vexing question for so many dog owners, and yet the answer is simple common sense. The amount of calcium that needs to be added to any dog's diet depends on only one thing. How much is already in there. If the food fed to that giant breed puppy contains adequate levels of calcium, [that is - somewhere between 1 and 2 percent] then no more needs to be added. Giant breeds do not need their diet to be any richer in calcium than the food you would feed to a smaller dog. They require their artificial diet to contain exactly the same percentage of calcium.

In other words you feed all growing dogs the same diet, but the bigger the dog, the more of that diet you feed. Common sense.

People who fail to realise this, and are feeding a commercial dog food, are probably feeding way too much calcium already. They compound that problem if they choose to add even more calcium as is so very common.

However, the answer to that question changes dramatically when that so called 'complete and balanced diet' is supplemented with other foods such as copious quantities of meat [without bones] or masses of grain type foods.

Suddenly that dog is suffering a calcium deficiency. The problem is, there is no easy way to figure out how much extra artificial calcium is required.

However, there is a simple and obvious solution. Switch to the BARF diet - but more of that shortly.

Calcium 'Thumb Rules'

Breeders, owners and vets, in fact any one who has been fiddling around with dogs for more than a few years, and feeding or recommending the use of calcium supplements, will have developed their own set of 'thumb rules' regarding the use of calcium. Let's have a look at a few of them ...

Calcium 'Thumb Rule' Number One

When feeding lots of meat to your puppy, you will be told to feed two teaspoons of calcium carbonate for each kilogram of meat fed, which is one teaspoon per pound for those of us who are non metric.

Now that particular rule of thumb is fine so far as calcium goes, if meat is all you feed. If you are feeding other things, then that answer may be way out. Even if that answer by some fluke turns out to be correct, you still have a problem. You have not balanced the diet for all those other factors which are not found in sufficient quantities in meat. Things such as iodine, vitamin A, copper etc. If you would like to read more about the disaster that is an all meat diet, refer to chapters Four and Eight of **Give Your Dog a Bone.**

Calcium 'Thumb Rule' Number Two

A fairly valid thumb rule is that you can feed up to half meat and half dry dog food, and still not need to add calcium.

This is true for quite a few different brands of dry dog food. Particularly the cheaper ones. This gives you some idea of the excessive levels of calcium already present in some of those cheaper brands. It would not be true for all of them however.

The problem is you do not know which ones contain extra calcium without having them tested and who is going to do that? Particularly when the next batch may be different!

Then there are the highly expensive premium brands. Some have the correct calcium levels. If you add meat to those products, you would need to add more calcium to make up for the calcium deficiency you were causing.

However, if you do that, although the diet may be fine for calcium, it may still be unbalanced for those other factors missing from an all meat diet.

Some of the super premium puppy foods have been found to be excessive for calcium, calories and protein. These ones, particularly if fed to excess will cause skeletal problems. Add extra calcium or extra protein, or extra calories to these - and really mess your pup's bones! On top of all that , these foods have lots of other problems which over the long term will result in degenerative disease.

Calcium 'Thumb Rule' Number Three

Another type of thumb rule that people use is to feed so much calcium per lb or per kg of puppy.

Any rule of thumb like that one must be totally disregarded. It does not take into account the amount of calcium already present in the diet, which as we have previously pointed out may already be in excess of a puppy's needs.

Calcium 'Thumb Rule' Number Four

Yet another common thumb rule is to feed so much calcium depending on the age of the puppy.

Once again that thumb rule totally ignores the amount of calcium already present in the diet. In other words, ignore that idea as well.

The Calcium Phosphorus Ratio

I have already mentioned the importance of the ratio of calcium to phosphorus in a pup's diet. [1.1:1.0] That is, when feeding processed foods they should contain approximately equal amounts of calcium and phosphorus with slightly more calcium. If the diet you provide your pup strays too far outside those limits there will be skeletal problems.

If you are feeding artificial food, you can be reasonably sure that the manufacturers do get the calcium to phosphorus ratio right these days.

The problems start when you supplement that artificial food with extra meat or extra calcium as so many people do. This upsets that ratio. If you upset it too much your pup will be headed for skeletal problems. This is a very common mistake.

For example, if you decide to devise a diet based half on processed food and half on other things such as meat, or you decide to add a calcium supplement, you will have no idea what the ratio between these two minerals is. The idea of having a bet each way - "half natural and half processed - just to be sure" - is the method that is commonly used to unbalance that ratio and produce skeletal problems.

In other words, unless you are pretty sure of what you are doing - this can be a dangerous path to walk down. So if you do decide to go the processed food way - it is much safer to feed dog food only and not to supplement.

If You Must Feed Artificial Food To Your Puppies ...

.... Then do find one that by actual analysis has the correct ratio of calcium to phosphorus, and whose dry matter contains not more than 2.0% and not less than 1.0% calcium. Make sure that this food contains no more than 20% protein, with about 90% of that being composed of the essential amino acids. It should contain between 5% and 10% fat. That fat should have a high percentage of the essential fatty acids with the correct ratio of Omega-3's to Omega-6's - about 1:3. These should not have been been damaged by heat, and they should be stabilised by vitamin E in adequate amounts.

Even more important is to make sure that you have seen the results of feeding trials which have demonstrated the adequacy of this diet in producing healthy puppies, that grow into healthy long lived adults with no bone problems and a minimum of degenerative diseases as they age.

Preferably, find one that has been trialled against the biologically appropriate diet that dogs evolved over centuries to require - the BARF diet. Choose that commercial diet which is found to be at least equal to the BARF diet.

If you cannot find such a commercial diet, let me give you a much simpler alternative.

There Is a Simple Solution To The Calcium Dilemma

If the sound or the idea of all that fuss about calcium bothers you, do not let it. I shall let you into a secret. There is a much simpler way. You do not need to be bothered with all those problems I have outlined for you. Nor do you need to be a scientist to be able to feed a puppy or an adult dog properly. Nor do you have to go through years of heartbreaking trials trying to get it right. It is very easy to achieve the correct balance of calcium to phosphorus, together with the right amount of calcium in your puppy's diet, without measuring a thing and without analysing anything either.

The food you feed to achieve this miracle is commonly available, it is cheap, it is very rich in calcium, it has the perfect balance between calcium and phosphorus and it can be fed in abundance without causing problems. If you feed this food, no matter how much your pup eats, it will always receive the precise amount of calcium it requires. Your puppy will never receive a calcium excess, or a calcium deficiency. This food will produce perfect bone growth.

Solving the calcium dilemma

What is this magic food - this miracle food? It is called ... **Raw Meaty Bones.** Raw meaty bones should form about 50% to 60% of the diet. It is impossible to cause the calcium problems I mentioned above when you supply calcium to your pup in the form of raw meaty bones.

If you supply your pup[s] with such a diet **you will find that there is simply no way you can feed excessive calcium to your pup** That is a thumb rule you can believe. It is valid, it is scientific, it is natural, obvious, useful, not difficult to understand, and anyone can do it.The calcium and phosphorus will be in the correct ratio, and the diet will never result in an excess of calcium. Nor can you cause problems with other minerals and you will not cause hormonal problems either. It is so simple.

There is not a complete explanation as to why bones do not cause these problems beyond the very obvious fact that they are nature's food for the dog, which means in scientific terms they are what the dog as a pup evolved to eat in order to grow its bones properly.

From a purely technical point of view however, we do have some explanations as to why raw meaty bones work so well. For example, a most important point is the fact that the calcium compounds in bone do not become attached to other minerals in the same way that cooked artificial forms of calcium do when commercial pet foods are produced.

This means other minerals are not made unavailable because of the presence of calcium in the food as bone. A related factor is the chemical form of the calcium in the bone. The organic form of calcium in the uncooked bone is nature's way of releasing the other minerals in the digestive tract instead of binding with them. In other words, this form of calcium actually aids in the digestion and absorption of other minerals rather than binding with them and preventing their assimilation into your dog's body. In short this raw organic form of calcium is more likely to allow other minerals to be available rather than cause them to be unavailable.

Equally and possibly more important is that **in this organic form, your pup's body is able to absorb only what it needs** as opposed to the artificial soluble forms of calcium, where the body is actually forced to absorb more than it needs, leading to the problems I have already outlined.

The bottom line with bones is that they are the perfect calcium source for growing puppies

Only bones have all the ingredients in perfect form to build bones. They contain all the proteins, fats and minerals that are required - no excesses and no deficiencies. Of course, this is hardly surprising - **dogs have been building their bones from other animals bones for millions of years.**

.

THE CALCIUM DILEMMA IS SOLVED!

However, you must do it right. So read very carefully **and then follow** the very simple programme I outline in Chapter Twenty Two - The BARF Programme For Pups.

A final word about Calcium

In the chapter[s] which deal with treating skeletal disease, there will be mention of occasions when people have been feeding a diet which is excessive for protein and calories, but deficient for calcium. The supplement I almost invariably recommend in this instance is Dolomite which is composed of magnesium and calcium carbonates.

The next chapter deals with the 'Excess Food' way to wreck your pup's bones.

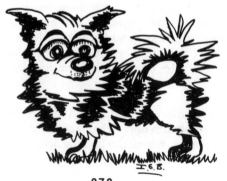

CHAPTER NINE

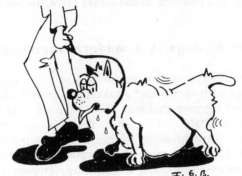

I. 6. B.

THE 'EXCESS FOOD' WAY
TO WRECK YOUR
PUP'S BONES

Over feeding pups and growing them rapidly ...

... Is a foolish management idea. Numerous scientific studies have shown that overfeeding - and all the problems stemming from it - is one of the most important predisposing factors in causing skeletal disease. This has been reported in horses, cattle, pigs, poultry and dogs. As puppy growers, we need to know how damaging over nutrition is, and then have the will to regulate the quality and restrict the amount of food we feed our puppies.

Throughout its life a dog is continually remodelling its bones ...

... in a ceaseless process of replacing, reusing and repairing the cells, the collagen matrix, the minerals, the blood vessels and nerves of which the bone is composed.

In a growing puppy this process is very rapid and very dynamic. It can be explosive and that is when it is dangerous. Bone growth must be kept in check. If it runs at maximum pace, by being over supplied with protein, fat, carbohydrates and calcium, those bones can grow too fast and become diseased.

Over nutrition of dogs is a modern phenomenon

We seem to have developed an insane desire to promote an early and sustained rapid growth rate, in fact a maximum growth rate in pups which are ill designed to be grown that way. Why have we done this? Ignorance of the dangers is probably one reason. The desire for rapid show ring success is another. The availability of the so called super premium growth foods is another. **However, more than anything the problem has come about because processed food and calcium supplements have replaced the humble raw meaty bone as the basis for canine bone growth.**

Most skeletal disease today is caused by excesses

The techniques used include over-feeding in general, or excessive feeding of particular nutrients such as fat or protein or carbohydrate, and - as we have seen - excessive supplementation of calcium. The problem often involves a commercial diet fed in **huge quantities**. Sometimes a commercial diet **heavily supplemented** with people food is the problem.

No matter which excessive diet is chosen, when pups are fed on very rich foods which are high in energy, and/or protein and/or calcium, we see a rapid growth rate and an overweight pup. **The pup's growth outstrips its ability to support itself. This produces Osteochondrosis. Modern Osteochondrosis.**

These techniques, designed to produce skeletal problems...

... work particularly well with puppies of the larger breeds, and most especially the giant breeds where they will practically guarantee bone and joint problems. This is because **in general, the larger the breed**, the more genes it has for fast growth. This rapid rate of growth is a major part of the reason that the large breeds of dog are so prone to Juvenile Bone Disease.

Over nutrition produces Modern Osteochondrosis which in turn leads to such bone diseases as Osteochondritis Dissecans, Hip Dysplasia, Elbow Dysplasia, Panosteitis, angular limb deformities, Wobbler Syndrome etc., and possibly slipping patellas and Legg-Perthes disease in the toy and miniature breeds.

The bad news is that by the time many of our pups are showing signs of being in trouble, permanent damage has already occurred.

The good news is, if you own or are about to own a new puppy, such problems are totally preventable.

It is quite easy to promote skeletal problems in pups

Over feed them. Take particular care to ensure the food you feed them contains lots of calories. That is, a high level of sugar, protein and most especially fat. Many people use the so called super-premium puppy foods as an easy way to do this. These products have high levels of sugar, protein and often fat as well. These foods, if fed to excess will promote a rapid growth rate and/or obesity. Other people just use lots of high calorie food scraps to achieve the same goal.

Just be aware that you do not have to try all that hard to produce fat puppies. All you have to do is allow the pup to be fed ad lib on any reasonably good quality 'growth type' food regime, and this can include a raw meaty bone based diet where lots of fat and lots of carbohydrate are fed to excess. The result is those fat and shiny roly poly puppies.

Common ways that over feeding and excessive growth rates happen

Often it happens in pups owned by new puppy owners - keen to have the best pup ever. People who try 'too hard.'

These people make sure that their puppy is never hungry, they buy their puppy the best of everything, they are likely to give it huge calcium supplements and they would never feed their puppy something crude like bones. Their puppy is fat and shiny and roly poly. These people have no idea what they are doing. They just do it!

Quite a number of astute breeders HAVE realised the importance of limiting growth rate. Keeping their pups slim and hungry. Many of them are German Shepherd breeders.They grow their pups SLOWLY. This will cause a degree of early stunting. These pups look like the patients at an anorexic clinic. The maturity of such pups is weeks behind their litter mates grown at a more conventional rate. Breeders know that by doing this their pups will not develop Osteochondrosis. When the dogs from their kennels are radiographed, they want those radiographs to prove to the world that their stock is superior genetically. No bone problems of any description. Such breeders attempt to get their puppy buyers to do the same.

However, many of those new puppy owners can't or don't or won't grow their pups slowly. Skeletal problems begin when that new and inexperienced puppy owner gets the pup home and starts feeding it.

That puppy, having initially been held back, will undergo an enormous compensatory growth spurt. The owners are absolutely delighted - at first. Unfortunately, one or more of the skeletal conditions very rapidly emerges.

As a consequence those pups are labelled genetically inferior. This happens in an amazingly short period of time. Meanwhile - "back at the ranch" - the SLOWLY grown pups have excellent hips and joints and are labelled genetically superior.

It also happens because pups will often undergo a period of reduced growth rate after leaving the breeder for a new home. That period of self imposed starvation may last for several days to a week as the pup adjusts to its new home. If this reduction in growth rate is followed by a compensatory growth spurt, this may be sufficient to cause Osteochondrosis.

New puppy owner - be warned! Do not be in a hurry to get that pup growing at a rapid rate once it does start eating. Far better to hold it back, even though it does want to eat like crazy!

Many People believe you HAVE to grow them fast

An unfortunate fact of life is that when people get themselves one of the larger breeds of dog, they just love to grow it fat and fast. If it is not done for reasons of pride, it is done for reasons of supposed necessity. New puppy owners, particularly the owners of the giant breeds, often believe that a fast growth rate is an absolute necessity. They believe that unless they grow their pup at top speed - it will not grow properly. Often they have not really thought it out. They simply 'know' that their dog has to be grown in this way. Unfortunately, nothing could be further from the truth. They have got it dead wrong.

These owners feed their pup as much food as it can possibly eat. If they are really 'keen' to wreck its bones, they ensure that the food is not only huge in quantity, but also very high in calories [fat] and protein. They also throw in large quantities of artificial calcium - just to be sure.

One of the things I have noticed over the years is that the keener many owners are to do everything right by their pup, the more likely they are to get it absolutely wrong!

Many of you will be asking at this point - "Just how does excess food cause a problem?" So let's examine that question right now ...

... Excessive Energy intake during growth produces skeletal weakness

What we are talking about here is feeding a pup plenty of concentrated carbohydrates such as grain, plenty of protein and plenty of fat. These are the energy foods. Excessive energy intake during growth is disastrous for growing and developing bones. The problem is, the growth of the skeleton is unable to keep pace with the growth of the dog. **Compared to normal bones, these rapidly grown bones are much decreased in density. The bones of pups fed this way are not only less dense, they are also thinner than normal and have fewer minerals deposited in them; less calcium, phosphorus and magnesium etc..**

The bottom line is that the bones in such a puppy are softer and weaker than the bones of a pup that is grown more slowly. Not only that, those bones are forced to support a much heavier pup than they should have to.

Excess protein intake during growth produces skeletal problems

There are three ways a protein excess contributes to skeletal problems.

- Firstly, a diet with an excess of protein contains excessive energy intake. As we have seen, this will cause a rapid growth rate which in turn causes skeletal weakness.

- Secondly, an excess of protein will cause skeletal problems because high protein diets cause the body to eliminate large quantities of calcium in the urine. This can contribute to a calcium deficiency - no matter how much calcium is fed.

- The third way that a protein excess will cause skeletal problems is by unmasking some previously hidden mineral deficiencies. What do I mean by that? It is very simple. If protein in a diet is deficient, the growth rate is greatly slowed. This means that although this diet may be deficient in a number of minerals such as calcium, or zinc or copper, there are very few or no problems with the skeleton's development because of the slow growth rate. **However, once that protein deficiency is corrected, but not the mineral deficiency, the dog grows faster and suddenly shows signs of the mineral deficiencies. These are seen as skeletal problems.**

Unmasking previously hidden mineral deficiencies can be a major damaging effect of excessive protein on bone growth. Such a situation commonly occurs when a dog goes from the breeder to the owner, and the new owner places the dog on a high protein and high artificial calcium diet which ties up minerals such as zinc, manganese, selenium, and copper. A deficiency of each or any of these can have a direct affect on the skeleton. For example, a copper deficiency has been documented to cause lameness, stiffness and enlarged joints.

As a point of interest, although a zinc deficiency will cause skeletal problems, so will a zinc excess! Many enthusiastic dog owners, aware that zinc is necessary for many vital functions such as skin health, reproductive ability and growth will heavily supplement their dogs with zinc. A zinc toxicity or overload causes many problems including a decrease in calcium absorption, **resulting in inadequate calcium for normal bone growth.**

Another cause of a zinc toxicity has been where galvanised pipes were hooked to copper pipes causing electrolysis resulting in the release of zinc from the galvanised pipes.

Obesity is a major cause of Skeletal Disease in growing puppies

It is part of the excessive feeding method used to produce skeletal disease including the so-called hereditary diseases such as Hip and Elbow Dysplasia.

Fat, roly poly overweight puppies are NOT healthy puppies and they will NOT produce healthy adult dogs. It is during puppyhood that the NUMBER of fat cells an adult dog will have is determined. If you have ensured plenty of fat cells are produced in your dog as a puppy, then there are enormous numbers of fat cells to fill up when that dog becomes an adult. That is why dogs which were fat as puppies are much easier to make obese as adults, and much more difficult to make slim.

If you have kept an adult dog slim as a puppy, you have limited its number of fat cells. Being slim as a puppy is the best foundation a dog can have to help it remain slim and healthy as an adult.

Yet it is those massive overweight pups that so many breeders and puppy owners strive to produce and so many judges award prizes to. The end result is enormous health problems for any pup grown that way. Health problems that will follow it for the rest of its life. Problems that will involve every bodily system. The first system to be damaged is often the skeletal system.

The effect of a pup being overweight is both physical and physiological.

The Physiological Impact of Obesity on Your Puppies' Bones

Modern pups are fed on diets high in heat damaged saturated fats or oils, together with high levels of carbohydrates, usually in the form of simple sugars. These foods are very damaging to the health of puppies, particularly their skeletal health. High levels of fat and sugar in a puppy's diet will have two effects. The first is an effect on hormone levels and hormone activity, and the second relates to damage by free radicals.

The deranged and abnormal hormonal activity ...

... which results from high dietary sugar and fat levels and puppy obesity causes abnormal bone growth. This part of the Osteochondrosis story is not yet well understood. However, we do know that it is happening and that it is a major contributor to the production of the so called hereditary bone diseases in pups such as Hip and Elbow Dysplasia etc. etc..

Quite obviously the simple way to prevent this cause of Osteochondrosis is not to feed the damaging foods which produce the problem, and also to limit the total amount of food fed to ensure that puppies are kept slim as they grow. The BARF programme for puppies is the obvious solution.

The second physiological impact of obesity on a puppy's bone growth is the damage by free radicals ...

... which are generated by the masses of unhealthy fats present in modern foods - including let me repeat - the so-called super premium foods.

In some trials, the addition of vitamin C [a free radical scavenger] to the diet has had some success, whereas in other trials it appeared to make little difference. This may well have related to the levels of free radicals in those trials. The presence or absence of vitamin E which is a potent free radical scavenger would also have had an impact on these trials.

Are you now convinced about the role of over nutrition in producing skeletal problems? I hope so. The answer is to feed the BARF programe for pups as outlined in Chapter Twenty Two. But there's more! Now we move on to a most important topic, the impact of excessive exercise on skeletal disease, which can be equally devastating.

CHAPTER TEN

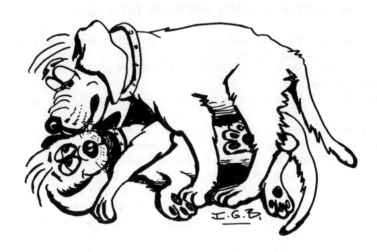

THE EXERCISE FACTOR
AND SKELETAL DISEASE

Bones should eventually become strong, tough, flexible structures, well able to support the weight and normal functioning of the animal they belong to. They should have a shape and size which is average for the breed, and the joints between them should allow the full range of healthy, effortless, pain free, unselfconscious movement.

Although that is what bones and joints should become, they are not that way while they are growing. During growth, bones and joints are structures which are relatively soft, fragile, malleable and highly vulnerable to physical trauma. What is vital for a pup's skeletal health is that the forces which work on its bones and joints should mould them into the correct shape.

If the stresses young bones are subjected to become too great or too jarring, both the bones and the joints are likely to become misshapen, deformed, painful, and less than normally functional. This is the the beginning of either Juvenile Bone Disease, or Osteoarthritis later on.

What is normal healthy exercise for pups?

What must puppy owners allow or do to give their pups' bones and joints normal stresses and strains? How do they avoid prolonged and extreme pressures being placed on bones which are soft and malleable, and whose growth plates and joints are so fragile? What sort of stress should be applied to young bones not yet ready to withstand the rigours of adult life?

A pup requires to be a normal weight and it requires to be subjected to the stresses of normal exercise, and that includes eating exercise. If the puppy is overweight and over exercised, or exercised in an inappropriate way, or not exercised during vital early days, as is so common, muscles, bones, joints and associated nerves can fail to develop fully or they can develop abnormally. That pup may then develop Osteochondrosis which may then go on and become one of the named diseases such as Hip or Elbow Dysplasia.

The Twin Traumas - Excessive Exercise and Weight

The damage caused to a puppy's bones by excessive exercise and excessive weight is the damage of simple trauma. Because a puppy's bones and joints are relatively soft compared to an adult dog's bones, when excessive pressures of exercise and weight are placed on them, they become damaged, bent, misshapen or deformed. Unfortunately, modern owners use the twin pressures of excessive and incorrect exercise together with obesity to traumatise their puppies' bones and joints. The joints go from healthy, normal, functioning pain free joints to unhealthy, misshapen, crippled, painful, malfunctioning joints.

It has become very common to allow excessive exercise, combined with an overweight puppy to permanently alter the shape of a puppy's bones. This is particularly so in the case of pups of the large or giant breeds. The way in which large breeds of dogs are exercised from weaning to about eighteen to twenty four months, particularly during two critical periods can determine whether they develop bone problems or not.

The two critical periods for bone development in puppies are from birth through to weaning, and from four to ten months of age.

The period, from four to ten months of age is the period of maximum growth rate. Pups must never be grown at full speed, and this is the period a puppy owner has to be at their most vigilant. It is during this period that pups are very susceptible to the effects of ANY excessive or inappropriate exercise and/or excessive weight.

What Is Excessive Exercise?

It would not be possible to mention every possible thing owners do to physically damage a young pup's bones. However, excessive exercise usually means exercise past the point at which a puppy wants to stop. It could be any exercise at all. It might include running a young pup to the point of exhaustion or any sort of jarring exercise such as allowing a pup to jump down from great heights - in fact **anything which is more than play** and which will put undue stress on a pup's bones.

If you have anything to do with raising puppies, you must understand how important it is to allow play only and try to leave everything else out - particularly where it involves exercising to exhaustion and any form of high impact. Even pups dancing around on their hind legs before their bones are mature can be dangerous to bone and joint health, particularly if the pup is overweight.

A common example of exercise which is designed to promote bone problems is where an owner drags his/her pup for miles on endless boring walks. The sort of walks where the puppy is so tired it drags one leg after the other, tail down and miserable.

'HEALTHY' walks – how they wreck your pup's bones

When a puppy starts out on a walk it is bright and bouncy. The muscles are strong and hold the bones in the joints strongly apart. Those bones do not sit heavily on each other. By contrast, when a puppy becomes tired and bored the muscles are no longer strong. They no longer hold the bones apart. They have stretched and are now allowing the bones to sit heavily on each other.

This places undue stress and pressure on the bones and the joints

There is stretching of the joint tissues, making them sloppy and loose. This allows the bones which form the joints to grind against each other in a loose sloppy fashion and at odd angles. There is trauma to both the cartilage of the joint and the cartilage in the very fragile growth plate.

This trauma can result in minute fractures in the cartilage and bone ends, blood loss into the joint, and loss of blood supply to the cartilage both in the growth plate and in the joint. This produces Osteochondritis [broken down inflamed joints] in the short term and in the long term Osteoarthritis or Degenerative Joint Disease.

Yes, old age or adult arthritis starts right here. Meanwhile, what we see in the young pup is pain due to all the damage. If we take radiographs we see remodelling of the ends of the bones which form the joints. In some dogs, the joint surfaces change their shape to something abnormal and eventually crippling to the dog. One very common example of this is Hip Dysplasia where the joint goes from a tight ball and socket shape to a loose cup and saucer shape.

Damage to only part of the growth plate - will permanently alter the angle at which the bone grows and the shape of the bone. This we see commonly in those dogs with the deviated carpus [wrist]. By doing this to our dogs we are ensuring permanent damaging changes.

The Physical Impact of Obesity on Your Puppy's Bones

For the last few hundred thousand years or so, puppies have grown up lean and hungry. Rarely fat. **Their bones were never designed by evolution to take the weight of a heavy pup.** The bones of modern pups have not changed. A light weight pup is what your puppy's bones are expecting to carry.

The more obese you grow your puppy, the more weight your puppy's bones have to carry around, and as a consequence, the greater the trauma likely to be suffered by those soft immature bones and joints.

Unfortunately, **even a marginal level of overweightness can have major consequences.** The problem becomes far worse when the pup is one of the giant breeds. In an engineering sense, dogs are not designed to be that big. As the breed of dog increases in size, so the effect of a small increase in weight is magnified out of all proportion compared to a similar increase in weight in a smaller breed of dog.

That is why large breeds must be kept exceptionally lean as they grow if bone problems are to be avoided. Unfortunately it is these larger heavier breeds owners just love to feed in an excessive manner, just to see how fast and fat they grow. It's a sort of a status symbol.

Just like fast growth, where it is mostly the larger breeds, especially the giant breeds, which have the potential to grow too fast, **there are real differences between breeds as far as the tendency towards obesity goes.**

For example, it is difficult to persuade any of the Greyhound type breeds - the sight hounds - to become excessively fat as puppies. On the other hand, breeds such as the Labrador, the Beagle, the Golden Retriever, the Rottweiler, the Saint Bernard etc. give their owners a real battle in the fight to keep them slim.

Nevertheless, if you try really hard, and lots of people do, **just about any pup can be made obese,** and if it happens to be one of the larger breeds, you are almost certain of producing bone problems. On the other hand, by feeding the BARF diet, and by limiting the amount of food fed, anyone can produce a pup of any breed to be slim, which is one of the secrets used to produce healthy bones and joints.

The dangers of obesity as a pup are at least fourfold:

- Firstly, and most importantly, that excess weight is adding to the trauma being placed on the growing points of the bones and in that way contributing to Osteochondrosis.

- Secondly, that excessive fat, particularly the heat damaged fat from the modern 'super premium' pet foods, is making the pup more prone to free radical damage. That is - degenerative disease! These foods not only contain highly damaging fats, it is highly doubtful if they would contain the necessary levels of vitamin E to adequately stabilise those fats in your dog's body.

- Thirdly, excessive fat results in hormonal changes which contribute to present and future bone problems and ...

- ... fourthly, obesity as a puppy increases the numbers of fat cells that pup will carry for the rest of its life. These fat cells will almost guarantee that pup's obesity as an adult and therefore the possibility of future poor health in every department of its life, and that DOES include future skeletal disease or Osteoarthritis.

There is every reason to keep that pup slim, lean and hungry as it grows!

There has to be SOME stress on young bones

The right type of exercise has positive benefits on skeletal growth. Bones MUST be stressed, but only in an appropriate way. Exercise of the correct type and for the correct amount of time will physically enhance the development of a young dog's bones. The old saying "Use it or lose it," certainly applies here. Bones will actually shrink if they are not used.

Let us now examine the exercise that is just right for a pup's bones.

What is safe healthy exercise for a pup?

There are two safe and beneficial forms of exercise for a growing pup. Exercise that not only avoids bone problems, but actively promotes the formation of strong healthy properly formed and normally functioning bones and joints. Notice I did not say perfect bones. It is important to understand that in biological systems there can never be perfection.

The first healthy form of exercise is good old fashioned play, and the second one is eating exercise. Most people are aware of what play is. For many people, eating exercise is a foreign concept.

Eating exercise is the very strenuous and healthy exercise involved in wrestling with, fighting over, ripping at, tearing into and crunching through raw meaty bones.

Both these forms of exercise come naturally to pups. All you have to do is structure your management in such a way that such activities are encouraged rather than inhibited.

Let us look at the way pups are exercised from birth

Many modern pups start their lives with a few weeks of unhealthy exercise. They spend their time sliding around on newspaper. This can be the beginnings of problems such as Hip Dysplasia.

Pups should be raised on flooring which allows them to get a grip without sliding. Newspaper, which is slippery, denies pups any possibility of healthy play and eating exercise. This is one of the myriad techniques owners have developed to encourage the production of bone and joint problems.

These problems happen - quite naturally - as pups slide around rather than walk around their whelping area. At its worst, newspaper promotes 'swimmers' and Hip Dysplasia. At the very least it is the beginning of bone and joint looseness and weak muscles.

Clean soil is great, and many a bitch has whelped successfully in a hole she has dug for herself. If you cannot organise that, do as I do, provide your bitch with deep piles of aged, deodorised wood mulch and/or straw. A deep litter system for bitches. The bitch forms her whelping hole in any of these materials with great safety, and warmth for the pups, and great traction for young paws and legs. In addition, it provides great absorbency for all those unwanted liquids so prevalent at this time. The urine, and vaginal discharges etc..

Allowing pups to be raised in this type of environment provides the best start on the road to normal healthy bone and joint growth. Get rid of that newspaper - it is way too slippery!

For more details regarding this form of whelping box see Part Two Chapter Five.

Healthy play and eating exercise starts at birth with those initial struggles to establish who gets what teat. This form of exercise continues and intensifies over the next couple of weeks and is combined with climbing over mum, climbing out of the whelping hole, and in generally exploring their limited environment.

In the week following the opening of their eyes, pups need to play with and fight over raw meaty bones in exactly the same way that wild pups do. It is essential for their normal healthy development that they have fresh pieces of chicken or turkey or duck - whatever - wings, carcases, necks etc., every day.

Initially you will see pups lying with, then sucking, then pulling and eventually fighting over these lumps of raw meaty bones. Pups love them with their great tastes and smells, and bits that can be grabbed hold of and tugged at. This type of play-cum-eating will occur whenever they are awake and hungry. No matter how many pieces you put in with them, you will still see a 'tug of war' over that one "special" piece that just has to be wrested from another puppy.

The exercise part of all this is an essential part of developing a pup's bones and muscles to be strong and its joints to be tight. Eating exercise not only provides isometric exercise for every muscle in the body, it also stresses the bones and joints in a very healthy way. Pups fed the BARF way are also cutting teeth and building strong healthy teeth. Consider the physical benefits denied pups that eat slop. The weak muscles, the unstimulated bones, the failure to develop the maximum number of neurological connections, the loose joints. All of this caused by the failure to feed young pups their heritage of raw meaty bones.

The benefits of eating exercise to brain, heart, muscle, bones and joints will be with a pup for the rest of its life.

Another important activity for pups is to be handled as much as possible from the day they are born. This includes their feet, mouth ears, and every part of their body. The aim is to have them so that they lose all fear of being handled when they become adult dogs. Other activities include stroking, squeezing, stretching, and moving every joint in their young bodies. All of this should be done by as wide a range of humans as possible. The pups should also be introduced to the motions of cars, and as many of the sights and sounds they are likely to encounter in their life as is practically possible. What ever reflexes, activities, skills, foods, sights, sounds, and smells you can introduce to those pups in this early stage will be imprinted for life. The more these pups are stimulated at this early stage, the greater will be their intelligence quotient, and their usefulness to us and themselves.

This is the time they are developing an immense range of attitudes, memories, loves, skills, and associations that will play an important mental and physical role, in every aspect of the rest of their life. This physical and neurological development, the nervous connections, conditioned reflexes which are developing throughout that pup's brain, spinal cord and body will be with that pup for the rest of its life. They are very much part of a dog's intelligence.

If a dog does not experience all of this as a pup, it will be all the poorer in every department of its life, and that includes the development of its muscles, bones and joints.

It is a pup's heritage to be introduced to life this way

It is an essential part of their education as a future member of the human/canine family. It ensures that these pups will be calm and socially adjusted as adults. This ensures they will be able to mingle freely and easily with both dogs and humans. They will not be the the anti-social dogs which have to be destroyed due to intractable anti-social behaviour. The added bonus to all of this will be pups that have sound bones and joints.

This whole programme of raising pups is simple and common sense. Yet it is largely ignored or unknown, or simply not practised out of either laziness or the weak excuse of a lack of time.

Most modern pups are largely ignored by their owners and weaned onto sloppy food.

Our poorly conceived and illogical methods of growing our pups, our failure to exercise our puppies' brains, spinal cords, nerves, muscles, joints, and bones in any adequate sort of way, means we are encouraging weak bones, weak bone to muscle connections, weak tendons and ligaments, poor neurological connections and sloppy joints. This is the beginning of skeletal problems including such problems as Hip and Elbow Dysplasia.

Other unrelated problems seen in pups raised with sloppy concoctions such as baby cereals or soaked and mushed dog food include the development of diarrhoea or other gastrointestinal problems. These cause nutritional, physical, psychological and immune system problems that will follow these pups for the rest of their lives.

As a final word on the importance of how you choose to raise pups till weaning, just remember that muscle, nerve, bone and joint health - begins or ends - right here in the whelping area.

Eating exercise does not end at weaning

It is vital for a pup's ongoing normal development after weaning that it continues to be daily involved in eating exercise.

Where raw meaty bone eating is persisted with all through a pup's growing days, [weeks, months and years], that pup has the greatest chance of developing sound bones and joints because of the combined effects of proper nutrition, the correct type of isometric exercise, and maximum development of neurological connections.

Pause and consider for a moment the enormous benefits pups are deriving from eating this way. A pup which obtains a large proportion of its nutrition from raw meaty bones is exercising its whole body in the process. To achieve this it is imperative that at least some of the bones it chews on are the large ones. The bones it has to spend many hours gnawing on.

Picture that pup with both front legs braced on a large meaty bone. As it rips and tears away at the meat, cartilage, tendons, and ligaments , it is helping to cut and clean its teeth. It is also developing strength in all its bones, muscles, and joints from its jaws, neck, shoulders, front legs, and spine, right down to every joint in its hind legs. This is healthy isometric exercise, carried out every day. This is exercise which strengthens these structures without giving them damaging stress. This exercise is an indispensable part of its proper development. Without this form of exercise, the pup will not develop to its full potential and has a much greater chance of developing Osteochondrosis. And there is more. A pup fed this way has far less chance of over-eating, another huge bonus. How else could this be achieved - and with no effort to the owner. The answer is - there is no other way.

But there is even more! Recent research shows that the consumption of cartilage on a daily basis, as dogs do when they eat the ends of the big bones, contributes in a fantastic way to joint and general health. A lifetime spent eating enormous volumes of cartilage is one of the major reasons dogs on the BARF programme rarely develop arthritis or cancer!

This whole programme is cheap, simple, fundamental, and has the end result of a normal happy healthy dog with no bone or joint problems.

The way it should be. Very sadly the vast majority of modern dogs in affluent societies have never experienced the joys of eating this way. Being denied the advantage of the BARF programme, they receive almost zero exercise as they eat their food. Just about the only exercise they receive when eating processed pet food is a bit of chewing, and precious little of that. Their poor teeth are filthy from day one - but that is another story! These dogs are condemned from the start.

If you don't raise your dogs this way, **let me challenge you to start doing this for your pups right now and notice the incredible difference.** Nothing could be simpler, easier, safer or healthier. Keep it up all through their growing days and allow it to continue into their advanced and very healthy old age.

Play, the other beneficial exercise

Play is the only exercise - apart from eating exercise - an immature dog with immature bones should be subjected to right up until it is an adult with fully matured adult bones.

Ideally a young pup should spend its days wrestling and play-fighting with other pups and gentle adult dogs together with free running over several acres of ground. Playing with humans is also healthy so long as the humans do not push the pup[s] too hard.

As the bones mature - in the period following puberty - more vigorous exercise can gradually be phased in.

The time of bone maturity varies for every breed ...

... and the larger the breed, the longer this maturing process takes. Dogs like Great Danes and Saint Bernards may have immature bones until they are about two years of age, particularly when they have been grown slowly as they should be.

In other words, the potential to cause damage with incorrect or excessive exercise depends very much on the pup's breed.

Another related breed factor is the pup's size and weight

Note that excess weight and excessive exercise in a small breed has much less impact on bone growth than in a giant breed. But no matter what the breed, if those stresses are excessive, and occur before a pup's bones have matured, altered or abnormal bone growth - Osteochondrosis - will occur.

Another breed related factor is muscle size, strength and hardness

Some breeds have very 'soft' muscles as young teenage dogs, whereas others seem to harden at a fairly young age. Those softly muscled dogs are much more vulnerable to bone damage than a dog of equivalent age and size with harder more developed muscles.

The bottom line is that before a pup's bones are mature, any exercise other than play has the potential to be highly damaging.

Another factor that needs to be considered is the possibility of accident or trauma. This will also have a major impact on future bone and joint health. It is a common cause of problems. In fact it can be difficult to differentiate between accidental trauma and the effects of excessive weight and exercise on a pup before its bones are mature and strong. Quite often they act in combination.

The simple answer to all of this

A pup's bones must become a support and movement system which will serve a dog well for the rest of its life. Their initial fragility means that the **only reliable and healthy forms of exercise a pup should have until its bones are mature,** are eating exercise, short walks, free running and play. A pup must never be allowed to become fat, or to be exercised or walked or run until exhaustion. A pup must always stop when it wants to. Before it becomes excessively tired. Before it becomes sore. It must never have any jarring sort of exercise where it is constantly jumping down on things. On the other hand, it should not be encouraged to dance around on its hind legs. That activity should not be encouraged until the bones are mature.

For all pups, raw meaty bone eating must be commenced at about three weeks and continued for the rest of that dog's days.

This is very simple but vital information. Dogs raised this way are so healthy. This has been going on for thousands of years and not a second thought has been given to it. People who do this simply expect and get healthy dogs. Today's dog owner by contrast expects and so often gets unhealthy dogs.

If you remember anything on the exercise score, remember the importance of play and eating exercise, as the only permissible form of exercise. If you are involved with one of the larger breeds which are far more susceptible to bone trauma than the smaller breeds, all of this applies - but even more so.

What programme will you choose to follow with your pup[s]?

In the next chapter we look at how people use old fashioned mismanagement to produce the 'ricketty' type of alterations in Endochondral Ossification or skeletal disease.

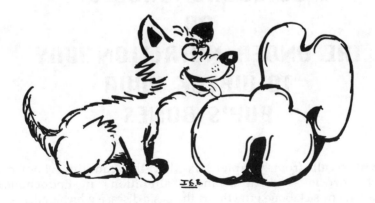

CHAPTER ELEVEN

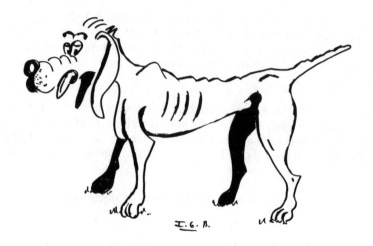

OLD FASHIONED
OSTEOCHONDROSIS
OR
THE UNDER-NUTRITION WAY
TO WRECK YOUR
PUP'S BONES

You will recall from Chapter Six that the condition known as Osteochondrosis - which means "alterations in Endochondral Ossification" or sick bone growth - is the basic disease which underlies all of the skeletal diseases we see in young dogs, and that these alterations in bone growth are caused by either excesses or deficiencies in nutrition and by excesses or deficiencies of exercise or trauma.

You will also remember that "Modern Osteochondrosis" is the term used to describe the basic disease process caused by excessive management practices of diet and exercise. These I have discussed with you in the preceding chapters. They lead to the modern skeletal diseases, including such problems as Hip and Elbow Dysplasia.

In this chapter, I want to halt the discussion of modern Osteochondrosis and move back in time to discuss Old Fashioned Osteochondrosis. This is a type of alteration in Endochondral Ossification which is caused by undernutrition or nutritional deficiencies rather than nutritional excesses.

Undernutrition leads to a group of problems collectively known as Rickets.

Undernutrition has become an uncommon way to ruin a puppy's bones. Twenty to thirty years ago in Australia, it was by far the most popular method. The most popular nutrient to be undersupplied back then was calcium. This was usually achieved by feeding an all meat diet. The results of course were disastrous.

In our modern world where most people feed their pets with processed food, there has been a swing in the opposite direction. Undernutrition is now a far less popular method of wrecking a pup's bones. However, there are still enough people keen to wreck their pups' bones with deficient sorts of diets and produce Rickets to make this chapter worthwhile.

Many of the people who unwittingly choose under-nutrition do so because of their concern regarding the dangers of processed food, excessive food and supplementation with artificial calcium. Unfortunately, out of a lack of knowledge, they exchange one bad method of raising pups with another, mainly because nobody has bothered to tell them anything different. Let's change that right now.

RICKETS is the name given to skeletal problems caused by a lack of calcium, vitamin D, or phosphorus.

A lack of any of these will cause failure of mineralisation of the growing points in the bone. Those growing points remain as cartilage.

293

This means there has been an alteration to Endochondral Ossification, which you will remember, is the basic process of bone growth. The bone has not mineralised, because without either calcium or phosphorus or vitamin D, mineralisation is not possible. I have called this problem 'Old Fashioned Osteochondrosis.' It is also known as Rickets.

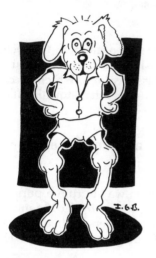

Pups suffering with Rickets have swollen bones at the growth plates. This makes them appear to have swollen joints. They will usually develop bent bones as well. If this is not corrected when the puppy is young, the adult dog will be left with a permanent deformity

Let us quickly run through the basic causes of Rickets starting with ...

Calcium Deficiency

This used to be the most common nutritional deficiency in young dogs. It goes under the impossible name of **Nutritional Hyperparathyroidism.** Don't be concerned about the name. It is just the scientific way of describing how the problem develops.

This syndrome is caused by a diet high in either meat or organ tissue - or both. Such a diet contains sufficient phosphorus but not enough calcium to allow mineralisation of the pup's bones. So the bones tend to remain as cartilage. If the pup's nutrition is normal in other respects - which is highly unlikely - the bone matrix or template continues to be formed normally. It just fails to become mineralised.

The problem occurs because low calcium in the diet initially causes the levels of calcium in the blood to drop. This causes the pup's body to release parathyroid hormone. This hormone takes what calcium there is out of the bone to maintain the blood calcium levels. Where the calcium is pulled out of the bone, the bone is replaced by fibrous connective tissue.

At first the affected pup will appear normal. That is, until **the bone is weakened to the point it fractures**. Commonly there are fractures of the vertebrae which may cause paralysis. Fractures of the femur in the hind leg are also common. **The teeth may become loose.**

If the problem has not gone too far - for example paralysis - the prognosis is good. Just get that poor creature onto a good diet. Preferably the BARF programme. The only modification required will be to mince the raw meaty bones because those poor rickety jaw bones are pretty weak. After a couple of weeks this will not be necessary.

Uitamin D Deficiency

This also is rare these days. This is because prepared pet foods and human foods usually contain enough vitamin D. Vitamin D is involved in the absorption of calcium from the intestines and its incorporation into bones. **The clinical signs and problems seen in the pup are similar to calcium deficiency**. The major difference is that the bony changes are not as dramatic. From a veterinary point of view another difference is that with a vitamin D deficiency you DO get a drop in blood calcium levels which is not seen with a calcium deficiency. The treatment is exactly the same as for a calcium deficiency. Switch that pup to the BARF diet!

Phosphorus Deficiency

This, like the other two is rare in dogs. A phosphorus deficiency is in fact the true or pure form of rickets. The problem comes about because of excessive calcium supplementation with a calcium supplement that does not contain phosphorus. For example - good old calcium carbonate!

This calcium supplement is then added to a high cereal diet. Although that cereal contains good levels of phosphorus, it is in the form of phytate which the pup finds difficult to absorb.

The high proportion of calcium which has been added to the diet further inhibits the intestinal absorption of phosphorus. Such a diet contains sufficient calcium but not enough phosphorus to allow mineralisation of the pup's bones. So the bones tend to remain as cartilage.

The puppy fed this diet will show problems that are similar to a calcium or vitamin D deficiency. Failure of mineralisation of the bone. However, in its pure form, the progression of this disease is much slower. Unlike the other two a phosphorus deficiency does not affect the teeth. Treatment? Exactly the same - feed that BARF diet.

There are a few other problems caused by undernutrition which are not strictly speaking Rickets. However, they are alterations in Endochondral ossification - or sick bone growth. They include ....

Vitamin A deficiency

An absolute deficiency of vitamin A is uncommon in pets fed with modern pet and human foods. However, because supplementation with cod liver oil - which is a rich source of vitamin A - proves beneficial time and time again, that seems to indicate most modern diets are still lacking sufficient levels for maximum health. Of course when you supplement with cod liver oil, you are also supplementing with vitamin D and essential fatty acids - all of which in my experience are of enormous benefit to the modern animal raised on 'junk' food.

Vitamin A has enormous responsibilities. Its presence is essential for a healthy immune system, for normal reproduction in both sexes, for the health of all internal surfaces including skin, respiratory system, digestive system, urinary system, reproductive system, for normal vision and **for normal skeletal development in growing animals.**

The skeletal problems we see with deficiencies of vitamin A are related to a retardation of bone growth and perhaps a reduction in bone resorption. The result is a shortening and thickening of the long bones and abnormal skull development. If the problem is very severe there may be neurological complications because of a pinching of nerves. These problems become very obvious with absolute deficiencies of vitamin A.

On the other hand an excess of vitamin A will cause excessive bone production which brings its own problems. The sort of diet which produces this problem is an all liver diet. Such a diet is much more common in cats than dogs.

However, given the improved overall health including skeletal health of pups fed the BARF diet - which includes lots of Beta Carotene the precursor of vitamin A, as well as supplementary cod liver oil - **there is little doubt that marginal deficiencies of vitamin A contribute in no small way to the numerous skeletal problems we see in modern pups.**

Uitamin C Deficiency

A vitamin C deficiency will affect the functioning of all cells within the body by stopping cell division. Nowhere is this more noticeable than with bone growth.

A lack of vitamin C will prevent the cartilage cells from dividing and from producing cartilage. The effect of this is to dramatically slow the growth of the bones. Because this lack of vitamin C does not affect mineralisation to any great extent, the bones are heavily mineralised but thin, weak, and easily fractured.

Dogs, unlike humans, do have the capacity to manufacture vitamin C in their livers. You therefore have to question whether it is possible for dogs to suffer a deficiency of vitamin C. Or to put that another way, would they benefit from supplementary vitamin C?

Firstly, do realise that vitamin C supplementation at the rate of 20 mg per kg daily can only ever be of benefit and will not under normal circumstances be toxic.

Secondly , if for some reason that ability to make vitamin C is impaired, as can happen on poor quality deficient types of diets, or the animal is heavily stressed which uses up vitamin C, or the animal is assaulted by masses of free radicals which also uses up the vitamin C stores - all of which is possible in our modern world - there may be a marginal deficiency of vitamin C. That is, there may be insufficient vitamin C to allow normal bone growth. This may, with other factors, contribute to skeletal disease in modern pups.

Thirdly, there is a body of literature which suggests that skeletal disease did drop dramatically when vitamin C was supplemented - as part of a natural diet.

For those reasons, a moderate supplement of vitamin C - as part of the BARF programme for pups, say 10 mg per kg twice daily - can only be of benefit.

Copper Deficiency

This mineral is essential for the normal production and strength of the cartilaginous matrix from which bones are formed. A copper deficiency will result in abnormalities of the growth of the ends of the bones which can become weak and deformed and may fracture.

The question is - "how could a copper deficiency come about with modern diets?" The answer is - "very simply - with modern diets!"

Many modern diets contain an excess of calcium. This will tie up the copper which has been added to these foods making it marginally deficient. If this happens there may be a marginal weakness of the ends of the bones. This is the sort of sub-deficiency which could help produce Hip Dysplasia, which is a disease involving a deformity of the end of the femur which forms part of the hip joint. There is no published data telling us to what extent a marginal copper deficiency produced by modern diets may interfere with the normal bone growth of modern dogs. However, by switching to a properly formulated BARF diet, you will ensure there are no problems with a copper deficiency.

Zinc deficiency

A zinc deficiency causes numerous problems in dogs. These include skin, coat and pigment problems, reproductive problems and growth problems. **The growth problems include include skeletal problems.** As has been explained in Chapter Eight of this section of the book, the most common way to produce a zinc deficiency is to over supply calcium. We don't know to what extent a marginal zinc deficiency produced by modern diets will interfere with the normal bone growth of modern dogs. However, the use of the BARF diet will ensure there no problems with a zinc deficiency.

Iodine deficiency

Iodine is necessary for the normal functioning of the thyroid gland and the production of the thyroid hormones, T4 and the more active T3. These are essential for the normal growth of the whole body and that includes the skeleton. **Where iodine is deficient there will be retarded growth of the growth plates and there will be failure of these plates to close when they should at maturity.**

We have absolutely no idea to what extent a marginal iodine deficiency produced by modern diets may interfere with the normal bone growth of modern dogs. However, the addition of kelp powder as part of the BARF diet ensures there are no problems with an iodine deficiency.

The concept of marginal deficiencies

If you have read through the above you will already have been introduced to this concept. Modern processed foods are so far removed from a dog's natural diet that we really have no idea of the extent to which they result in marginal deficiencies of a whole host of essential nutrients in our dogs.

What we do know is that pups fed these diets suffer a multitude of skeletal problems. We also know that when the BARF diet is implemented, we see radical improvements in the health of the skeleton. On that basis we can conclude that modern diets have the potential for a complex array of subclinical or marginal deficiencies, all working together to produce skeletal problems in our pups.

The solution? Get your pups off those 'awful' diets and swap to a biologically appropriate diet which will not allow marginal deficiencies to occur and will instead promote normal healthy bone growth.

What I want to do now is run through a number of common scenarios which are much closer to what we see in real life compared to looking at individual deficiencies which almost never occur as single events.

Rickets - using the all or mostly cereal diet

This method has many permutations and combinations, but the basic approach is to raise puppies on an exceptionally poor quality dry dog food, or a mostly bread or breakfast cereal diet.

This is a great way to ensure that a puppy becomes deficient in such things as protein, essential fatty acids, energy, copper, vitamin C, vitamin D, calcium, and possibly phosphorus. Some of these diets are so low in protein and other nutrients they severely stunt a a pup's growth. In many instances they lack some of the essential amino acids. They are always low in the amino acid Lysine. Lysine is an amino acid which is essential for normal bone growth.

Puppies fed these deficient sorts of diets develop Old Fashioned Osteochondrosis which if not corrected will eventually produce obvious signs of Rickets. If those obvious signs of rickets do not occur, damage is still occurring. It simply turns up later as arthritis or Legg-Perthes or slipping patellas. It is almost never linked to its true cause. Faulty nutrition. In this case under-nutrition during the growing stage.

Puppies that develop Rickets in an obvious form become generally unwell. They can be very weak, they often have diarrhoea, and of course there are the bony changes. The joints become exceedingly swollen and are weak and in the case of the wrist or carpus bend forward in a very characteristic way. See diagram. The other common change is bowed legs which will cause slipping [luxated or dislocated] patellas or kneecaps.

Rickets is more likely to be seen in the smaller breeds of dogs, particularly Chihuahuas or their crosses. However Rickets can be seen in almost any breed if it is raised badly on these deficient sort of diets. The nutritional factors mostly responsible for rickets are diets which leave out one or more of vitamin D, calcium or phosphorus. But note: they are all difficult to produce unless you really go out of your way to cause problems.

For example, a vitamin D deficiency is an uncommon cause of rickets in Australia because most dogs spend plenty of time in the sun. However, when puppies are raised indoors during the winter, are not fed any bones but are given mostly cereals, and are not fed a dietary source of vitamin D such as Cod Liver Oil, they can suffer from vitamin D deficiencies, calcium deficiencies and an excess of phosphorus. The net result is weak easily broken bones. This is because vitamin D has to be present before what little calcium there is in that diet can be absorbed from the intestines.

Phosphorus deficiencies are also rare as a cause of rickets because most of our doggy diets are very high in phosphorus, particularly diets which contain lots of meat or organs such as heart and liver.

However, it can be done. If you are really keen to create Rickets using a phosphorus deficiency, then feed a badly done vegetarian diet without any bones. Any sort will do, but the most common one people use is a diet consisting mostly of cereals, or a very cheaply made dry dog food, or in the case of dog owners who favour the macrobiotic diet, lots and lots of rice.

Other people will do it with a diet consisting mostly of breakfast cereals, and feeding these as the major part of the diet. However, by themselves these diets will not create a phosphorus deficiency. To ensure you do have a problem, it is essential to add lots and lots of calcium carbonate. This is a sure fire recipe for rickets due to a phosphorus deficiency.

The reason a lack of phosphorus causes rickets is because phosphorus is necessary for bone mineralisation. The end result is the same as a calcium deficiency. That is, thin weak easily fractured bones. The only difference being that with a phosphorus deficiency, the problem develops more slowly.

However, do not concern yourself. If you feed your puppy a raw meaty bone based diet there is no way any of these problems can happen.

The simple solution when a puppy is found to have this type of bone problem is to switch it to a properly balanced diet based on raw meaty bones. Because these puppies have weak sore bones including their jaws, they have difficulty chewing bones.. at first. The solution is to mince up the chicken wings, bones and all.

Nutritional Hyperparathyroidism – or – the all meat diet

This diet is less common than it used to be. However, it is still common enough as a deficient sort of diet which will cause bone problems in pups to deserve a mention together with a strong caution - DO NOT DO IT!

The all meat diet is the easiest and most popular way to produce a puppy diet which is deficient in a wide range of nutrients, including calcium. This is because puppies absolutely love it. They often become addicted to it. This encourages their owner to continue feeding it, in the firm belief that a puppy's instincts could not be wrong. Many people believe it is a puppy's "natural food".

Unfortunately, puppies that eat only meat are receiving a diet which is so unbalanced, so unnatural, it can only end in disaster. It is quite possible to totally ruin a sound puppy in about a month, by feeding it this way.

Those puppies do not grow. They fail to develop sexually. They are weak and sore if touched. They are pot bellied, anaemic, stunted, thin skinned, with very little pigment in their hair or skin. Their bones are paper thin and so fragile that the slightest bump, or even their own weight can cause a fracture.

AND PLEASE - do not fall into the following trap!

Puppies fed meat on the bone - MUST eat the bones - not just the meat!

It is absolutely essential when feeding puppies raw meaty bones that they actually eat the bones. If those puppies eat only the meat and leave the bones untouched as can and does happen, **they are on a meat only diet.** In other words, it is possible to produce an all meat diet by feeding raw meaty bones!

A common scenario is a little dog fed big bones or very hard bones, usually with lots of meat on them. Be warned, these little dogs often eat the meat only, leaving the bones for the owner to throw away! Those puppies MUST EAT THE BONES - not just the meat.

That is one of the reasons I recommend chicken necks and wings which are eminently suitable for little dogs. They will eat them whole with no problems, consuming both the bones and the meat!

Why Does An All Meat Diet Cause So Many Problems

Meat is great food for dogs, including growing puppies, as part and part only of a balanced diet. However, by itself, meat lacks many of the nutrients essential for a growing puppy.

An all meat diet supplies more than enough protein, no carbohydrate, no fibre, variable amounts of fat, only some of the vitamins a puppy needs, only some of the minerals a puppy needs, and that includes a severe deficiency of calcium. It only contains four percent of a puppy's calcium requirements.

For your puppy to get enough calcium for strong healthy bones it would have to eat seventy five of those meat meals every day !

Fortunately most people raising pups these days are aware that meat by itself is deficient in calcium. What many of them do not realise is that even if they add sufficient calcium to balance that diet for calcium, their puppy will still be eating food which is grossly deficient in iodine, copper, and vitamins A, D, and E and some of the water soluble vitamins including vitamin C and some of the B group. It is probably also deficient in other essential trace minerals such as chromium and selenium.

By adding vitamin and mineral supplements and with a lot of fiddling about, we could in theory correct all those deficiencies. In reality that proves an impossible task to get exactly right. **Dog owners who attempt to balance their dog's diet by adding various supplements - and plenty have tried over the years - find that their puppy still shows all sorts of health problems associated with nutrient deficiencies and excesses, not the least being problems with their dog's skeleton.**

For example, if we indiscriminately supplement with calcium this will depress the uptake of other minerals, particularly zinc. If we try to correct this problem by adding extra zinc to the diet, we run the risk of depressing the uptake of a whole host of other nutrients - including calcium, selenium, chromium etc. etc.. And so the problem compounds.

On top of all of that there are many 'unknown' nutrients present in a natural diet. We do not yet have the knowledge to be able to replace them by adding supplements to modern artificial diets.

As I have mentioned, the impossible technical name for the bone problems caused by an all meat diet is **Nutritional Hyperparathyroidism.** Forget the name. It is not important. Just remember that an all meat diet causes heaps of problems, not the least being weak bendy calcium deficient bones.

For the record, if you have produced such a puppy, the best diet you can use to correct the problem [with your vet's help of course], is the properly balanced diet based on raw meaty bones.

Bone problems and deficient diets in the smaller breeds

A common reason that smaller breeds of dogs develop bone problems is because they teach their owners, who are often [but not necessarily] elderly, to feed them badly. Commonly a calcium deficient high protein, mostly cooked meat diet. Cooked meat is even worse than raw meat when it is all that is fed. Vitamins are lost as are the amino acids lysine and methionine during the cooking process.

The nutritional problems are made worse when such pups spend most of their time indoors, out of direct sunlight. This means they miss out on their vitamin D which is absolutely essential for normal bone growth.

In place of nice healthy bones to chew on, many of these pups often live a life filled with an endless round of sweet biscuits, chocolate treats, cups of tea, and possibly weekly doses of paraffin oil "to keep them regular".

Eventually, or perhaps invariably, these pups suffer from a number of deficiencies, including calcium, and vitamins A and D. This is commonly accompanied by obesity. I have also seen pups fed this way become very thin and develop severe bowel problems such as inflammatory bowel disease.

All of this is further complicated by either no exercise or incorrect exercise ...

... including a complete lack of chewing exercise [they do not eat bones]. Such pups are always being picked up. These pups suffer an almost complete lack of such activities as **aerobics, body building and anything that might remotely be construed as healthy play, except unfortunately for the following.**

The owners of these small dogs being fed deficient diets which encourage skeletal disease, often further encourage skeletal problems by ensuring that the only consistent exercise allowed is jumping around on the hind legs. This will contribute in no small way to bowed legs which may ultimately result in slipping patellas. See Chapter Twenty for a full description of this problem.

The other common problem which can result from a combination of one of these deficient sort of diets and excessive trauma to the hind legs, is damage to the growth plate in the femoral head. This may unfortunately result in degeneration of the femoral head, which is known as - Legg-Perthes Disease. See Chapter Twenty One for a full description of this problem.

Between kneecaps that won't stay in their groove and femoral heads that want to disintegrate and rot away, many small dogs eventually end their puppyhood with totally deformed hind legs which require drastic corrective surgery.

In summary, the best way to produce bone problems in the smaller breeds is to make sure your little dog is overweight and then combine that with the following: an all meat calcium deficient diet with insufficient sunlight and therefore no vitamin D, lots of standing on hind legs with very little other exercise, general malnutrition, including lots of sweet biscuits, and finally lots of cooked and processed meats. This is a sure fire recipe for skeletal problems, particularly in the hind legs.

Now of course, all this happens to varying degrees in different households. It all depends on the pup's genetic background, the diet of its parents and the dietary ideas of the owners involved, including the types of bones fed. For example feeding lamb shanks often leads to an all meat diet in smaller dogs because they just eat the meat off them without actually eating the bone.

Other contributing factors include the sort of things the owner allows or encourages the puppy to do by way of running, jumping etc., the weight of the pup, and whether those pups ever get out into the sun. Not only that, where pups are given a regular dose of paraffin, this further depletes their vitamin A, D, E and K intake.

However, the most basic cause of all these problems may be stated as a failure to feed raw meaty bones as the basis of the diet. The practice of bone feeding compensates for a wide range of feeding, exercising and genetic errors.

The final point I want to make about these little breeds of dogs is that the bandy legs and the slipping patellas are said to be inherited. As I have said elsewhere in this book, heredity does have a vital underlying role in every one of these Juvenile Bone Diseases. However, the vast majority of bone disease is caused by accumulated errors of management which have as the basic error the failure to feed raw meaty bones. These bandy legs are also very much influenced by diet and exercise as well as heredity.

A happy conclusion

The good news is that it is possible for a puppy to completely recover from the alterations in Endochondral Ossification or deranged bone growth caused by deficient diets, if those diets are corrected early enough.

However, BE WARNED! Do not start a stunted puppy on high quantities of food, even if it is the correct diet. Keep the growth rate down, because a stunted puppy allowed to grow at maximum growth rate will undergo a compensatory growth spurt. This is a sure way to cause bone problems due to a too rapid growth rate - to be described shortly.

Further good news is that as I have already mentioned, not too many people do this to puppies these days. This is particularly true of the larger breeds. Unfortunately many owners of the smaller breeds continue to feed these highly deficient diets. This is not done out of malice of course. They are completely unaware of the harm they are doing, in fact it is almost always done in the name of love and kindness.

One good thing about these deficient diets is that with the smaller breeds, you can get away with feeding them badly - for much longer than is possible with the larger breeds - without too much damage done. It does eventually catch up of course. If not during the puppy stage, then later as an adult dog, when arthritis rears its ugly head, often accompanied by severe obesity, and a multitude of related problems.

We now leave Old Fashioned Osteochondrosis and move on to examine the disease Osteochondritis Dissecans, which is the first of a number of skeletal diseases that develop from the basic skeletal disease of Modern Osteochondrosis.

CHAPTER TWELVE

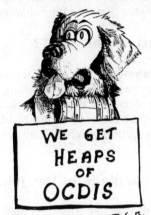

WE GET
HEAPS
OF
OCDIS
I.G.B.

OSTEOCHONDRITIS DISSECANS
OR
OCDIS

What is Osteochondritis Dissecans or OCDIS?

Osteochondritis Dissecans is a worsening or further development of the basic skeletal problem of Osteochondrosis. It is a problem which can affect a large number of joints and is a common cause of lameness in young large breed dogs. Pups are not born with this problem. They develop it after birth. This means that ...

... OCDIS is a developmental disease

In common with all other alterations in normal skeletal development, it is a result of excesses of nutrition and exercise. A disease of faulty management. Like all the skeletal problems in growing pups there are genes which predispose a growing dog [pup] to this problem. They include the genes for large size, heavy weight, fast growth, small muscles, obesity, and bad engineering.

307

There may be other genes which act independently of management, The direct genes. Their existence is unproven, however, if they exist, it is these genes which must be eliminated. The bottom line to preventing OCDIS is that it is best controlled by management rather than genetic manipulation.

What actually happens to the joint?

You will recall that Osteochondrosis involves a thickening and a failure of the mineralisation of the growing points in young bones. The growing points become abnormally thick and soft and weak. If Osteochondrosis is not halted by rectifying the excesses of nutrition and calcium and exercise which cause it, one of the conditions which may result is Osteochondritis Dissecans. OCDIS.

OCDIS occurs in the cartilage in the joint .....

..... That sick cartilage becomes sicker and develops small fissures which penetrate to the underlying bone. This means that Osteochondrosis has gone one step further and become Osteochondritis Dissecans [OCDIS].

When the thickened non-calcified cartilage fissures, it results in joint inflammation, pain and lameness. A piece of that sick cartilage now begins to break away from the underlying bone leaving a raw and gaping hole in the bone.

The flap of cartilage which tears away can become partially or totally detached from the underlying bone. Next to this thickened joint cartilage there develops extra bone and next to the extra bone you see bone thinning. This form of OCDIS was first described in the shoulder.

The damage done to the cartilage in the joint by this process will in the long term result in degenerative joint disease [Osteoarthritis] and may even result in permanent lameness. This is seen as joint swelling. If radiographs are taken at this later stage, extra bony growths or osteophytes are seen in the joint.

The lameness is hardly noticed – at first

It usually starts between 7 and 10 months of age, although it can be seen earlier. Once lameness has started it is usually constant - i.e. present every day, and can be slowly progressive.

The degree of lameness is mild to moderate, and may be most obvious when the animal gets up to walk or run. Lameness is usually present on both sides, although one side is usually worse than the other. In fact, owners usually report to their vet that the dog is lame on one side. The problem does not cause the animal to run a temperature or become ill in any way. Males are affected more commonly than females.

What Joints or bones does OCDIS affect?

OCDIS has the potential to affect most of the major joints of the limbs. **The joints commonly affected are the shoulder, the hock or ankle, the knee or stifle, and the elbow.** Other, less common sites include the wrist or carpus, the hip and possibly the vertebrae and ribs.

The joint in which OCDIS was first described and which is still the one most commonly affected is the shoulder joint. Here, it will damage not only the humerus, but also the opposing scapula. Where owners follow the BARF programme for pups, and strictly adhere to the limited food approach, this problem, in common with other skeletal problems, disappears.

OCDIS in the elbow joint is receiving much attention as a major part of the Elbow Dysplasia complex. As with Hip Dysplasia, Elbow Dysplasia is being labelled a genetic problem.Unfortunately, while ever we rely solely on genetics to get rid of Elbow and Hip Dysplasia, we cannot expect any great success - not in the short term anyway. In fact, getting rid of the problem that way will be almost impossible.

The problem of Elbow Dysplasia is discussed in Chapter Fourteen.

Diagnosing OCDIS

Early diagnosis is vital. The earlier skeletal problems can be diagnosed, the greater the chance of a successful treatment and a return to normality. This is particularly true with OCDIS.

Too many puppy owners ignore the lameness until it is severe, unrelenting, and major damage has occurred to the joint. With any skeletal problem, it is best to detect it early in the Osteochondrosis phase - before it turns into something worse such as OCDIS.

Pressure on the growing points can be detected in a lame dog long before there are physical changes which are able to be detected by radiographs.

This is the ideal time to detect and put a stop to the possibility of OCDIS.

As OCDIS worsens, pain will be detected by hyperextending or straightening out the affected joint. At this stage you will also note that the muscles of that limb have begun to waste due to lack of use. By palpating or feeling the joints of the elbow, hock [ankle], or stifle [knee], it may be possible to detect a thickening of the joint capsule or a swelling of the joint due to extra joint fluid. These are not always found and cannot be detected with a deep joint such as the shoulder.

Radiography

Once the OCDIS has advanced sufficiently in a given joint, radiography will clinch the diagnosis. Once you have a radiographic diagnosis you know that the problem is advanced and serious. Let me emphasise the importance of not ignoring any pain or lameness in young pups, particularly pups of the giant breeds. Once these problems start, they must be detected early so that positive steps of diet and exercise can be taken BEFORE we have a radiographic diagnosis.

Treating OCDIS

Treatment may involve surgery, it almost certainly will involve drugs such as pentosan polysulphate, and it should most definitely involve adoption of the BARF programme for Skeletal Disease.

Surgery is only necessary when the problem is advanced

The immediate aim of surgery is to explore the joint and seek out and remove any fragments which may be contributing to the dog's pain and lameness. These fragments are either still attached or running around free within the joint. A piece that runs around free within the joint is known as a joint mouse. This is a piece of cartilage which can eventually become calcified, or it may reattach, or migrate within the joint. Depending on their location, joint mice will cause periods of pain followed by freedom from pain.

The long term aim of surgery is to slow down progression of the disease process by removing the dead and damaged tissue and scraping the bone back to fresh healthy tissue. This will help prevent the development of Osteoarthritis or degenerative joint disease.

However, if surgery is not teamed with a regenerative diet - the BARF diet - the progression of degenerative joint disease is highly likely. This is particularly so where one of the dry foods - especially the super premium foods - is employed. With their high levels of damaged fats and their high levels of grain, they are a perfect recipe for promoting arthritis and therefore continuing the problem.

With OCDIS of the shoulder, surgery is the usual remedy except for small lesions, caught early with no flap and only mild lameness. The advantage of surgery is that the patient is usually sound within two months. Also, by operating you are avoiding future degenerative joint disease.

With Stifle OCDIS - surgery is mostly of benefit, with seventy five percent returning to normal after surgery. This particular form of OCDIS is moderately difficult to detect without radiography. There are not many clinical signs to help its detection.

OCDIS of the hock joint is a problem seen commonly in the Rottweiler and Labrador Retriever.The result will not be good, whether surgery is done or not. There will be a lot of lameness which ever way you go. So let me say once again, that by managing our pups correctly, this problem should not appear. The best results are obtained when the surgery is done early, hopefully before degenerative joint disease has set in. However, even if surgery is done, the probability of degenerative joint disease or Osteoarthritis appearing is very high.

If surgery is performed after one year of age, it is usually too late because degenerative joint disease is already present.

Sometimes, when hock OCDIS has been left to proceed to a really advanced stage of degenerative joint disease, it becomes necessary to fuse the whole joint together. This is called arthrodesis. Such a procedure is termed a salvage procedure. This is only used when all else has failed - apart from euthanasia.

Treatment of Elbow OCDIS

This is part of the Elbow Dysplasia complex and is dealt with in Chapter Fourteen.

With mild cases where surgery is not indicated ...

... conservative therapy must be started as early as possible. This means abandoning the current method of feeding, and adopting the BARF programme as outlined in Chapter Twenty Two.

In a nutshell the modified BARF programme for OCDIS involves the high vegetable low calorie BARF diet, total rest, weight loss and the use of drugs such as pentosan polysulphate. This means a decrease in raw meaty bones [compared to the usual BARF programme] and an increase in crushed vegetables. Naturally all calcium supplementation will stop, and exercise will be almost totally curtailed. This modified BARF programme will continue until the dog has been sound for a couple of months. Then return to the normal BARF programme for pups.

Let me stress once again that if the BARF programme is used in place of the conventional dietary programme, the prognosis is much improved.

What can we conclude about OCDIS?

- Firstly, let's avoid it all together by adopting the BARF programme to raise our pups.

- If the problem is already in existence, let's detect it early before any great damage is done.

- If the problem does occur, no matter whether surgery is required or not, give the dog maximum chance of recovery by switching it to the BARF programme for skeletal disease.

Our next chapter deals with the dreaded HIP DYSPLASIA!

CHAPTER THIRTEEN

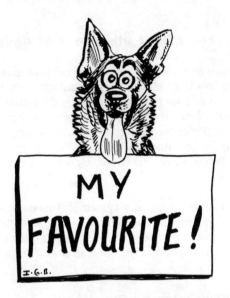

HIP DYSPLASIA

The word "dysplasia" means badly formed. Dogs with Hip Dysplasia have badly formed hips. These badly formed hips are the direct result of a loose fit between the head of the thigh bone or femur, and the socket in the hip bone.

Dysplastic hips can give birth to a host of problems

Eventually those loosely fitting or sloppy hips become badly shaped. More like a cup and saucer and less like a ball and socket. Such hips can severely reduce a dog's usefulness and happiness, with the dog in constant pain. This can intensify to become severe and crippling. There may be a reduction in mobility, with the consequent development of arthritis or Degenerative Joint Disease. Eventually there may be total immobility.

For the owner of a dysplastic dog there is a sharp rise in the costs associated with keeping the dog. These include not only medical and surgical costs, but also emotional costs.

Hip Dysplasia can affect all breeds of dogs

However, it is **more commonly seen in the large or giant breeds**. It is not common in breeds less than 11 kg. It is particularly common in dogs having endomorphic features. That is, dogs which tend to smaller, weaker, softer muscles. Dogs with lots of body fat that gain weight easily and have trouble losing it, such as Saint Bernards, Rottweilers, Labradors, Golden Retrievers etc. It is less common in the more heavily muscled breeds - the so called ectomorphs such as Great Danes, Doberman Pinschers or Greyhounds.

Hip Dysplasia does not cause any systemic illness. It affects both sexes equally. The problem may be detected as early as eight weeks, although abnormal walking patterns are not usually seen before 5 or 6 months of age. It can also appear at any later stage of life.

No puppy is born with Hip Dysplasia

Hip Dysplasia is a problem which develops after birth.

Pups that develop Hip Dysplasia have hip joints that become progressively sloppier or looser, and the muscles surrounding the hip become poorly developed and do not hold the hip joint firmly in position.

Puppies which do not develop Hip Dysplasia are seen to have well developed muscles surrounding the hip joint. These muscles hold the nicely rounded ball part of the hip joint deeply and firmly within the socket part. There is no pain and there is complete freedom of movement of that whole limb, of that dog's spine and associated muscles, in fact of its whole body. This is a healthy dog with healthy hips.

There are two basic kinds of Hip Dysplasia

The severe acute form and the mild chronic form.

The severe acute form of Hip Dysplasia ...

... occurs early in life. It produces pain, weakness, extreme muscle wasting of the hind limbs, an abnormal gait with a wide rump that sways from side to side, a refusal to walk very far, bunny hopping at the run, and a reluctance to climb stairs. There may even be a clicking sound when walking.

Unless the problem is due to trauma in one leg, both hind legs are usually affected, although it is not uncommon for one leg to be more lame than the other. The disturbance to an animal's gait can vary from almost no disturbance to badly affected. It rarely causes total immobility in a young dog. The back is arched rather than flat. The hips appear to be broad, but the hind legs are held close to each other, much straighter than normal.

Most of the weight is taken on the front legs with the hind legs tip-toed. The elbows point outwards. Stretching the hind legs out in any direction can be painful. For that reason your vet may have to use sedation or anaesthesia to physically detect that the joint is loose rather than being a tight snug fit.

Initially, these disturbances of gait may not be easy to detect, but with time they become difficult to ignore. Sometimes the signs of Hip Dysplasia can occur quite suddenly. All at once the pup is in pain, is not able to stand easily and is reluctant to join in walking or running. It will not climb stairs. In the young dog, the problem is mostly one of weak hind legs. The pup or dog with Hip Dysplasia fatigues rapidly.

So what is going on in those hips to make them loose and dysplastic?

There is little doubt that some breeds, the larger breeds, have a genetic tendency to looseness of the hips. However, there is also little doubt that much of that looseness is environmental. It does not have to be.

Those loose hips begin in the whelping box with a heavy pup sliding around on slippery newspaper. They become progressively looser as that puppy eats slop and receives no isometric exercise because it does not eat raw meaty bones. This is where not only loose hips are encouraged, but weak and small muscles are developed.

The looseness of the hips is amplified by rapid growth, excessive weight and overly exuberant and prolonged exercise which is combined with excessively soft and malleable bones. From this point it is all downhill.

A combination of the sloppy fit between the femur and the hip, together with the weight and movement of the pup, and very easily moulded young bones causes the joint to become progressively more like a cup and saucer, rather than a ball in a socket.

As this happens, the muscles and supportive tissues which surround the joint become weaker and stretched. This occurs partly because the bones grow faster than those tissues, stretching them, and partly due to a deterioration of those tissues.

Accompanying these changes is pain and reduced mobility. There is microscopic damage to the muscles and growing parts of the bone combined with chiropractic or spinal mobility faults. Sometimes the whole back end of the dog fuses into an immobile mass. With reduced use, muscles, bones and joints continue to deteriorate.

Radiographs may show loose hips, shallow sockets, flat femoral heads, and bony growths round the joints. Paradoxically, some dogs show very little change from normal. Some quite reasonable looking hips on radiographs are very painful for the dog, while awful looking hips can be found in a dog that is functionally quite normal.

Much of this damage is healed by the time the dog is 12 to 15 months of age. Such dogs will appear to be much sounder although not fully normal. At about eighteen months of age, radiographs will show little bony growths round the edges of the hip joint. Degenerative joint disease has begun. As time passes, these dogs progressively lose joint cartilage and develop further bony growths round the joint. They show increasing pain, stiffness and mobility problems. They are moving into the ...

... chronic form of Hip Dysplasia

In many dogs, Hip Dysplasia will not appear to be present, or be diagnosed, until old age. At this time it will appear as chronic degenerative joint disease. This is the more common form of Hip Dysplasia. It starts as difficulty in rising, restricted movement of the hind limbs, pain, stiffness and lameness after either unaccustomed activity or periods of rest.

In time all of these signs will worsen with the condition progressing to become severely debilitating. The unfortunate dog will have extreme muscle wasting and hind quarter contracture. Now we have crippling degenerative joint disease.

This dreadful disease – Hip Dysplasia – can go today!

... if we go about getting rid of it correctly. Unfortunately this is not happening. We have been attempting to get rid of Hip Dysplasia for about fifty years with very little success.

The veterinary profession has a programme which aims to identify animals with loose hips. We assume that such animals have genes for Hip Dysplasia, while dogs diagnosed as having sound hips don't have these genes. The dogs with the loose and/or dysplastic hips are then culled from the breeding programme, the aim being to get rid of the genes which cause Hip Dysplasia. It is assumed that the dogs with sound hips do not have these genes.

Unfortunately, all of the dogs we kill or cull have precisely the same number and type of genes for Hip Dysplasia as the dogs we keep. The mere presence of genes for Hip Dysplasia does not cause the problem to occur. There are other factors involved. This is the key which unravels the mystery of why Hip Dysplasia sometimes appears and at other times not.

Whether the Hip Dysplasia lies dormant or surfaces as clinical disease depends on how pups are managed during their growing period. If they are managed well, it lies dormant. If they are fed badly and are exercised incorrectly, the problem surfaces.

Unfortunately, as this happens time and time again, this feature of the disease is ignored. The highly suspect assumption continues to be made that the problem is entirely genetic.

That is why the eradication programme is not working. As a profession we have not realised that Hip Dysplasia is in essence a management problem. While ever we seek a genetic solution, AND seek to keep our breeds as they are - ie large, heavy, fast growing, obese, and badly engineered - the problem will not go away.

Hip Dysplasia is often thought of as a 'special case'

That it is a disease 'quite different to all the other skeletal diseases we see in young dogs.' That it bears very little relationship to them.

In fact the origins of Hip Dysplasia are precisely the same as all the other skeletal diseases we see in young dogs.

That being the case, the problem is solved. Hip Dysplasia can be prevented and therefore eliminated in exactly the same way as these other diseases by using sound management.

Once this is understood, our extensive Hip Dysplasia schemes will become almost redundant.

Let me begin the case for this point of view by asking the question ...

What causes Hip Dysplasia?

Hip Dysplasia is a worsening of the basic problem of alterations in Endochondral Ossification or Osteochondrosis. In other words it is no different to - but is simply a particular example of - all the other skeletal problems we see in young, large, fast growing dogs.

This makes Hip Dysplasia a problem caused mostly by faulty management.

Underlying this disease is the presence of predisposing genes. Genes which I have labelled indirect genes. These are the major genes associated with this disease and they only function to produce Hip Dysplasia in the presence of excessive dietary regimes and incorrect exercise. These indirect genes include the genes for large size, heavy weight, rapid growth, obesity, poor muscling and bad engineering.

There may be other genes which act independently of management, which I have labelled direct genes. Their existence is unproven, as is their role in the production of this problem.

However, what I have just told you - is not the official view.

Unfortunately, most vets say ... "Hip Dysplasia is a hereditary disease"

This is the official veterinary view and it is our greatest stumbling block when it comes to eradicating the disease. That label prevents the dog world from solving the riddle of Hip Dysplasia which was first reported as a rare disease in the 1930's and has since spread through our dog population, until today it is one of the most frequent and vexing problems our dogs suffer. **We have not beaten it. It keeps coming back, despite massive campaigns to eradicate it.**

To control a problem we must know the precise cause. That is, all the factors involved. Not just some of them. Although we have amassed an enormous body of data on this disease, and know more about it than most other problems facing our clients' animals, we have not pin-pointed the cause with crystal clear accuracy. As a profession we have not put this 'jig saw puzzle' together. That is why we are no closer to eliminating the problem than we were fifty years ago.

Nowhere is this situation made more clear than in the April 1993 edition of 'Veterinary Practice Nurse.' In this publication, veterinary surgeon John Foster, who is a member of the panel for the British Veterinary Association Kennel Club Hip Dysplasia Control Scheme, heads an article on Hip Dysplasia with this provocative title ...

'HIP DYSPLASIA - HERE TO STAY'

He states that it is a "big problem" and that it will "never be eliminated." He points out that in many breeds, if the strict breeding criteria his panel recommends for eliminating the problem were adhered to - "many breeds would cease to exist."

If we continue along the same path we have trod for the last fifty years, I would have to agree with this gentleman. However, there is a simple solution. To get to that solution, let me begin by asking the question ...

... Does the veterinary profession believe that genes are one hundred percent of the problem?

No it does not. We know that management is involved. We acknowledge that diet and exercise can influence the development and course of Hip Dysplasia. However errors in these two areas have never been regarded as the major cause, or the means by which the problem could be controlled or eradicated. **This is despite the fact that these factors are responsible for 60% - 80% of the problem while genes control only 20% - 40% of the problem.**

The only thing we do not currently realise is that the 20% - 40% cannot be eliminated without making drastic alterations to the breed. [See Chapter Seven for a full explanation of this statement.]

It gets worse. Even if we did realise the pivotal importance of correct management, as a profession we have no worthwhile management alternatives. All we have to offer is commercial dog food and calcium supplements. Because we have only these to offer, we cannot help clients make worthwhile managerial changes. It seems we have no option but to stick to our gene theory. **But it gets worse ...**

We cannot even tell accurately which dogs have Hip Dysplasia!

Numerous studies have shown that except for the PennHIP method, not one method we currently use to detect Hip Dysplasia or predict its future occurrence, has any useful degree of accuracy. The PennHIP method could - if it replaced the other methods - tell us which dogs do actually have loose hips, and therefore do actually have the ability to develop Hip Dysplasia. **The problem is, that is about all it will tell us.**

We still cannot distinguish Genotype from Phenotype

Even if we do adopt the PennHIP method and and can with a fair degree of confidence decide which dogs do in fact have loose hips - that is have the potential for developing Hip Dysplasia - **this does not tell us whether the basic cause of those loose hips was genetic [genotype], or environmental.**

In other words, just because we can measure something, that does not automatically tell us what caused it.

Just because we can say - yes - this dog has loose hips - that does not automatically tell us that the problem was caused by bad genes!

Yet that is the assumption we vets - as a profession - automatically make! This is very bad science. This is a very poor application of our knowledge of genetics.

When the radiographs of a dog's hips show that dog to be dysplastic - with very few exceptions, those radiographs are simply demonstrating the end result of poor management in the presence of genes which allow skeletal problems to surface.

Hip Dysplasia is fundamentally the same as any other bone problem in growing puppies. It is a disease caused by poor management. That is - faulty nutrition and faulty exercise.

The point at which a puppy's genes become involved in producing skeletal disease is where the decision is made as to which particular type of juvenile bone disease is going to evolve. Even that decision is a 'joint' one between the genes and the type and extent of the **mismanagement** a puppy owner perpetrates.

Could Hip Dysplasia have been prevented in this pup?

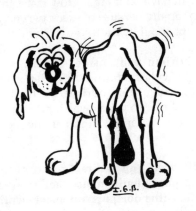

To help you see the absurdity of labelling Hip Dysplasia as being solely genetic, I want to take you through the development of this problem in a young puppy that has been diagnosed with reasonably bad Hip Dysplasia.
See over the page.

Would Hip Dysplasia have been prevented in this pup if it had been grown slowly on a natural or biologically appropriate diet based on raw meaty bones without any calcium supplements and without being over exercised? That is, raised on the BARF programme. Or was it inevitable?

Why DID its hip joints become sloppy and painful? Did the puppy have genes which said "these joints WILL become sloppy and painful" or did the joints become that way because of external pressures such as a very heavy pup doing lots of hard exercise, combined with internal weaknesses due to poor nutrition?

Why ARE the tissues which surround the joint stretched and weak? Is it because that puppy had a set of genes which said "these tissues WILL become stretched and weak", or did they become that way because of an over-weight heavily exercised pup whose bones were growing very rapidly, but were not strong enough to support a body that was far too heavy?

Why DID the muscles which surround the hip joint become poorly developed? Is it because the puppy had a set of genes which said "the only way these hip muscles will develop is poorly"? Or did the muscles develop poorly because of inadequate exercise from birth, together with pain in the hind legs which resulted in less use being made of these muscles?

Why DID the bone grow faster than the muscles? Did this poor puppy have a set of genes which said "this puppy will have bones that grow faster than its muscles"? Or did that bone grow too rapidly because of excessive energy in the diet, and hormonal changes brought about by excessive calcium?

Why ARE the bones which make up the hip joint badly made? That is, either softer or more malleable than normal, particularly during the earlier stages of the problem, or harder and less malleable than normal, particularly during the later stages of the disease? Is it due to genes which say "this is the way it will be no matter what," or is this abnormal situation once again due to inappropriate diet and exercise?

In other words, are those sloppy malformed hips a direct result of that unfortunate puppy inheriting a mass of poor quality genes 'hell bent' on wrecking its bones, or does the answer lie with poor puppy management?

These questions are obvious, fundamental and vital, yet not one person involved in the Hip Dysplasia eradication schemes ever bothers to give them a thought.

There is little evidence to support the theory that a mass of genes hell bent on wrecking a dog's bones will cause Hip Dysplasia come what may. Come good nutrition or bad nutrition. Appropriate exercise or excessive exercise.

To help you understand this let us briefly review the two types of genes which cause Hip Dysplasia , the indirect genes and the direct genes .....

The genes which indirectly cause Hip Dysplasia are very common

Indirect genes are the genes for large size, fast growth, heavy weight, obesity, small muscles and poor engineering.

Indirect genes are the the major genetic cause of Hip Dysplasia, and are the genes we have been trying to remove - so unsuccessfully - with our radiography, hip scoring and culling. Unfortunately this has been a pointless exercise for two reasons.

Firstly, the indirect genes will not produce Hip Dysplasia without the presence of triggering environmental factors including - incorrect nutrition and inappropriate exercise.

Secondly, the indirect genes are also the genes which make a breed what it is. They are responsible for the major characteristics of the dog in which they are found. Given time, they could be removed, but the price would be unacceptably high. The price would be the loss of the breed and its replacement with something very close to a breed like a greyhound.

The genes which directly cause Hip Dysplasia are relatively rare ...

... if they exist at all, yet these are the genes we - the veterinary profession and dog breeders - should be trying to remove. Why? Because if these genes exist, they will most definitely cause Hip Dysplasia - with or without faulty management. The only problem is, we are not totally convinced that these direct genes exist!

As a profession we also have no idea how to diagnose which dogs might have these direct genes, and if they do have them, as a profession we have no idea how to differentiate these direct genes from the indirect genes.

So how do we get rid of Hip Dysplasia?

Because Hip Dysplasia is one of the many forms of modern Osteochondrosis, and   modern Osteochondrosis is a developmental disease related to physical and dietary excesses, all we need do is stop these excesses, and the problem disappears!

By raising pups as Nature or God or Evolution intended on a biologically appropriate diet - the BARF diet - in limited amounts with appropriate exercise, most pups of any breed will grow to be free of Hip Dysplasia.

Where a dog develops the problem when raised this way - THAT IS THE TIME   to eliminate that individual. It carries   those directly acting genes. The ones we do not want. The problem is solved!

We are quite capable of eliminating Hip Dysplasia - along with the vast majority of the other skeletal diseases in young dogs today, including Elbow Dysplasia - by adopting the oh so simple BARF programme.

These very simple, very obvious and very practical facts have been staring us in the face since the disease was first recognised. Sadly, we have ignored them.

Much of the evidence to support the view that management is the key to eliminating Hip Dysplasia is found in the preceding chapters. However, because Hip Dysplasia is such an important disease, we need to revisit some of that   evidence, and also consider other pertinent research that relates directly to Hip Dysplasia itself.

I will briefly present some of my experiences with Hip Dysplasia, the role of diet, the role of physical damage and then we will look at what a number of breeders have 'discovered' regarding the control of both Hip and Elbow Dysplasia.

These breeders have discovered that management is the key to solving the problem. However, for reasons politic, that knowledge is being suppressed, and is being used to prop up the genetic theory instead.

My experience with this disease .....

I have been involved in breeding Great Danes, Rottweilers, Fox Terriers and Toy Poodles. I have raised several hundred other puppies across a wide spectrum of breeds and crosses. I have supervised the growth of thousands of puppies owned by clients. I have questioned the owners of other dogs whose growth I had not supervised. This I have combined with my training as a veterinary surgeon and my research into commercial and natural diets.

This mass of data has convinced me that although Hip Dysplasia - and other skeletal problems in large breeds - has a hereditary basis, there is no way breeding is going to eliminate it in the foreseeable future......

That is why I have for the last 16 years approached all skeletal problems in pups as if they were not inherited, but caused by improper feeding and improper exercise. The results have been seemingly miraculous.

The problem has largely disappeared when this approach is taken

When I switched my dogs from processed food to a BARF type diet, their skeletal problems quietly disappeared. I went from experiencing and observing numerous problems including Osteochondrosis and Hip and Elbow Dysplasia, to seeing pups with no bone problems whatsoever. The management changes had been mostly dietary, together with a reduction of exercise, so that play and eating exercise was all that was allowed.

This has been demonstrated time and time again. Any puppy can grow to be totally free of skeletal disease by being managed correctly while growing, or it can develop skeletal disease including Hip Dysplasia by the use of poor management. It is that simple. Hip Dysplasia or one of the other skeletal diseases can be produced at will or prevented at will by simple alterations in management.

Diet and Hip Dysplasia

The common dietary errors which produce modern Osteochondrosis also produce Hip Dysplasia. They include feeding excessive calcium and overfeeding with diets containing excessive protein and calories to produce rapid growth and obesity.

Many of the super premium puppy foods fed to excess are used to produce these conditions.

Any breed, but more particularly the larger or giant breeds, grown at their maximum growth rate , will become too heavy too quickly. Their bones become unable to properly support them. This results in skeletal disease which can include misshapen hips - Hip Dysplasia.

Overfeeding puppies to produce obesity will by itself, or combined with excessive exercise, cause weak hip muscles and stretched joint capsules. Both these errors will also result in hip joints that become misshapen - leading to abnormal mobility of the hip joints and pain. Those pups have Hip Dysplasia.

Experiments have shown that Great Danes fed a commercial diet which was balanced in all respects except that it had excessive calcium [and this was only at a level equal to that found in most of the popular brands of dry dog food], all developed numerous bone problems including Hip Dysplasia. The control group with levels of calcium that did not exceed 2% of the dry matter - did not develop the disease.

Another group of Danes fed a well balanced commercial diet ad lib [that is **they were over fed**] all developed bone problems including Hip Dysplasia, whereas those dogs who ate the same food but in limited amounts, which resulted in a slower growth rate and no obesity, did not develop any bone disease.

The severity of existing Hip Dysplasia can be altered drastically and easily by changes in management. The Hip Dysplasia can be made to either disappear or worsen, depending on the changes made. If the change is to more food, more rapid growth, greater calcium supplementation, greater obesity of the pup and a sharp increase in heavy exercise, the problem will worsen.

The most popular method currently being used to promote bone disease including Hip Dysplasia in pups is to feed the specially formulated super premium growth foods for pups. The high calorific value and the high protein levels in these awful products together with their damaged essential fatty acids is a sure fire recipe for bone problems. Some of them also compound the problem with excessive calcium.

If pups are to grow up to be free of Hip Dysplasia they must be held back, kept slim, grown very slowly so that they reach their mature body weight many months later than is the currently accepted norm. This must be done with a good diet - not with a poor quality diet as has become accepted practice in some circles

In other words, to avoid Hip Dysplasia, the diet we should be feeding will be one that actually encourages healthy bones and joints, prevents a rapid growth rate, prevents obesity and does not allow the consumption of excess calcium. This turns out to be the BARF diet - for pups - as outlined in Chapter Twenty Two.

Physical damage as a cause of Hip Dysplasia

Hip Dysplasia has been produced experimentally by loosening the hip joints of young puppies. The pups were three days old when they had their hip joints loosened, and they were kept that way for six months. Every one of those pups developed Hip Dysplasia. Other pups from the same litter had their hip joints kept nice and tight for the first six months of their lives. The disease did not appear in those pups.

It is now well accepted that if you can keep a pup's hip joints properly formed and tight and therefore free of Dysplasia for the first six to nine months of its life, no matter how good or bad its parents' hips were, it will not develop Hip Dysplasia.

If a puppy is observed to have developed loose hips, no matter what the cause, and is caught early enough, the clinical signs of Hip Dysplasia can still be eliminated.This has been achieved by keeping the puppy slim and keeping it confined to a small cage or similar till six months of age.

In other words, even if the Dysplasia process has started, its progress can be arrested. To do this, it is vital to keep exercise to a minimum. Puppies treated this way will develop much tighter hips and have only slightly dysplastic or near perfect hips as an adult.

The most popular and practical method of wrecking a young pup's hips with physical trauma is to take it on long boring exhaustive walks. This will help mould those loose hips into that nice familiar cup and saucer shape of the dysplastic dog.

If you wish to avoid damage to a young dog's hips through correct exercise ...

... the exercise you must encourage is - **play and eating exercise. The play must not** be too boisterous. It must be play that will stop when the pup wants it to. That way, no abnormal or excess pressures will be placed on growth plates or joint cartilages or tissues surrounding the joints - including the muscles. That means no chance of causing Hip Dysplasia by traumatic means.

If you wish to start a dog on the right track to sound hips, then you must start in the whelping box. Pups must be weaned using a surface that gives them traction, such as earth or wood shavings. Definitely not slippery newspaper.

If you wish to grow a pup's bones and joints strong and tight, then wean them using raw meaty bones, starting at about three weeks of age, and continue that practice of feeding your dogs raw meaty bones for the rest of their lives. This eating exercise which starts in the whelping box is the beginning of sound strong normally functioning bones and joints.

Breeders' momentous discovery

What I want to do now is look at what a number of breeders have 'discovered' regarding the control of this problem.

These breeders have discovered that management is the key to solving the problem However, that knowledge is largely being suppressed, and is being used to prop up the genetic theory instead. The story begins with statistics ...

Statistical research implies degrees of apparent improvement recorded by kennels participating in Hip and Elbow Dysplasia eradication schemes.

Participants in these schemes agree to cull any animal with radiographic signs of Hip Dysplasia. The statistics from these schemes show that puppies derived from parents with bad hips are more likely to develop Hip Dysplasia than puppies from parents with normal hips and that parents with normal hips are more likely to produce pups with normal hips.

In other words, the Hip Dysplasia Eradication scheme appears to be having some sort of success.

This moderate success appears to confirm that Hip Dysplasia is indeed a problem that can be solved using genetics. That the programme is making some genuine genetic headway.

However, it pays to be cautious when dealing with statistics.

Statistics are used by many people in much the same way as a drunk uses a lamp post. Less for illumination and more for support.

Things in the dog world are not always as they seem. Hip Dysplasia schemes are no exception. **The generally better hips submitted for evaluation,** which indicates an increasing soundness of succeeding generations of dogs, are not necessarily due to genetic improvement.

Please explain!

It does not take breeders in Hip Dysplasia schemes long to recognise which of their dogs is dysplastic. Those dogs are never radiographed. That produces an instant improvement in the statistics **AND** the status of their kennel. It also eliminates individual dogs with the problem. This would be fine if that method eliminated unwanted genes. But it doesn't. It simply removes a dog which developed Hip Dysplasia because it was raised badly.

We see more of the same turning up in the next generation. They too are disposed of but the problem remains.

However, breeders do more than this

Serious breeders striving to eliminate Hip Dysplasia will not only seek to use genetics to improve their stock. Many other approaches are examined. As a result, many breeders have discovered the importance of management. They discover in whole or in part such things as the role of supplementary calcium, growth rate, calorie and protein content, and the role that exercise plays in the production of skeletal disease.

From their discoveries they evolve a system of management that becomes their trade secret.' Naturally that system is rarely discussed or shared with any one outside that particular kennel. They do not even tell their vet.

The only people those breeders share their "management secrets" with are the new owners of their puppies, particularly if those pups are going to be show dogs and carry on the name and reputation of the original breeder.

When the new owners are advised on feeding and exercise, that advice, based on long experience, is handed down with strong conviction and dire warnings. For that reason those ideas are usually followed to the letter. The new owners are told just enough of the 'secret' method of feeding and exercise to enable them to produce a pup with reasonable to good hips. As a result, the new owners produce dogs with about the same degree of soundness as the breeder's dogs

Sometimes the breeder will not let the pup go to its new home until it has passed the rapid growth phase, and its hips [and elbows] are out of danger. Part of the contract with the new owner involves desexing and non showing should the pup show clinical or radiographic signs of unsoundness.

The result is that the next generation of pups is about as sound as the parents, because the management has been roughly the same.

That is the reason for such a strong correlation between sound parents and sound offspring. And the statistics look great! **It appears as though the breeding programme is producing genetic improvement, when in reality, the improvement is due to sound management!**

And what do the breeders talk about? Do they say "We have stock with lousy genes, but their hips are good because of our great management?" Of course not! What those breeders are happy to talk about is the **GENETIC** soundness of their stock and the radiographs which prove that point. Breeders know that **if it is believed** that their stock is totally free of the genes responsible for Hip Dysplasia, they will sell puppies, win shows, and in general attract applause and envy.

And so the myth continues ...

... that dysplastic hips or sound hips are something a dog inherits. The reality is, the state of those dogs' hips is very much the product of either sound puppy management or poor puppy management, with the emphasis being on nutrition and exercise.

What is even more interesting is that having evolved this method of management which produces pups with sound hips [a lot of the time], quite a few breeders begin to believe the myth themselves. Either that or they 'play the game' and pretend the improvement is all due to a change in genes. It is much easier to play the genetic game than to tell the truth and buck the system.

On the other side of the coin, kennels who regularly produce puppies with unsound hips do one of two things. They either pass on no advice, or very poor advice. In this way they unwittingly supervise the production of dogs with unsound skeletons, and that way the statistics confirm that unsound dogs produce unsound offspring.

Then there is the role of the novice in producing Hip Dysplasia

The offspring from so called 'Hip Dysplasia free lines' which ultimately develop Hip Dysplasia, are usually the ones which have been raised by an enthusiastic novice.

Somebody who is determined to have the fastest growing, most calcium rich, most exercised, 'most best' dog that ever existed. The sad truth is, they are going to have one of the worst. This is a very common pattern of events. A common method of producing Hip Dysplasia - or some other skeletal problem.

Let's get this news out there!

I want breeders, owners and vets to realise that these simple management tools will make an immediate and dramatic difference to the individual dog TODAY and that they are available for anyone to use. Sadly, instead of this happening, what we are seeing is just the reverse. The origin of these improvements is being ignored. The improvement is being labelled genetic and is being used to prop up the very shaky genetic theory.

In fact we can probably go further and say that in many ways, the breeders are fooling the vets. The breeders know what is going on, but they keep the vets in the dark.

I am looking for honesty from breeders and vets who do realise what is going on

Let us spread the news. Let us make this 'secret breeders' business' common knowledge amongst all breeders and dog owners.

This will enable all dog owners to take the simple steps necessary to prevent Hip Dysplasia and the other skeletal problems without believing they have only the genetic myth to fight the problem.

What should we do with our hip scoring schemes?

Should we keep them or abandon them?

One of the problems we have with these schemes is that we have no idea which genes we have or have not eliminated when we cull an animal diagnosed as having Hip [or Elbow] Dysplasia.

Have we removed indirect genes, which most animals have, and which we actually want to keep, or have we removed the very rare directly acting genes, which do need to go?

Because all dogs have the indirect genes, that is what we mostly remove. This achieves very little. As we get rid of these genes we have a breeding programme which selects animals which possess them because these are the genes which make our breed what it is.

This means, as currently practised, our culling has not achieved a whole lot. We are mostly culling animals that have developed Hip Dysplasia because of faulty management! The faulty management was the trigger which allowed the indirect genes to express themselves.

The only genes we should be attempting to eliminate are the direct genes. They are the ones which, if they exist, will cause the problem no matter what. As to whether we have removed any of these - **we have absolutely no idea! Apart from not being sure if they exist, we have no idea which dogs carry them.**

How can we make sure we get rid of the direct genes?

To check whether a dog carries these directly acting genes is very simple. It involves growing the dog properly with the BARF programme. If it develops skeletal problems it has direct genes - so cull it - Simple!

That works because the BARF programme provides no predisposing factors for skeletal disease. If the dog has only indirect genes, no skeletal disease will be seen.

On the other hand if there are direct genes present, then that dog will almost certainly develop one or more skeletal problems. **We must cull this dog. It has genes that absolutely must go.**

Therefore we may conclude that keeping our radiography and hip scoring is a good idea ...

... so long as it is based on eliminating the direct genes. As we have seen, attempting to eliminate the indirect genes is largely a waste of time.

Unfortunately our hip scoring schemes have two basic flaws.

The first flaw is that the the current methods used to score our dogs' hips do not appear to be valid. There is very little agreement between methods currently used. There is very little agreement between radiographers, and if a radiographer is asked to reinterpret a series of radiographs, there is very little agreement between the two assessments.

The second flaw is that a radiograph of a dog's hips tells us nothing about what sort of genes that dog carries for Hip Dysplasia. It simply tells us how well or how badly that dog was managed as a pup. As has already been demonstrated, phenotype - how a dog looks - does not necessarily equal a dog's genotype - its genetic inheritance.

If our hip scoring programmes are to have any validity, we first have to ensure that we are using **USEFUL** methods of diagnosing the problem.The new PennHIP method does appear to have some worth. It would appear to be far more reliable than anything else we currently do. By comparison, every other method is practically useless.

Until a method such as the PennHIP method becomes standard, all our efforts to determine which animals actually have dysplastic hips will be to very little avail.

However, even if we can validly assess the hip status of an animal, what does that tell us? Very little in genetic terms UNLESS we also know HOW that animal was raised. This is the perennial genetic problem of trying to separate genotype from phenotype.

The only way we can make real genetic headway with our hip scoring and killing, culling or keeping schemes, is to standardise and idealise the conditions under which we raise our dogs. That is, we must use the BARF programme - nationwide/worldwide. That is the only way we will separate the individuals with real genetic problems from those that are developing Hip Dysplasia due to poor management. Only then may we Keep, Cull or Kill with confidence!

If we do not adopt such a programme, but continue to assume that all bad hips are the result of bad genes, then I am strongly suggesting that for all the reasons I have mentioned, there is very little genetic gain being made in terms of bone and joint health.

In the meantime there will be a continuing loss of valuable genetic material with the loss of the animals killed or culled for having "Radiological Hip Dysplasia."

Having said all of that let me also say that these schemes have a use in that they focus a breeder's attention on producing sound pups. They give breeders insight into how well they are doing in their management programme. What this also means is, if they follow the BARF programme, they will very quickly discover just how sound that management process has become.

Some conclusions about Hip Dysplasia

Most puppy owners do more than one thing to wreck their pup's bones. In the case of Hip Dysplasia, the problem is usually associated with commercial pet food, particularly the super premium pet foods with their inflammation-causing heat damaged fats. The ones designed for 'growth.'

When these are fed to excess or the owner supplements the diet and causes that diet to be generally excessive, or excessive in specific nutrients such as carbohydrates, protein, or fat, the pup will commence to grow rapidly and may become obese. Not uncommonly this is teamed with excessive and inappropriate exercise. The exercise regimes designed to produce the skeletal diseases include long boring walks and overly exuberant punishing exercise, particularly very jarring exercise.

The other common skeletal-problem producing practice is to throw in loads of artificial calcium. And there you have it. The very simple and very common, universally practised recipe for skeletal disaster.

Just be aware that for the maximum chance of producing juvenile bone disease, including Hip Dysplasia, all these factors should be combined together. That is, excessive calcium, excessive food, super premium foods and inappropriate exercise.

Although Hip Dysplasia does have a genetic basis, the problem cannot be eliminated by breeding without making drastic changes to the breed. Final mature weight, size, obesity, engineering and growth rate are THE most important genetic factors involved in producing Hip Dysplasia.

That being the case they are the only features it would be worthwhile breeding out. However, they are the ones we are least likely to want to breed out. By doing so, we lose our breed.

So if you do not wish to convert the large breeds into small breeds or into Greyhounds, you must concentrate not on breeding the problem out of the breed, but keeping the problem out of the individual through simple measures of correct management while that puppy is growing.

The only way we can have any immediate, consistent and major impact on Hip Dysplasia, is to raise animals using a controlled regime of diet and exercise. The BARF programme. If that is done, and the animal still becomes dysplastic, it has direct genes for Hip Dysplasia and must be culled. This is valid and scientific.

If your dog is one of the giant breeds, it may may have inherited maximum possible genes for Hip Dysplasia, but if it is fed properly and exercised properly as a puppy, you will have minimised its chance of developing Hip Dysplasia or any other skeletal problem.

If your dog is a member of a breed whose medium to small size, lack of obesity, relatively slow growth rate and well muscled body would tend to guard against it developing skeletal disease, it is still not immune from such problems. If it is fed badly enough and exercised sufficiently in an incorrect fashion, there is a strong chance that it will develop Hip Dysplasia or some other sort of bone or joint problem.

That is why we may conclude that while genes do play a major role in the production of Hip Dysplasia, they may for the most part be ignored - because the extent to which genetic manipulation can be used to eliminate this problem is almost non existent compared to what can be achieved with sound nutrition and sensible exercise regimes.

The indirect genes largely responsible for causing Hip Dysplasia have been present since our breeds were developed. When we started to mismanage our dogs in the mid thirties those genes began to exert their effects. They began to produce all the skeletal diseases we are now seeing in ever increasing numbers. If we restore appropriate diet and exercise, the genes will cease to exert those effects.

While it will take untold generations to alter the genetic structure of our dogs, it takes only take one generation to alter the management.

We may therefore conclude that no matter what genes your dog has inherited, it will in the vast majority of cases develop either sound hips or dysplastic hips because of what it is fed and how it is exercised as a puppy. If you get the feeding and exercise part right, the genes become relatively unimportant in the vast majority of cases.

While ever the veterinary profession seeks only genetic solutions for problems such as Hip Dysplasia, when clearly the problem is for all practical purposes one that involves exercise and diet, Hip Dysplasia will remain with us and continue to cripple our larger breeds while we waste enormous amounts of time, money and genes in a useless attempt to be rid of the problem.

There is every reason to believe Hip Dysplasia could be eliminated world wide in one generation. At the very least we could bring it back to the 1930's level. All we have to do is educate owners and breeders to adopt the simple but sound management practices of diet and exercise that nature intended dogs to have.

Unfortunately, many people find this idea so naively simplistic, they refuse even to think about it, let alone try it. They want to believe there is no simple solution to such a complex and challenging problem.

The key to eliminating Hip Dysplasia is education

Any programme that seeks to eliminate Hip Dysplasia must educate puppy owners to concentrate on reducing to a minimum all the factors OTHER than the genetic factors which predispose to Hip Dysplasia. In other words they MUST be educated in those correct management techniques which are essential to the elimination of skeletal disease from dogs.

**The BARF programme for pups
is the cornerstone
of this management programme.**

Until such an ideal and standard method of raising dogs is adopted, I doubt we shall make much headway with reducing the incidence of Hip Dysplasia or any other modern skeletal disease of dogs.

Treating Hip Dysplasia

Most Hip Dysplasia cases have other skeletal problems - at varying stages of development. That is a further reason it is imperative that they be treated with the BARF programme which has been modified for early skeletal disease - see Chapter Twenty Two. This programme of diet and [non] exercise may be combined with pentosan polysulphate, analgaesics, acupuncture, chiropractic manipulation and anything else which your vet or natural therapist may recommend to slow the progression of all these problems.

There are numerous surgical procedures which are being used to treat both early and more advanced cases of Hip Dysplasia. It is not my intention to go through all of these.There are plenty of standard veterinary texts which deal with such procedures. The main aim of this book is prevention - not treatment.

If you do have a dog with Hip Dysplasia that has tight pectineus muscles - with or without degenerative joint disease, and cannot afford expensive surgery, such as a bilateral hip replacement, then I strongly recommend bilateral pectineus muscle removal.

Performed properly, I find that this procedure DOES produce long term benefits, even with advanced degenerative joint disease. However, for best results it must be teamed with the BARF programme.

For more information on treating Hip Dysplasia and other skeletal problems please read Chapters Twenty Two and Twenty Three.

Note to Ueterinary Surgeons

When removing the Pectineus muscle[s], use clamps on each end of the muscle, remove as much of the muscle as possible, drop amoxil powder into the wound, and **do not** sew any fat into the wound. You must leave that dead space open. **Note**: if you close off that dead space, you encourage the formation of scar tissue. If scar tissue forms to replace that muscle - the end result will be worse than before you performed this procedure.

Close the subcutaneous tissue with a continuous absorbable suture. Follow that with a sub-cuticular if necessary, then skin sutures as normal. Discourage all activity till the skin sutures are removed after ten to fourteen days.

I find that in my hands, this procedure produces long term benefits to dogs suffering from Hip Dysplasia. This is particularly so in older dogs - where the pectineus muscle is tight and ropey, and because of this has been keeping the hind legs in a state of constant adduction.

As you read the next chapter which deals with Elbow Dysplasia,
do realise that to prevent, control and eradicate that problem, requires
exactly the same approach as you have just read concerning Hip Dysplasia.

CHAPTER FOURTEEN

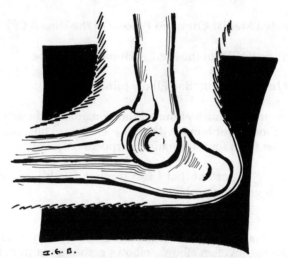

THE ELBOW DYSPLASIA COMPLEX

Elbow dysplasia occurs mostly in large breeds such as the Labrador, the Bernese Mountain Dog, the Rottweiler, the Golden Retriever, the Newfoundland, the German Shepherd, the Flat Coated Retriever, the Saint Bernard etc. etc..

Elbow Dysplasia usually results in lameness which is seen between four and eight months of age. The problem is usually seen in both front legs, is more common in the male, and usually, though not necessarily, appears or starts slowly, rather than suddenly appearing as a severe crippling disease.

The lameness will start as a a mild gait change. The elbows may or may not be held out from the body. This can progress to swollen elbows, front legs that will not bear weight and a dog that is reluctant to move. The problem becomes worse with exercise and is relieved by rest and pain killers.

The Elbow Dysplasia Complex consists of a group of four syndromes or diseases which include

The Ununited or Fragmented Anconeal process [UAP]

The Fragmented Medial Coronoid Process of the Ulna [FCP]

Osteochondritis [OCD] of the Medial Humeral Condyle

Elbow Joint Incongruity or 'Bad Elbow Joint'

Now don't worry too much about all those names or the actual anatomical location of those problems within the elbow. They are not all that important. I list them for information purposes only.

It is much more important that I run through with you some important facts about this growing problem.

All these diseases present with much the same set of symptoms. Clinically you see lameness, swollen elbows, elbows pointing out from the chest, and painful elbows, especially when they are extended.

The term Elbow Dysplasia means incorrect growth of the elbow joint. This incorrect growth of the elbow, in common with most of the skeletal diseases seen in growing dogs, is a problem which develops some time after birth, and most probably after weaning. **Dogs are not born with it.**

As a result of these growth defects, the elbow joint becomes unstable. This results in abnormal contact of the bones within the joint and incorrect weight distribution. There is damage to the bones involved which ultimately leads to degenerative joint disease.

Elbow Dysplasia is a group of diseases which are all linked inextricably

Where one occurs you will usually see another. Commonly, you will see problems in other joints as well. This is telling us they all have a common cause. **Poor management and predisposing or indirect genes.**

The indirect genes only act when incorrect nutrition and incorrect exercise are present. The combination of indirect genes, incorrect nutrition and incorrect exercise results in alterations in Endochondral ossification or Osteochondrosis which ultimately leads to the Elbow Dysplasia complex.

We now know that the Elbow Dysplasia complex is mostly due to two forms of Osteochondrosis. Firstly Osteochondritis Dissecans with its fissuring and fragmenting of cartilage, and secondly mismatched or unequal bone growth.

There is a mismatch in growth between the radius and the ulna. The end result is unusual pressures within the joint.

Looking inside the joint, you will see erosion of the cartilage, you will see fissuring of the cartilage [Osteochondritis Dissecans], you will see bone erosion or worse you will see bone fractures under the cartilage with displacement of the fragments.

The reason for the pain with this group of diseases ...

... is the fragmenting cartilage and also the enormous pressure within the joint which is caused by the mismatching. The lameness seen is due to the pain.

The diagnosis is made ...

... on the basis of a number of radiographs whose positioning is critical.

These radiographs reveal new bone formation in the joint. This new bone formation reflects the damage that has happened to the joint and the subsequent inflammation that has followed.

The damage seen on the radiographs is a direct result of poor nutrition, excessive exercise and mismatched growth between the radius and the ulna.

The current conventional veterinary view ...

... is that this syndrome or group of diseases has a genetic basis where the mode of inheritance is polygenic, multi factorial, and in fact inherited in a similar fashion to Hip Dysplasia.

That is why Elbow Dysplasia, like Hip Dysplasia is attracting the attention of orthopaedic experts who take the view that the only way to eliminate the problem is to breed it out. As a consequence they have developed ...

The Elbow Grading System

The grading system is used to determine which animals should be culled and which should be allowed to breed. The basis of the grading system is the amount of new [pathologic] bone formation with grades going from 0 to 3.

O is no bone formation, 1 is less than 2 mm, 2 is between 2 and 5 mm and 3 is greater than 5 mm. Animals graded either 0 or 1 are permitted to breed but not 2 or 3.

This may well be an exercise in futility. The only logical way to get rid of this problem RIGHT NOW is to minimise skeletal damage by correct management. In other words, this scheme is likely to have all the problems seen with the Hip Dysplasia schemes.

Nobody is even considering the role of management in the prevention or production of the Elbow Dysplasia Complex.

Not one person involved in this scheme is looking at this problem and realising that like Hip Dysplasia, the ability of genetics to eliminate the problem may well be close to zero. That like Hip Dysplasia, we have to look at the role of management!

The Elbow Dysplasia complex is only or mostly seen in those breeds of dogs with the indirect genes for skeletal disease. That is, genes for fast growth, obesity, large size, heavy weight, poor muscling and bad engineering. These are the the genes which predispose a pup to develop bone problems. They only cause these problems when the the management is poor. You will also recall that these are the genes which make a given breed what it is.

Every disease in the Elbow Dysplasia complex is due to poor management of the growing pup. Because modern puppy management is so poor with its nutrient damaged processed foods, excesses of nutrition including excess fat, protein, carbohydrate and calcium, and excessive exercise, the incidence of Elbow Dysplasia like that of Hip Dysplasia is rising.

Another clue to the origins of all these problems is that they respond - if caught early enough - to alterations in management. That is - to a reduction in all those factors of diet and exercise which exacerbate modern Osteochondrosis.

It is interesting to note that more than 50% of the animals submitted for evaluation show the problem radiographically but only 15 % are clinically lame. There are a lot of dogs out there that are being raised very badly!

What this means is that no matter what genes a pup has inherited, in the vast majority of cases, the Elbow Dysplasia Complex is completely avoidable by using correct management. How do you do that? Just follow the BARF programme.

Let us now look at the individual diseases in this complex starting with ...

The Ununited or Fragmented Anconeal Process

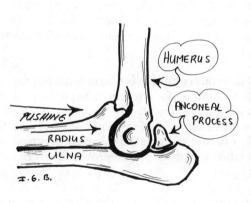

The anconeal process should unite with the ulna at five months [twenty weeks] of age. If the anconeal process has not joined with the ulna by this time it is considered to be diseased or pathological.

Radiographic studies have shown that the cause of this non-union is a pushing effect by the more rapidly growing radius. The radius becomes too long relative to the ulna. The pressure from the radius prevents the joining of the anconeal process to the ulna. This makes the joint both unstable and painful.

Let me emphasise that this mismatch in growth between the radius and the ulna is another manifestation of Osteochondrosis or disordered skeletal growth.

It is the result of poor management of the growing pup.

The ununited anconeal process is seen particularly in German Shepherds and also in Bassets - a breed where it is also common to see angular limb deformities. It is more common in males than females and there is no systemic illness. Again these last two features are consistent with it being a problem caused by poor diet and trauma.

Two of my earliest cases of UAP were a rapidly growing male Bull Mastiff and a young female German Shepherd. They were being over fed and over supplemented with calcium. They had had their early growth held back and when presented at my surgery they were going through a compensatory growth spurt. Both dogs had very advanced Elbow Dysplasia and neither fared well following surgery. Both ultimately developed Degenerative Joint Disease.

With Ununited Anconeal Process - the lameness usually begins subtly and if not corrected with a change in management, the prognosis is poor. It can be seen in one or both legs. Pain occurs with hyperextension. As the problem becomes chronic the joint becomes thickened and there is usually grating or crepitus with movement. There may be excessive joint fluid. The elbows will be turned out or abducted. As time passes Degenerative Joint Disease becomes more evident.

It must be realised that by the time this condition is diagnosed it has usually reached an advanced stage. It is common for owners to hope the problem will go away if treated with a tincture of time. By the time they realise this is not going to happen, the problem has passed the point of no return. On the other hand, if caught early - before any great damage has occurred and the correct management procedures instituted - the problem will in most cases quietly disappear.

Radiographically the best picture is taken with the elbow flexed. A mediolateral view. Once the diagnosis has been made ...

...Treatment options include ...

1. The removal of the ununited anconeal process. This was the original treatment. This is not a good treatment. It will lead to joint instability which in the long term will result in Degenerative Joint Disease and lifetime lameness.

2. To use a screw to fix the process back in place. This is a technically difficult operation, but even if it is successful, the problem remains. That is, you are trying to screw the anconeal process into a place where it does not fit because the radius is still too long!

3. You must consider this third option which is called ulnar osteotomy. That is, cut through the ulna just below the elbow joint - using a wire saw and leave it unstabilised. This takes the pressure off the elbow and allows union of the Anconeal Process. So far the statistics have demonstrated excellent success. Where this operation has been used 90 to 95% of the processes have healed, the dog has become sound! In the case of the ulna, it does finally heal, but slightly bent.

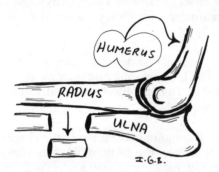

Note: Cutting through the ulna [ulnar osteotomy] is not successful once you have Degenerative Joint Disease, in which case all you can do is remove the Anconeal process.

Let us now examine the other three parts of the Elbow Dysplasia Complex.

Fragmented Medial Coronoid process of the Ulna, OCD of the Medial Humeral Condyle and Elbow Joint Incongruity.

Don't let the names scare you. Just realise that these more complex manifestations of the Elbow Dysplasia Complex are becoming increasingly common. They are seen in the larger breeds such as the Rottie, Retriever, Bernese Mountain Dog etc.. They are commonly seen together.

Most importantly **they all stem from two basic forms of Osteochondrosis. That is, mismatched growth between the radius and the ulna and Osteochondritis Dissecans.** In other words, they are all caused by poor management of the growing puppy. **They are all preventable!**

The results of surgery for these parts of the Elbow Dysplasia complex vary with breed and age, but many dogs will improve after surgery. The clinical signs usually begin at six to ten months of age. If they are seen later in life, it is usually as a result of progressive degenerative joint disease.

All these conditions are difficult to definitely diagnose - they require special radiographic techniques. Lameness may be seen in one or both forelegs. Affected dogs will resent the joint being manipulated. They will particularly dislike direct finger or thumb pressure applied over the medial [to the inside] aspect of the joint. Excess joint fluid can vary from considerable to non existent.

With all of these conditions the onset of lameness is usually insidious or subtle, but occasionally a traumatic event may cause the sudden appearance of the problem.

At this early treatable stage there is usually no detectable muscle atrophy or restriction of elbow movement. The lameness may be intermittent at first, becoming more severe with time. The lameness is usually unilateral although the problem is usually bilateral.

As these conditions advance, the elbow joint may be swollen and will have a reduced range of movement. When the radiologist sees new bone formation, not only is the diagnosis made, you also know that there is Degenerative Joint Disease.

In general surgery to remove fragmenting bone is best avoided particularly where the dog is more than 12 months of age. However, if a calcified flap is found - usually between 5 and 9 months - then surgery is essential.

The surgeon will get in there and remove the broken off fragments and scrape out all the dead and sick tissue and get back to a clean healthy surface. Unfortunately, if that is all you do the final outcome is still Degenerative Joint Disease. The difference in bone length has not been resolved. **For that reason, in these advanced cases, it is still necessary to remove a piece of the ulna to fix this basic problem.**

The cutting of the ulna should only be used in selected cases. That is, cut the ulna in advanced cases of the problem, but where not too much degenerative joint disease has occurred.

There will be no need to cut the ulna if the problem can be caught early before any real damage is done. In this case treatment will consist of the BARF diet, drugs such as the non steroidal anti-inflammatories and pentosan polysulphate, together with rest and weight loss.

This type of so called conservative treatment is used with either very young animals in the early stages of the problem -with only mild signs - or with older dogs suffering from advanced Degenerative Joint Disease when it is much too late to operate.

Secondary Degenerative Joint Disease ...

... is a common sequel to Elbow Dysplasia. This is partly because no one is looking to improve the diet of these animals once they have the problem, and also because of the extensive damage that has already occurred before these cases are diagnosed.

Let me emphasise - do not ignore lame young dogs! Catching the disease in its early stages and treating it with rest and a change of diet provides the best outcome.

Better yet, avoid the problem altogether. When raising pups abandon modern foods, do not use calcium supplements and do not submit the pups to excessive exercise. Instead, substitute these with the BARF programme for pups.

It is imperative that once these dogs are diagnosed, their diet is changed

So many dogs continue on the same damaging diet that caused the problem, the only difference being that the diet is fed in more limited amounts and the pups are rested. Now limiting the diet is fine - as is rest - until the bones heal. However, for long term control of the problem and to reduce Degenerative Joint Disease it is imperative that the modified BARF programme for skeletal disease as detailed in chapter Twenty Two - page 392 - be followed.

The BARF diet contains high levels of anti-oxidants, phytochemicals, enzymes and anti-inflammatory omega 3 essential fatty acids etc.. These healing and health promoting nutrients are entirely absent from modern foods which contain damaged and damaging components.

The modified BARF diet for skeletal disease is very low in energy, protein, calcium and phosphorus, but high in raw crushed vegetables. This diet should be continued until such time as the pup's skeleton has returned to normal - which means it no longer has Osteochondrosis - or if permanent damage has occurred, that modified diet must be continued until the condition has stabilised. At that time, the normal BARF programme of food and exercise should be gradually reintroduced. You will need your vet's during this time to assist you in deciding what stage of the disease your dog is at.

What should we do with our Schemes to eliminate Elbow Dysplasia?

Fortunately, it would seem that our methods of assessing whether a dog or pup has this problem are in fact valid compared to the current highly suspect methods being used to diagnose Hip Dysplasia.

However, as with Hip Dysplasia, even if we can validly assess the status of the elbows of an animal, what does that tell us?

Very little in genetic terms UNLESS we also know HOW that animal was raised. The way things are with animals being raised in a wide variety of ways, we still have the problem of being unable to separate genotype from phenotype.

Should we abandon our radiography and elbow scoring?

Not at all, if we can use it to make some genuine genetic headway. To do that it must be based on eliminating the direct genes. As we have seen, attempting to eliminate the indirect genes is largely a waste of time.

As with Hip Dysplasia, those radiographs and the rating of the elbows that follows are valuable because they focus a breeder's attention on producing sound pups.

They give breeders insight into how well they are doing in their management programme. What this means is, if breeders follow the simple methods I outline, they will very quickly discover just how sound that management process has become.

The only way we can make real genetic headway ...

... with our scoring and culling schemes, is to standardise and idealise the conditions under which we raise our dogs. That is, we must use the BARF programme. That is the only way we will separate the individuals with real genetic problems from those that are reacting to poor management.

If we do not adopt such a programme, but continue to assume that all bad elbows are the result of bad genes, then I am strongly suggesting that for all the reasons I have mentioned, there is very little genetic gain being made in terms of bone and joint health.

In the meantime there will be a continuing loss of valuable genetic material with the loss of the animals killed or culled for having 'Radiological Elbow Dysplasia.'

If you have not read the previous chapter on Hip Dysplasia, please do so. Much of what it says about the origins and prevention of hip Dysplasia applies equally to Elbow Dysplasia.

The final word on Elbow Dysplasia is that the only way we can have any immediate, consistent and major impact on this problem, is to raise animals using a controlled regime of diet and exercise: the BARF programme. If that is done, and the animal still develops elbow problems, we can be certain it has genes for Elbow Dysplasia that must go. It must be killed or culled. This is valid and scientific.

In the next chapter - we look at the Wobbler Syndrome.

CHAPTER FIFTEEN

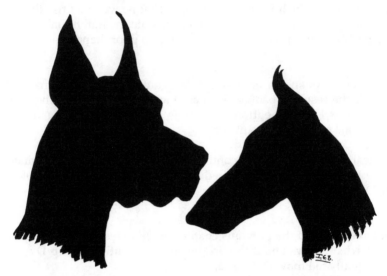

THE WOBBLER SYNDROME

The Wobbler Syndrome is also known as Cervical Spondylopathy, Compressive Myelopathy or the Cervical Vertebral Instability Syndrome. However, you can forget all these difficult names - I have thrown them in for information purposes only. Just remember - **'Wobblers.'**

The Wobbler Syndrome is caused by improper growth of the cervical or neck vertebrae. Like the other skeletal problems seen in growing dogs, this is a problem of the large and giant, fast growing breeds There are two breeds that are commonly affected - Great Danes and Doberman Pinschers. The problem usually occurs in **young** Great Danes and **older** Dobermans, but it is not uncommon to see exceptions to this 'rule.'

This disease occurs because vertebrae in the neck area - and their joints - are badly formed. Mostly it is the last three neck vertebrae - cervicals five, six and seven which are deformed.

This poor formation of the neck vertebrae involves several defects ...

... the first defect is a narrowing of the spinal canal which puts pressure on the nerves of the spinal cord.

The second defect is that the joints between these last three vertebrae are not formed properly. They allow excessive movement - in fact a partial dislocation of the spine. This also puts damaging pressures on the spinal cord.

The end result of these two problems is damage to the nerve tracts responsible for normal strength and the ability to stand and move normally.

What you see in the dog with this damage ...

... is incoordination, lameness, pain, and sometimes paralysis. The problem is usually most noticeable in the hind legs.

If the skeletal changes are only mild, when the animal is young it may appear normal. However, as the animal becomes older the damage will slowly worsen. Eventually, a combination of degeneration and pressure on an intervertebral disc may cause it to rupture. A ruptured disc places immediate and much heavier pressure on an already mildly compressed cord. Now we have an acute problem which needs urgent attention.

With young great Danes

the most common picture is a slowly developing, progressive, incoordination and paralysis of the hind limbs. The problem is not associated with any known injury to the neck. It usually starts some time between three and twelve months, although many dogs are not presented to the vet until they are ten to twelve months of age. The owner just assumes they have a young animal with a clumsy or wobbly gait.

Commonly the pup adopts a crouched posture with the toes of the hind limbs 'knuckling' or dragging when walking. The pup will adopt a wide based stance to keep balanced. Owners notice there is swaying of the hind legs with longer strides than normal. Their pup is clumsy or 'wobbles.'

The pup may find it impossible to walk on smooth or slippery surfaces. The problem is particularly noticeable when the pup is made to turn. The pup may fall. Eventually the front legs will become involved.

Affected dogs will show a characteristic 'goose-stepping.' As the problem progresses the toes on the front feet will also start to knuckle and drag.

Neck pain can vary. Commonly it is not usually pronounced, in fact the neck may be pain free. Other dogs have have been known to resent their neck being manipulated and may even drop to the ground when this happens.

Because the damage to the spinal cord only involves the particular functions we have been describing, the dogs with the Wobbler Syndrome remain normal in all other respects including demeanour, eating, defecating etc..

With Doberman Pinschers ...

... the problem is more likely to occur later in life. Commonly between years five and seven. These dogs will wobble when they walk. The front legs are usually involved from the start, with short choppy steps. Untreated the condition will only become worse. The dogs will appear 'arthritic.'The head will usually be carried low because of the pain. This syndrome can be acute and in this case the neck will be much more painful because it is due to a 'slipped disc' [cervical disc rupture] in the neck area.

The diagnosis ...

... is based on the breed, the age, the clinical signs and confirmed by radiographs. Sometimes a myelogram is used to show exactly where the pressure is and whether the cord is inflamed and swollen.

At this time there is no reliable method of predicting the problem from radiographic signs, although common-sense tells us that a severe problem radiographically would indicate the potential for problems.

Osteochondrosis and the Wobbler Syndrome

There is little doubt that an underlying genetic tendency to develop the problem exists.

Nevertheless, the Wobbler Syndrome in common with all the other skeletal diseases which occur in young dogs is very much the product of modern mismanagement. That is, the Wobbler Syndrome is due to excessive growth rates on diets too rich in protein, energy, phosphorus, calcium and overly exuberant exercise of the wrong type. It is another example of Endochondral Ossification gone wrong. The end result of one basic problem - Osteochondrosis.

Several factors usually work together to produce this syndrome. Let's look at the nutritional insults which help produce this problem.

The excessive blood calcium caused by overloading pups with calcium results in an excess of the hormone calcitonin being released by the thyroid gland. The role of calcitonin is to retard the resorption of calcium from the bone. This is to drop the blood calcium back to its normal level. Unfortunately this also stops the spinal canal from enlarging and so we have increased pressure on the spinal cord as it grows.

Excess food producing an excessive growth rate that outstrips the ability of the under mineralised cervical vertebrae to support a heavy head can also result in damage to the vertebrae. This in turn will result in nerve damage.

Malformation of the joints in the spinal cord - will occur because of hypernutrition and inappropriate exercise. This can result in improper alignment of the spine which in turn can lead to nerve damage.

Treatment

A 'slipped disc' can be a medical emergency

It may cause paralysis. It requires both medical and surgical treatments. **The medical treatment** - given initially and temporarily - is aimed at stopping any further damage by reducing inflammation and swelling. This involves anti-inflammatory drugs including corticosteroids, diuretics such as mannitol and anti-oxidants such as vitamin C and E to protect the nerves from damage by free radicals.

The second or surgical stage of treatment aims to relieve the pressure on the cord by removing ruptured disc material and pieces of vertebrae - then fixing them so they will heal in a stable position. This allows the return of oxygen and nutrients to the spinal cord which prevents further damage.

If the dog is treated immediately - including surgery to remove the disc material - the prognosis for a return to reasonable health is good.

However, if too much damage has occurred or the surgery is delayed too long - there may be permanent damage to the cord.

If the problem is not so acute, treatment will involve rest and anti-inflammatory drugs etc. If there is no improvement - surgery will be needed.

Following surgery, the best that can be expected will be the ability to perform normal functions such as eating and defaecating etc., but almost certainly the dog will be left with the 'Wobbles.' The best case is the dog that has been steadily getting more ataxic and suddenly goes down. These animals have ruptured a disc. Surgery to remove that disc material will probably have a good outcome.

The use of a harness instead of a lead to prevent harsh pressure on the neck is useful both to prevent the problem occurring in the older dog and also to prevent further damage once the problem has occurred.

Great Danes which usually do not suffer the acute form of the disease may respond to conservative treatment without the need for surgery - if the problem is detected early enough.

Conservative treatment consists of total rest - e.g. in a cage - together with anti-inflammatory drugs including corticosteroids, diuretics such as mannitol and anti-oxidants such as vitamin C and E to protect the nerves from damage by free radicals. That is - as for the acute form. Some vets will recommend a neck brace to help relieve pressure and to stop further damage caused by movement. The diet must be adjusted to bring down the protein levels, the energy levels and the calcium levels. That is simple. Go to the BARF diet as outlined in Chapter Twenty Two.

If these measures can be adopted early enough, damage to the vertebrae may be halted with normal growth from that time onwards. Unfortunately, if this slow progressive form is discovered late, and a lot of damage to the spinal cord and associated nerves has already occurred, surgery may not achieve a lot in terms of a return to normal, although it may prevent further damage.

In other words, early detection is vital. However - even better is to prevent the problem in the first place.

So let's prevent the Wobbler Syndrome rather than have to treat it

This is the important bit. The answer lies with correct management. That is - use the BARF programme for pups properly from birth and be certain of not producing Wobblers or any of the other skeletal diseases and have a healthy long lived dog as well!

Feed your pups individually. This is vital. It will be the 'dominant greedy pups' which develop skeletal problems. They will be the ones that grow fast because they get the 'lion's share' of the food.

What about breeding?

If the problem occurs AND you have been using the BARF diet properly, then that dog DOES have direct genes which absolutely must go. Now is the time to cull.

Prognosis

The prognosis or final outcome with the Wobbler Syndrome depends on the amount of damage that has occurred to the spinal cord. Further damage after medical and surgical treatment will depend on careful management. This will involve the BARF diet, and attention paid to how the neck is moved for the rest of the dog's life.

The diet part is easy. The movement part you must discuss with your vet. It will depend very much on how much and what sort of damage has already occurred to the spinal cord and the vertebrae in the neck.

CHAPTER SIXTEEN

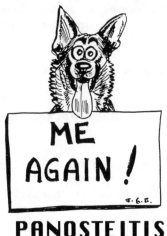

PANOSTEITIS

If your pup has to get one of the skeletal diseases, this is probably the one it should get. It is self limiting and usually leaves the pup relatively unharmed.

Panosteitis is seen in young large breed dogs. It is a further development of the basic problem of alterations in Endochondral Ossification or Osteochondrosis involving the growth and resorptive areas around and inside the shaft of the long bones of the limbs.

It almost certainly has a genetic basis, and the genes involved are probably the indirect genes which only function in the presence of certain environmental factors including excesses of diet and exercise.

Because this problem involves inflammation of the growth areas of the shaft, the feeding of high levels of heat damaged polyunsaturated fatty acids as found in the super premium growth foods for puppies could well be one of the triggering factors. Keeping all of that in mind, it is fairly obvious that Panosteitis is best prevented by management rather than genetic manipulation. The modified BARF programme is the ideal diet both for prevention and treatment.

Panosteitis or 'Panno'

Panosteitis is a self limiting, inflammatory condition of the long bones of young, growing, large breed dogs, such as German Shepherds, Basset Hounds, Doberman Pinschers, etc.. Some regard it as 'doggie growing pains.' It has had quite a few names over the years including Enostosis, Eosinophilic Panosteitis and a few others. **Dogs with Panosteitis often suffer from other skeletal diseases such as Hip Dysplasia.**

The disease occurs spontaneously causing pain and lameness. The onset is usually acute, sometimes after strenuous exercise or play. The pain and lameness is due to inflammation within the bones and inflammation of the membrane surrounding the bones of the legs. It has long been regarded in official circles as having no known cause with many different causes being proposed including viral, genetic and dietary. I believe that this disease, like all the other skeletal diseases in growing dogs today, owes its origins to our modern methods of raising pups. In other words ...

Diet and exercise is the major cause. This includes the usual high protein, high calcium, high energy, puppy diets which people use to push a pup to grow too fast. In particular, the heat damaged polyunsaturated fats of the super premium foods deserve our attention as a possible major cause, because of their promotion of the inflammatory process. Indirect genes play a predisposing role in common with all skeletal disease in young dogs, and the problem may be induced or worsened by stress.

Panosteitis is usually diagnosed between five and ten months of age, although the disease has been reported in dogs as young as two months and up to twenty four months. Isolated cases have been seen in German Shepherds up to five and even seven years of age.

The disease may last for up to twelve months. The average duration is two to three months. It may persist for less than a month. Recovery is normally spontaneous and complete.

German Shepherds appear to be the most commonly affected breed. Males are 4 times more likely to be affected than females. In one study, 86% of dogs with Panosteitis were found to be German Shepherds. Are they more predisposed to it or are there simply more German Shepherds than any other large breed of dog? Probably the latter!

Panosteitis commonly affects the shaft of the long bones

That is, the radius, ulna, and humerus of the front leg, and the femur and tibia of the hind leg **The bones most commonly affected** are the bones of the limbs nearest the body. That is the humerus and femur. It may also affect the ilium or hip.

The disease will vary from mild to severe and is characterised by a shifting lameness, that is seen in different bones at different times. It can vary from a subtle lameness to a reluctance to bear any weight on the limb. It is almost always accompanied by other signs of illness. The so called systemic signs. E.g. lethargy and lack of appetite. Lethargy and food refusal may accompany very painful lameness. With the disease itself, there is pain with pressure on bones which can be quite severe.

Typically, one or the other front leg is affected first. It may appear in just one limb or all simultaneously. The lameness and pain will move, shifting from leg to leg. It may shift from day to day, or stay for a couple of weeks before shifting. Commonly there are periods of improvement and worsening of the symptoms. Improvement may only last a couple of days before the lameness appears in another limb. This may go on for as long as eighteen months, but rarely past two years of age. There may be muscle atrophy.

The cyclical nature of this disease makes it difficult to assess the response to treatment. There is a typical pattern of dogs recovering with or without treatment, followed by a relapse. When lameness recurs in a previously affected limb, it involves a different bone within that limb. Pain and lameness can begin before there are any signs on a radiograph and can be gone long before the radiographic changes have returned to normal. Panosteitis will eventually go away, with or without treatment.

Diagnosis of Panosteitis

X-rays are used to rule out other causes of lameness or confirm Panosteitis. Panosteitis can be confused with fungal or bacterial Osteomyelitis, some forms of bone cancer or Hypertrophic Osteodystrophy.

Radiographically you will see ...

... bones with greater density than normal together with the formation of bone within the marrow cavity. There have also been reported changes in the growth plate. These are alterations in ossification. In other words Panosteitis is a form of modern Osteochondrosis.

The bone with less radiographic changes is usually the more painful one, because early in the disease is the period when there is great inflammation but the body has not yet laid down the bone in response to that inflammation. The bone which shows the greater radiographic changes is often less sore because the inflammation has subsided.

When pressure is applied to the affected bones, there is usually pain. The dog will pull its leg away. They will also be seen biting their legs. Bad pain usually persists for one or two months. However, it may keep returning for up to eighteen months.

Treatment of Panosteitis

During the acute phase the dog must be totally rested. Exercise will worsen the condition. However, severely affected dogs will be reluctant to move anyway, so this is not usually a problem. Exercise should also be restricted during the non painful times because severe and prolonged exercise is one of the factors which helps the problem return. Before allowing a dog to return to normal exercise, I would recommend that at least one month should have elapsed since the last attack, and the exercise should be phased in gradually.

The pain, if severe enough, should be treated with analgaesics. However, pain control is debatable. While it is important to make a dog feel more comfortable, painkillers are not necessarily for the good of the pup. If the pain is masked too much, it may result in damaging exercise and the condition will worsen. In other words, only use them when the pain is severe. At other times it may be best to let some pain remain to reduce the dog's natural inclination to be active. Drugs used include aspirin, or Bufferin or phenylbutazone - or some of the newer non steroidal anti-inflammatories. If these drugs are not working and severe pain remains, corticosteroids may have to be used.

Treating Panosteitis with Diet

Take the pup off the damaging food it is eating and switch to the BARF programme.

Panosteitis will disappear much more rapidly when the patient no longer eats processed food. Food which is so pro-inflammatory. Exercise must be limited and the puppy must be switched to low protein, low calcium and low energy food. The pup's new diet should ensure that its weight is kept low, and growth rate is reduced.

To do this there is only one diet I recommend. The BARF diet. Modified for skeletal disease. See chapter Twenty Two. This will ensure a reduction in protein, calories, calcium and phosphorus. It will ensure your dog loses unnecessary weight to reduce the stress on the legs and ease the pain. It will ensure anti-inflammatory and anti-oxidant nutrients such as Vitamin C and the omega 3 essential fatty acids are fed.

Fresh linseed oil - not damaged by heat and not rancid - is an essential component of this programme because of its strong anti-inflammatory action. This must be accompanied by a vitamin E supplement.

By following the BARF programme, you will ensure the greatest chance of a successful outcome.

Prevention of Panosteitis

This could not be more simple. Grow your pups on the BARF programme from the word go. Most particularly **don't feed the super premium puppy foods, or the ones promising a super shiny coat.** These products promote skeletal disease because of their excess protein, energy and possibly excess calcium. In particular these **diets contain the heat damaged omega 3's which promote inflammatory processes such as Panosteitis.** Do make sure the only exercise is play - but not too boisterous - particularly during rapid growth spurts.

CHAPTER SEVENTEEN

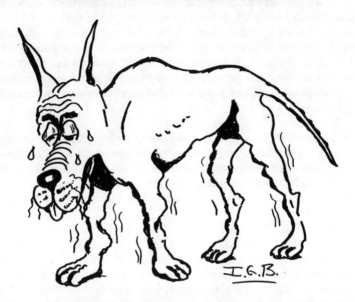

HYPERTROPHIC OSTEODYSTROPHY
OR
HOD

HOD has had a number of names over the years including Metaphyseal Osteopathy and Skeletal Scurvy. All of these names are pretty difficult to remember, so just think HOD, which also happens to stand for...

"the most Horrible Orthopaedic Disease that we see in young dogs."

I say this because HOD is a nasty disease!

Affected dogs can be very sick. Showing high fever, lethargy, inability to stand, excruciating pain, diarrhoea, decreased appetite, salivation, and sometimes problems with the lungs.

What is HOD?

HOD is a moderately uncommon multi bone lameness that occasionally affects the limb bones of large heavy breed dogs such as Great Danes, Setters, Retrievers, German Shepherds, Dobermans and Weimaraners. It has occasionally been seen in small light breeds. It is a disease of uncertain cause which probably has both a genetic and viral basis. The virus is the Distemper virus, and the genes are more than likely the same indirect genes which predispose to the other skeletal diseases we see in young large breed dogs.

Like all the other skeletal diseases we see in young pups it is probably - at least in part - a further development of the basic problem of alterations in Endochondral ossification or Osteochondrosis. The growing points that are affected include the growth plates and the membrane surrounding the shaft. Some authorities say more males are affected than females while others say not.

The onset of HOD is sudden. It usually begins as lameness which starts somewhere between three and six months of age but it can begin as early as two and as late as ten months. In many cases the onset has been linked to vaccination. The signs are often episodic or cyclic. They subside and flare up again. Each relapse drags the often very sick pup further downhill.

All four limbs are usually affected. Pups are inactive due to the pain, and any movement is stiff, tentative and deliberate. Affected dogs will often stand with the back arched and with all four limbs tucked under the body.

The disease causes bony thickenings near the joints - particularly in the ends of the forelegs. It is the bones which are sore rather than the joints. The pup is sore in the growth plate area. Those front legs are swollen hot and painful. For the technically minded there will be swelling at the level of the growth plates in the distal [nearest the ground] end of the radius and the ulna - and also the tibia in the hind legs. We now know these growth plates are not only inflamed but they can also be pus-filled!

All of this is associated with a high white blood cell count. **Latest research has demonstrated the presence of the distemper virus in these sick growth plates.**

As the disease progresses the pup will develop angular limb deformities because of weakened pasterns, together with splayed feet, and stunting of the long bones.

The diagnosis will be made on the basis of all of these signs and confirmed with radiographs. Radiographs will show a characteristic set of distortions in the affected growth plates. In some dogs, the picture looks more like Osteomyelitis, and in others it looks more like skeletal scurvy in humans.

Also there will be a dramatic appearance of new bone laid up and down the shaft of the affected bones producing grotesquely enlarged bones, particularly the radius, ulna and tibia. Some dogs develop pneumonia with mineralisation of the lungs. In smaller breeds the mandibles [jaws] have become involved.

When attempting to diagnose HOD, the diseases it must be differentiated from include Hereditary Neutropaenia of Border Collies with secondary Osteomyelitis, Panosteitis, and bacterial bone infection or Osteomyelitis.

With the exception of Panosteitis, all of these can be confused radiographically because they all affect the growth plate and they are all pus producing.

However, dogs with either Panosteitis or HOD can start off looking pretty much the same, on a clinical examination, so it is a good idea to know the major differences and similarities.

Panosteitis will usually be seen at six to eight months while HOD is seen earlier between two to eight months, but usually three to four months.

Panosteitis will continue for longer and may show recurring bouts up to eighteen months of age, while HOD will last a few days to several weeks and no more than two or three months.

They can both show acute lameness, although of the two, HOD is usually far more painful. They will both show improvement followed by relapse.

With Panosteitis the problem shifts from limb to limb, while with HOD all limbs are consistently affected.

Both conditions can show fever and reluctance to eat. Both will have sore legs.

With Panosteitis, the soreness is in the shaft while with HOD the pain and swelling is seen more in the growth plates at the ends of the bones.

Both show the ulna, humerus, radius, femur, and tibia affected.

Radiographs of Panosteitis show changes in the shaft of the bone while HOD shows changes initially in the growth plates and then very characteristic changes in the shaft which include very dramatic and irregular new bone growth.

The cause[s] of both conditions are much the same - that is - diet, exercise, genetic predisposition and for HOD an additional factor - a viral cause - Distemper vaccination.

The treatment is much the same for both conditions and includes anti-inflammatories and analgaesics, rest and a change to the BARF programme for skeletal disease.

Although they are both self-limiting diseases, the prognosis is usually good with Panosteitis but guarded to poor for HOD.

Cause[s] of HOD

The causes of HOD include a combination of the following: genetics, nutrition, infection, trauma (over-use, over-exercise of soft young bones), hormone imbalance, reaction to vaccination,   auto immune disease, and the Distemper virus invading the growth plates and infecting them following vaccination.

HOD often follows **the pup's final distemper vaccination.** The cause is thought to be the distemper virus, possibly as a result of vaccination. Research scientists have isolated Distemper particles from the growth plates of affected animals. Note that the typical age of onset of HOD is four months of age. That is, after the final puppy vaccination!

Genetics. Some breeds are more commonly afflicted with HOD, namely **Great Danes, Boxers, Irish Setters, Weimaraners, and several other large, fast-growing breeds**

The disease is sporadic, usually affecting only isolated puppies in a particular litter or line. However, there are reports of **family clusters, entire litters, or significant numbers of litter mates being affected.** Some breeders have experienced consistently high percentages of pups with HOD in related litters, suggesting genetic influences. However, there has been no data kept on feeding or exercise regimes - so the data are not really valid, particularly when other matings using puppies that should have been carrying these genes did not develop the problem.

Nutrition and HOD

HOD has occurred in puppies over supplemented with calcium, or fed on diets with excessive protein, and calories. Numerous studies have shown that overfeeding highly palatable diets will cause bone growth abnormalities. However, no trial has demonstrated that over nutrition will consistently reproduce HOD in test puppies. This is because the condition also requires that viral - Distemper - infection.

In fact, pups in all nutritional states have been affected. Vitamin C deficiency has also been accused of causing HOD This is because one type of HOD has the radiographic appearance of human scurvy. Although dogs synthesise their own Vitamin C it has been suggested that certain breeds of dogs may be predisposed to faulty Vitamin C metabolism. However, controlled trials using **small** doses of supplementary vitamin C did not correct the condition. It may be that larger doses would be required together with other immune system boosting nutrients such as vitamin A , zinc, and herbs such as Echinacea and Pennywort, the latter being included for its anti-inflammatory properties.

Treatment

Of all the juvenile orthopaedic diseases seen in dogs, nothing causes the intense pain of HOD. **The treatment** involves instituting the BARF programme, rest and pain relief. Having - at least in part - a viral cause, there is no absolute cure. Treatment is aimed at easing the suffering with anti-inflammatory medications and analgaesics.

Drugs used are designed to control fever and relieve pain. Only minimal activity is allowed during the recovery period. If you have a pet with this condition, limit its activity to short walks outside for elimination.

Prognosis

It must be understood that these are sick dogs. A proportion of dogs will die from this problem. If the owners can tolerate seeing their pup so distressed and can battle through the problem, it will eventually resolve. However, in many cases the dogs are so sick and so sore, they either die, or euthanasia is requested.

Usually after a few weeks they will get better. Occasionally they will go for months before they get better, but the treatment is still the same. Note, at the end of the day, they may be very crippled animals because of the laying down of massive amounts of new bone.

It often takes several months before any permanent improvement is seen. Most pups will recover, but there may be some stunting or bowing of the affected bones. Severe cases usually result in permanent deformity of the legs. As already mentioned, a small percentage get progressively worse and die due to extreme fever and associated complications, or more commonly are put to sleep. The outcome of the problem seems unrelated to any drug based treatment.

Treating with Diet

Take the pup off the damaging pro-inflammatory commercial food it is eating and switch to the BARF programme.

Use the BARF diet modified for skeletal disease. See Chapter Twenty Two. This will ensure a reduction in protein, calories, calcium and phosphorus. It will ensure your dog has a reduced growth rate and loses unnecessary weight. This will reduce the stress on the legs and ease the pain. It will ensure anti-inflammatory and anti-oxidant nutrients such as Vitamin C and the omega 3 essential fatty acids. Fresh linseed oil - not damaged by heat and not rancid - is an essential component of this programme because of its strong anti-inflammatory action. This must be accompanied by a vitamin E supplement. By following the BARF programme, you will ensure all of this.

Prevention of HOD

This could not be more simple. Grow your pups on the BARF programme from the word go. That programme not only slows growth and avoids excesses, it also builds a strong immune system, so important in preventing viral and other diseases.

Most particularly don't feed the diets with the heat damaged omega 3's in them - that is -the super premium puppy foods, or the ones promising a super shiny coat or the growth foods for puppies. These are the foods which contribute so markedly to these skeletal diseases involving inflammation. They also have excess protein, energy and possibly excess calcium. Make sure the only exercise is play - but not too boisterous - particularly during rapid growth spurts. **Exercise must be limited.**

As is usual with all these diseases based on alterations in Endochondral Ossification or Osteochondrosis, if the problem appears in pups raised on the BARF programme, it would be prudent not to breed with such pups, because such an occurrence would strongly indicate the presence of direct genes for this problem. What about close relatives? All I can say here is, if certain lines consistently produce the problem - when being raised properly on the BARF programme - then cull them.

My final word on this disease is - Grow your pups on the BARF programme from the word go. Most particularly don't feed the diets with the heat damaged omega 3's in them. Make sure the only exercise is gentle play. Keep your puppy well fleshed, but not fat. Slow steady growth is best. The puppy will eventually reach its potential, but without bone problems. Avoid excessive proteins, calories, calcium and anything which claims to be designed as a puppy growth food.

CHAPTER EIGHTEEN

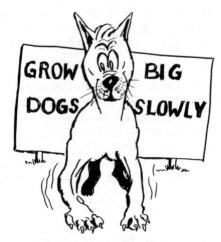

THE CARPAL
INSTABILITY/FLEXION
SYNDROME

This relatively harmless - if treated correctly - skeletal disease, originates at least in part from Osteochondrosis and is probably caused by both indirect and direct genes. The indirect genes may be the only ones involved and they certainly play the major role in producing the problem.

The problem only appears to arise when certain environmental factors including excesses of diet and exercise are suddenly thrust upon newly weaned pups. For these reasons, it is best controlled by management rather than genetic manipulation.

The Carpal Instability/Flexion Syndrome is seen in pups between eight and sixteen weeks. It is seen mostly in the larger breeds including Dobermans, Shar-Peis, Rottweilers, Rhodesian Ridgebacks, and Australian Cattle Dogs. Officially it does not discriminate between the sexes, but my experience sees it occurring mostly in males.

The problem appears very suddenly!

The pup stands with its carpus [one or both] bent forward. If any weight is placed on the limb, the carpus or wrist gives way and buckles forward. It commonly quivers at the same time. The pup walks on the outer edge of the paw which tends to turn inward. The condition is not painful, and there is no swelling. Upon examination there is no detectable instability. Sometimes only one leg is affected. Radiographs do not show any abnormalities.

Officially the cause is unknown

However, in my experience, this is another condition that is caused by incorrect management. Principally it is a problem that occurs with early stunting followed by an excessive growth rate, combined with a sudden increase in exercise. This happens when a pup, previously held back nutritionally and confined to a small area with its litter mates, is given upon arrival at its new home, unlimited food and space and over exercised with free and hard running and jumping. Such pups undergo a compensatory growth spurt. When this growth spurt is combined with minor damage to the growing bones, ligaments and tendons of the carpus or wrist, we see this Carpal Instability and Flexion syndrome.

Some cases will spontaneously recover after two to four weeks. However, many cases if not treated will remain permanently deformed.

The treatment ...

... is to slow that growth rate and splint the legs. This involves instituting the BARF programme of restricted diet and limited exercise.

Food intake should be moderately to severely restricted depending on how excessively the pup has been fed. It is essential to restrict calories, protein and calcium. The two front legs should be splinted in an extended position. The splints are left on for up to a week and reapplied after two or three days. This may have to be done three or four times. If the diet has been corrected to the BARF diet - modified for skeletal disease - this will usually result in a full recovery.

Do note that this condition can occur with ANY diet fed to excess - including the BARF diet.

Prevention involves the BARF programme ...

... taking special care to prevent new puppies from over eating or over exercising when they arrive at their new home. Particularly puppies of the larger breeds, and particularly when the breeder has deliberately [or otherwise] held that pup back and not allowed it to grow fat and fast.

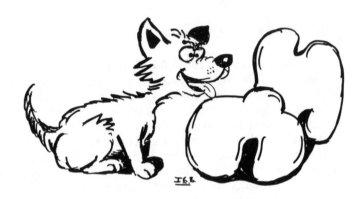

CHAPTER NINETEEN

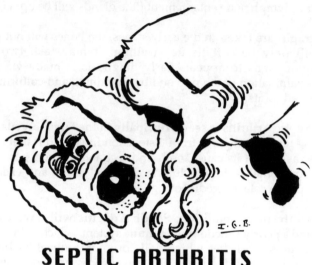

SEPTIC ARTHRITIS

What we are talking about here is lameness due to an inflammatory condition involving infectious organisms - usually bacteria - **within the joints of young dogs.**

It appears to occur spontaneously, apparently without prior injury, surgery or severe trauma, although teething has been suggested as a point where bacteria may gain entry.

The problem may involve one or more joints. It is usually seen in dogs of the larger breeds and may occur as young as six to eight weeks of age. Neither sex is affected more than the other. This is a condition which may be confused with other lamenesses in young dogs such as Panosteitis, Osteochondritis etc.. It is important to make that distinction because a suitable anti-microbial drug will be necessary as part of the treatment.

The onset is usually sudden and the pup is found to be severely lame. The infected joint[s] are found to be swollen and painful. If more than one joint or leg is affected, the pup may be reluctant to walk.

The pups will usually show signs of systemic illness. They will often have a high temperature, be lethargic, reluctant to eat and depressed. Commonly there will be lymph node enlargement ['the glands will be up.']

If radiographs are taken in the early stages, the bones will not show much. There will only be soft tissue swelling. It may take two weeks for radiographic signs to appear. Early diagnosis is made via a thorough physical examination of the pup and by examining and culturing joint fluid from affected joints.

Because Septic Arthritis is seen principally in the larger breeds, it probably originates - at least in part - from Osteochondrosis and if that is the case, it will have as part of its cause, both indirect and direct genes. This means that environmental factors including excesses of diet and exercise almost certainly play a role as predisposing factors.

Being an infectious condition, Septic Arthritis will have as part of its background a poorly functioning immune system which is the end result of being fed the sort of diet which will promote unhealthy inflammatory processes. That includes being fed any processed foods, which in my experience are all poor in their ability to promote a healthy immune system.

Products which should particularly be avoided are the ones high in the heat damaged fats such as the super premium puppy growth foods, or the products which promise a shiny coat. The heat damaged fats in these products all have the potential to promote unhealthy inflammatory conditions.

Puppies denied the health enhancing benefits derived from eating raw meaty bones, may develop mouth, tooth and gum problems - a great focus of infection. That combined with a poorly functioning immune system, and damage to joints due to modern Osteochondrosis, is the most likely background to these problems. Other factors which cannot be ruled out include raising pups in sub-standard, poorly ventilated, never cleaned, generally unhealthy conditions

In common with all the other skeletal conditions seen in young dogs, the BARF programme is ideal both as a preventative and as an essential and vital part of the treatment regime.

Other aspects to the treatment will be rest, **appropriate anti-microbials**, any improvements in hygiene required, herbs such as Echinacea, together with Cod liver oil, and zinc - to help boost the immune system - and possibly analgaesics.

Please note that it is essential that your vet takes a sample of the joint fluid from an affected joint and has it examined by a pathology laboratory to determine which organism[s] is/are present and which anti-microbials will be suitable for treating this condition.

For long term prevention of septic arthritis in pups, look to management rather than genetic manipulation. It is essential that dogs be raised in a clean healthy environment on an immune enhancing diet. The BARF diet. Note that this includes the teeth and gum 'health enhancing' process of being weaned with - and therefore teething with - raw meaty bones.

When using the deep litter system to raise pups, it is essential to replace the litter between whelpings and to thoroughly disinfect the whole area as well, before putting in the new material.

CHAPTER TWENTY

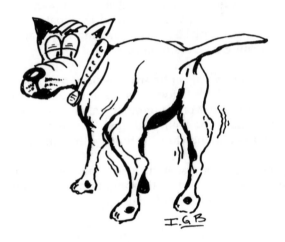

PATELLAR LUXATION
OR
SLIPPING PATELLAS

This is a problem of the knee or stifle. The leg becomes bowed, and the patella or knee cap, instead of staying in the groove at the end of the femur, slips out of that groove, usually to the inside of the leg. Sometimes the patella slips in and out of its groove causing intermittent lameness - or rides on the edge of the groove. This will cause pain and eventually degenerative joint disease.

Patellar Luxation is a common cause of lameness in young, mostly small breed dogs. It is particularly common in breeds such as the Chihuahua, the toy and miniature Poodle, the Papillon, the Yorkshire Terrier, and Maltese Terriers etc..

It is occasionally seen in larger breeds such as the Bichon Frise, the Keeshond, the Bull Terrier, the Staffordshire Bull Terrier etc. It can also be seen in association with Hip Dysplasia - e.g. in Labradors. Not uncommonly the condition occurs as a result of trauma to the knee. When this occurs, it is only seen on the traumatised side. There is no tendency for either sex to be affected more than the other.

It is usually considered to be congenital, i.e. present at birth, and possibly genetic. However, apart from the cases caused by trauma, my experiences with the condition tell me that in many cases, the problem is either made worse or initiated by poor management of pups. **In other words it is in part at least, another manifestation of Osteochondrosis: either modern or old fashioned. That is because ...**

The poor management can involve ANY type of feeding errors. Bowed legs and slipping patellas can be produced by deficient diets or excessive diets, by low calcium or high calcium diets.

Perhaps the most important factor is excessive exercise and very often wrong exercise. For example, the situation where overweight pups, already suffering some nutritional bone problem, are encouraged to dance around on their hind legs at a very young age.

The conditions conducive to producing bowed legs and slipping patellas begin when pups are whelped onto slippery surfaces such as newspaper. They will develop much stronger straighter legs if they are raised on clean soil or suitable deodorised aged shavings. That allows young paws to get a firm hold. The next error is the failure to supply good eating exercise and this is followed by weaning onto either a calcium deficient all meat type of diet such as mince, or a calcium excessive diet such as processed food and a calcium supplement.

In other words, we may summarise all of this as a failure to raise pups properly as nature intended with the BARF programme for puppies.

Many dogs with the problem show no signs of being lame. Quite often the problem can be controlled by keeping the dog slim, particularly while growing - and keeping it that way as an adult. Excess weight causes the leg to bow out further. The knee does not usually appear swollen or deformed. Unless the problem was due to trauma, both legs are usually affected.

If the condition is allowed to become severe and is not arrested before the legs have finished their growth, the legs WILL become permanently deformed.

The onset of lameness is usually very slow unless the problem was caused by trauma.The usual picture is one of intermittent lameness. Once the patella becomes permanently out of joint, the lameness also becomes permanent. Where the problem is severe, due to severe bowing of the legs, with the knee cap or patella not actually contacting the end of the femur, such dogs can walk awkwardly, but without undue pain. The dogs show no signs of illness.

Assessing the condition with radiographs is usually not necessary. Palpation with fingers is usually all that is required.

The smaller the breed, the greater the number of genes an animal may inherit for this condition, and therefore the greater care that will have to be taken with management during the growing period.

Severe cases will have to go to surgery for correction to avoid future mobility problems involving deformed legs, degenerative joint disease, and permanent shortening of the quadriceps group of muscles.

The best preventative measures involve the BARF programme, which includes not raising pups on slippery surfaces and instituting a raw food diet including raw meaty bones - where they actually eat the bones - from about three weeks of age. Discourage early obesity, rapid growth, processed foods, and dancing on hind legs before the bones are mature which will not be until after twelve months of age.

Where a young pup is diagnosed with the problem, it is important to correct the diet. Go to the BARF programme.

If the pup was on a rickets producing, generally deficient and calcium deficient sort of diet, and is undernourished and poorly, with bowed legs, then sunshine, cod liver oil, B and C vitamin supplementation and plenty of raw meaty bones such as chicken wings and chicken necks will be necessary to correct the condition. Don't over do it however. That is, do not grow the pup at a huge rate. Just quietly improve the diet and keep the pup improving steadily with moderate exercise and a vitamin C supplement of about 20 mg per kg of pup per day.

If the pup was on a high calorie, high protein, high calcium sort of diet, then go to the 'modified for skeletal disease BARF diet': the one with lots of vegetables and low in raw meaty bones. You have to drop the weight to get the bow out of the legs. Add a vitamin C supplement.

If the pup was on an all meat calcium deficient diet and is overweight - still go to the BARF diet modified for arthritis, but make sure the pup gets about 20% of its diet as chicken necks to ensure adequate mineralisation of those calcium deficient bones.

Surgical treatment of slipping patellas ...

... involves a number of different techniques depending on the severity of the condition.

If the patella is merely loose, tightening up the lateral ligaments and stabilising the patella in its groove may be all that is necessary. If the condition involves severe bowing of the legs and the channel in the end of the femur becoming shallow, more drastic measures will be required. However, that is something to discuss with your veterinary surgeon should the need arise.

The role of genes in producing slipping patellas

This is a problem that does have an underlying genetic predisposition. However, it seems to involve mostly indirect genes. That means incorrect diet and exercise is the most important cause of this problem in most cases.The good news which arises from that is - the condition can mostly be prevented by correct diet and exercise - which translates very simply to adopting the BARF programme.

The BARF programme of diet and exercise is the most important tool in treating and preventing slipping, or luxating, or dislocating patellas. Of the two management factors, exercise is by far the more important. Appropriate or inappropriate exercise is the major factor in either preventing or causing this condition.

Problems often begin in the whelping box ...

... as little legs try to stand, walk, and move around on slippery newspapers. The problem grows as little pups become obese and sit around eating soft mushy food without the benefit of eating exercise. The problem is continued and worsened as these tiny, obese, poorly muscled, bow legged, puppies are picked up to go everywhere with the only exercise they receive being their never-ending dance on hind legs - as they ask to be picked up yet again - and/or fed some inappropriate scrap of food. All of this is a sure fire recipe for patellar luxation!

You can begin the Prevention of Patellar problems in the whelping hole ...

... that is, with pups being raised on some form of deep litter system. This encourages strong straight muscled legs. This healthy limb formation is continued when those pups start their isometric whole body exercises as they struggle with raw meaty bones after about three weeks of age. That process must become an integral part of the rest of their lives. In particular, those pups must be fed and exercised appropriately until their bones are mature at around twelve months of age.

A vet check of the knees ...

... in susceptible breeds at four to six weeks of age - or earlier is a great idea. If the condition is diagnosed at this stage, it can often be corrected with daily massage and exercise carried out by the owner in conjunction with all the other aspects of the BARF programme.

This involves the pup's knee joint being extended and flexed very gently three or four times a day in five to ten minute sessions. At the same time, the quadriceps group of muscles [the tight muscles above the knee on top of the thigh] must be massaged daily to relieve spasm. Dancing on hind legs must not happen. Healthy gentle play is to be encouraged, as is isometric bone eating exercise. **Obesity must disappear!**

Above all, follow the BARF programme of feeding and sensible exercise from a pup's earliest days and continue that programme for the rest of that pup's life.

CHAPTER TWENTY ONE

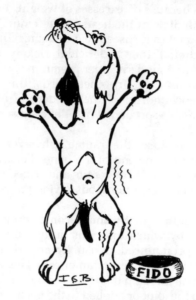

ASEPTIC NECROSIS
OF THE FEMORAL HEAD

This disease is also known as Calve-Legg-Perthes Disease - or simply Legg-Perthes Disease. It is seen in young small breed dogs such as the Poodles, Miniature Pinschers, various terrier breeds and so on. It usually strikes between four and ten months of age. It seems to affect each sex equally.

What is Legg-Perthes Disease?

This problem could be described as the small dog version of Hip Dysplasia in that it is a deformed hip problem and involves problems that arise during the growth of the dog. However, the problem is not due to loose or sloppy hips.

As the name implies, the problem does not involve infection but does involve a **necrosis or atrophy of the ball part of the ball and socket hip joint.**

The problem occurs because of excesses of weight, exercise or straight out trauma to the growth plate of the head of the femur. That weakness of the growth plate which makes it susceptible to damage may well be related to an inappropriate diet. Either a deficient rickety sort of diet, a poor processed food diet, or a modern super premium sort of diet with excesses of protein, fat, calcium etc.. In other words, this is another condition springing from Osteochondrosis: either modern or old fashioned. That is, due to either an excessive sort of diet or a deficient sort of diet.

The damage occurs because the trauma, whatever it may be, causes the growth plate to shear off the end of the bone. This results in a loss of the blood supply to the head of the femur and it begins to degenerate. The blood supply does eventually return, but the joint never recovers.

Lameness usually begins quietly and becomes progressively worse over three to five weeks, by which time it is quite obvious. Muscle wasting, which will become pronounced, is usually apparent within two to three weeks of the first appearance of lameness. The condition is painful, particularly if the leg is lifted up to the side or out to the back, or pressure is placed directly on to the joint or applied to the pectineus muscle.

The problem is usually seen only on one side, with ten to fifteen percent of cases having both legs affected. The problem does not make the dog ill in any way.

Radiographs taken in the early stages show only subtle changes. After two or three weeks there is a widening of the joint space with an apparent shrinking and change in shape of the head of the femur. The head becomes less calcified, less rounded, smaller and more irregular in shape.

Treatment is surgical and involves removal of the femoral head. Correct after care which is aimed at reducing Osteoarthritis of the hip joint involves the BARF programme.

Prevention involves raising that pup properly with the BARF programme and avoiding obesity, excessive exercise and trauma until the pup is twelve to fifteen months of age when the bones are mature enough to withstand the normal healthy exuberant exercise of these little dynamos.

CHAPTER TWENTY TWO

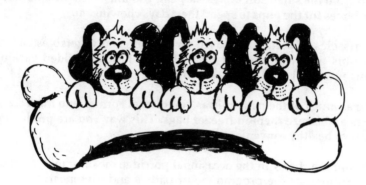

THE 'BARF' PROGRAMME FOR PUPS

If you have not already done so, please read Part One of this book which details the general BARF programme, and gives information on the basic ingredients used in the BARF diet.

The BARF programme for pups consists of two parts. Diet and exercise. First the diet.

The BARF diet for pups ...

... Is suitable for any pup after about four or five weeks of age.

- The BARF diet for pups consists of two basic parts. Firstly, the raw meaty bones, and secondly, the vegetable and mince patties or rissoles as we call them in Australia.

- The raw meaty bones will usually consist of chicken necks or chicken wings. These are chosen for pups because they are relatively soft and small. That is - suitable for pups. Whatever you choose, make absolutely sure the pups eat the bones and not just the meat.

- Apart from the small soft bones they eat, you must also provide some large bones for the pups to spend their days chewing on.

- The rissoles or patties are based on raw crushed vegetables and/or fruit plus raw lean minced meat. To this base are added various additives which I shall outline shortly.

- Make as much of the patty mix as you like to. Form it into meal sized patties and freeze them in freezer bags. This way you are producing your own healthy convenience food for pups.

For variety you can throw in the occasional porridge meal, or milk meal or meat meal. So long as the programme of patties and raw meaty bones I have just outlined makes up at least 80% of the total diet of the pup, then little additions of people food or whatever should not make too much difference. For more information read Chapter Seventeen - 'Feeding Your New Puppy' in **Give Your Dog a Bone.**

Making the meat and vegetable Patties

When making the patties it is essential that the raw crushed vegetable material should form at least half of the mix. The only time you want the patties to contain more mince would be when you have a pup that is [initially] reluctant to eat vegetables. However, do realise that the extra mince is only there for that reason. To persuade that pup to eat the patties. It must be reduced as soon as possible. The need to reduce the mince to less than half becomes most critical, particularly with the larger breeds of dogs where we need to limit protein and total energy intake.

The raw crushed vegetables will include such things as silver beet, spinach, celery, members of the cabbage family, root vegetables such as carrots and sugar beet. **Whatever is seasonally and locally available.** Many pups just love the taste of sugar beet. Use whatever fruit is in season - or whatever you can get hold of including such things as tomatoes, apples, oranges, mangoes, grapes, bananas - whatever.

The other half of the patty mix consists of raw lean meat - finely minced. That minced meat can be virtually any lean mince - chicken, beef, lamb, rabbit, turkey, buffalo, pork, crocodile, kangaroo, moose, bison, venison - whatever. It must be raw. Use whatever is readily and cheaply available. Remember, the mince should only form at the most half or preferably less than half of the mix. It may be minced chicken or turkey or duck wings or necks, in which case it will be more fatty and contain bone. This must be kept in mind when you are attempting to limit the calories in your patty mixture.

The following amounts of additives are added to a total mix of two kg of vegetables and mince.

Yoghurt - low fat and plain - say half a small tub.
Eggs - raw and preferably free range - about three.
Flax seed oil - 2 or 3 dessert spoons
Raw Liver - a quarter of a lamb's liver
Garlic - 1 or 2 cloves
Kelp powder - 2 or 3 teaspoons
B vitamins and vitamin C - a mega dose of each.

Plus other healthy food scraps

These might include small amounts of cooked vegetables, rice, cottage cheese, other left overs such as scrambled eggs etc.. These are more likely to be available for individual dogs in families rather than to large numbers of pups in a breeding or boarding kennel.

Blend the raw crushed vegetables, the lean raw minced meat and the additives together into a smooth homogeneous mix.

You can make as much or as little as you like

Let me emphasise that the above recipe may be scaled up or down. It all depends on how much you need, how much freezer space you have for storing it, how much you want to make and freeze ahead of time and what sort of equipment you have to produce it.

IMPORTANT

It is essential that your pup eats everything you have put in the mix, so make sure the whole lot is mixed into one homogeneous mass that your pups cannot separate and therefore pick and choose the bits they do and don't want.

Any surplus not fed on the day - should be formed into patties, frozen then thawed out and used as required.

Add vitamin E just before you feed the patties: e.g., for an 11 lb [5 kg] PUP, give 100 i.u. or 100 mg daily.

These patties can be fed alternately with the raw meaty bones. If your pup shows a preference for either the raw meaty bones or the patties, then feed whichever of these the pup likes least when it is most hungry.

Feed your pup cod liver oil every day: e.g., for an 11 lb [5 kg] pup give 1 to 2 ml daily.

You must also ensure that there are available the large bones - the dinosaur bones. The long bones from the limbs of cattle or sheep etc. The femurs and tibias of the hind legs and the humerus, radius and ulna of the front legs. These are for the pups to spend their days chewing on. The pups will only be able to chew the ends of these. However, these bones provide valuable eating exercise, particularly for the jaws, they help cut teeth, they clean teeth and the pup eats the valuable cartilage off the ends of these bones. That cartilage plays an enormous role in producing healthy disease free joints in the pups.

How much do you feed?

As you know by now, to grow pups with healthy bones it is essential that they be grown slowly, particularly the larger breeds of dogs, and most particularly the giant breeds.Numerous trials have demonstrated that pups of any breed grown in this manner - slowly - will not develop any of the juvenile bone diseases.

To achieve the desired rate of growth you must only feed enough food to support a moderate rate of growth. Sufficient food and no more to have that pup growing at about sixty to seventy five percent of its maximum growth rate.

How do you figure out how much food to feed to support this reduced rate of growth?

There are two methods you can use to achieve this restriction in food intake and therefore in growth rate. You can either restrict the **amount** of food fed at each meal, or you can limit the pup's access to food to a specific period of **time**.

Feeding by meal SIZE restriction

The rule of thumb is to feed a pup two thirds of its possible maximum food intake. That is, two thirds of what it would eat if it were allowed free access to the food at all times. This is fine in theory, but often difficult in practice to know exactly what that figure would be. However, it can be done. All you need is an approximation.

Feeding by meal TIME restriction

With the time restriction method, you set aside a specific period of time in which the pups are allowed access to the food. Something like 20 minutes at a time. Or less. It all depends on how quickly they eat, and to what extent they are distracted during this period of time. Quite often pups are like kids, play is more appealing than eating.

With both methods of feeding the number of periods allowed depends on their stage of growth. Younger puppies need feeding more often. As a general rule, three or four feeds a day until weaning, two or three feeds a day to six months of age, one or two feeds a day after six months, and one feed a day at maturity.

Feeding the BARF DIET with meal SIZE restriction

When using the BARF diet this way, you feed a pup two thirds of its possible maximum food intake. That is, two thirds of what it would eat if it were allowed free access to the food at all times. So how do you figure that out!

Start off by feeding - or offering your pup 10% of its body weight in food every day. How do you do that? Weigh your pup. Suppose your pup weighs 5 kg which is 11 lb. On a daily basis feed that pup food with a total weight of half a kg [500 gm] or a bit over 1 lb.

The basic puppy diet consists of 60% raw meaty bones and 40% of the patty mix.

Just to make the sums easy let's make it 50% of each. That means 250 gm of chicken wings or necks and 250 gm of patty mix.

Depending on the age of the pup this will be divided into between 2 and four meals. For most pups 3 meals is fine. For very young pups it might be four meals daily, and for older pups, it might be two meals daily.

Do this for several days. If the pup cannot possibly eat any more, then you have reached its maximum intake, so reduce the amount you are feeding by one third. One third less weight of wings and one third less weight of patties.

On the other hand, if the pup is still hungry after eating 10% of its body weight daily keep adding a little more food each day until the pup cannot eat any more. Now you have maximum food intake, so drop it back to two thirds of that.

An example

Suppose your pup weighs 22 lb or 10 kg, and its maximum daily food intake was 2 lbs 13 ounces or 1.3 kg. That means it was eating 13% of its body weight daily. It only needs to eat two thirds of this, which is 8.7 %. If you do your sums you find that 8.7% of 22 lb is 1 lb 14 ounces, or of 10 kg is 870 gm or 0.87 kg.

You can use that figure of 8.7% to figure out how much to feed as the pup grows. You just need to keep weighing the pup once a week and do the sums. Do keep a record of what your pup weighs together with his or her age. You might even like to plot your pup's progress on a graph.

However, weighing your pup[s] and doing the sums is only half the programme.

The other half of the programme is watching the pup[s]

If you notice that the pup is becoming excessively thin ...

... and does not appear to be growing properly - then you are probably not feeding enough, or you are feeding too much vegetable material and not enough raw meaty bones. So what do you do? It is very simple. You feed it more. The big question is - how much more and do you change the proportions of patties to raw meaty bones? The first thing to realise is that you do not want to feed the pup too much more. If you did, you may cause a compensatory growth spurt and that pup would then become prone to developing OCD.

One approach would be to go through the process of gradually increasing the food fed until you reach maximum intake, and then drop back by about a quarter or a fifth instead of a third. At the same time you could also increase slightly the level of raw meaty bones being fed. Do not drop the amount of vegetables being fed however.

Watch the pup's growth rate over the next week. This is the art of it all. There should be steady weight gain, but the pup must not be too fat or roly poly. You must keep it slim and hungry.

Another approach would be to increase the food slowly and when the pup is looking better, ease back and just make daily adjustments, keeping a close eye on that pup. Keep weighing it. Keep graphing its progress. Is the pup still hungry when it has finished? Is the pup picky with its food? Is it so full it can hardly move? If it is - then it is not hungry and needs to be fed less.

The adjustments you make will involve varying the levels of vegetables [low calorie foods] and raw meaty bones, oils, fatty meats and other high calorie foods as well as the amount fed. Preferably you will have the pup still a little hungry when it has finished each meal.

The important message is still the same, whatever you do - be careful. You do not want a previously slowly growing dog to suddenly spurt ahead and grow rapidly.

If you notice that your pup is becoming roly poly and plump ...

... and you notice on your graph that the growth rate is rising sharply, then you are feeding too much food and maybe too much high calorie food and not enough of the vegetables. So what do you do? It is very simple. If the pup is growing too rapidly, cut back the total food fed by one third, and reduce the proportion of raw meaty bones to only 20% of the total food fed. This means 80% of the total intake is the vegetable patties. At the same time, increase the proportion of vegetables in the patties to about 80%

Feeding the BARF diet by meal TIME restriction ...

... **is not really feasible.** However, if the method appeals to you - feeding the BARF diet this way involves allowing the pup[s] a specific period of time in which to eat its [their] food. That is, something like fifteen or twenty minutes at a time, or less. The number of periods allowed depends on their stage of growth. Younger puppies need feeding more often. As a general rule, three or four feeds a day until weaning, two or three feeds a day to six months of age, one or two feeds a day after six months, and one feed a day at maturity. However, let me repeat, this method does not work well when feeding the BARF diet.

If raising several pups together ...

... you have to make sure that each pup is only allowed to eat its allotted share. If not, the shy and timid pups will starve while the more aggressive/assertive bullies will eat their food and over time achieve that unwanted maximum growth rate as they eat as much as they possibly can. This is particularly so when feeding bones.

Dogs can become very possessive over bones, and fights are to be avoided at all costs. The simple solution is to feed growing pups on their own. This will ensure they eat only what you give them. Even if you have to provide separate quarters for each pup, or have each pup tied to a stake whilst eating, it is certainly worth the effort. Each pup eats the optimum amount desired. No starvation and no over eating.

Individual variations between pups are important when you are deciding how much to feed. The amount fed will be different for each breed and each stage of growth, it will depend on the puppy's sex and it must also take into account individual variations between pups. This means constant individual assessment of each pup. Its weight and its appearance. Is it too fat? Is it too thin? Is it becoming sore or lame? Is it a boy or a girl? Males will grow quicker than females. They are much more likely to develop problems because of this.

Whatever you do in the way of weighing and observing, the whole process is as much art as it is science. This is important. There is always going to be an element of judgement involved in growing healthy pups, especially pups of the giant breeds.

Another really valuable thing to do is enlist the help of an experienced breeder or vet. If you can find the right sort of person to help you, that is, someone who is experienced AND who is sympathetic to your aims with the BARF diet, this is great. Do not use someone who is trying to persuade you to use commercial food. With the help of the right sort of person, you will be able to safely modify the amount and balance of food fed.

Together, you and they will be looking for a steady weight gain, nothing rapid; always a waist present on the dog/pup when viewed from above, no obesity, being able to feel but not able to see the ribs, and always some hunger left.

Be patient with yourself. You will get the hang of feeding pups this way. All it takes is a bit of experience, some common sense, faith in the method and patience.

A final thought. If in doubt - if you think a pup is becoming too fat, but you are not sure, it is usually better to err on the side of feeding too little rather than too much. Good luck!

The above is a starting point and a guide only. It is up to you where you take your pup. Try and keep all the principles in mind that this book discusses, most of which may be summarised as follows .....

A summary of puppy feeding principles

Pups need to be fed a diet based on raw meaty bones - about 60%

Pups need a diet based on raw crushed vegetables - about 30%

Pups need some offal in their diet - about 5%-10%

Pups should be kept lean and slightly hungry, no matter what the breed

Pups should not be allowed to become fat

Pups should be grown slowly

Pups should never be grown at their maximum growth rate

Pups do not need extra calcium if they eat plenty of raw meaty bones

Pups do not need processed food

Pups do not need cooked grain meals - a little bit occasionally is OK

Pups do not need a feeding routine

Pups do not need each meal to be complete and balanced

Pups DO need their whole feeding regime to be complete and balanced

A pup should eat mainly raw food

Fresh frozen food [thawed] is fine for pups

Healthy soil or clay may be part of a dog's diet

An occasional short fast will not be harmful and may be of benefit

Pups should be exposed in a controlled manner to bacteria

If you can use the above as a check list and say yes - that is how my pups are raised - there is very little chance your dogs will develop skeletal problems.

Whatever you do, be aware of the basic errors that cause problems. **Too much food, an extra fast rate of growth, extra protein, extra fat and extra artificial calcium are all potential bone wreckers.**

The BARF programme of exercise for modern pups

From those first struggling moments to find a teat and begin sucking, through the many encounters it has with that teat and with its brothers and sisters as it struggles to find that teat again or that 'just-right-spot' to sleep or stretch, through its first walking steps, a young pup is constantly moving and stressing all its bones and joints. **That struggling/walking exercise will ideally begin in a saucer shaped whelping circle that mum creates in the earth or in deep litter of some sort.** This simple depression provides optimum traction or grip for young paws. This is vital. Young pups that slip and slide around on slippery surfaces are destined for bone and joint problems.

By the second week following birth, there is much definite wrestling and struggling. This play fighting is a vital part of the building of strong healthy bones and joints. Once again, a soil base is essential - providing good traction for those growing and developing legs.

As pups begin to walk, the soil or litter base base on which they live provides the perfect grip they require. This ensures optimum use and therefore development and strength of those little legs and their bones and joints. This will ensure that no pup ever develops into a 'swimmer.'

The next part of a pup's exercise regime is when it is introduced to solid food at about three weeks of age.Now those pups have something to fight over. Ever watched three week old pups fight over raw meaty bones? Ever heard them?! Now they are really working. Pulling, tugging, chewing, the whole body braced, to win possession of that precious morsel. Exercising jaws, necks, shoulders, back and legs. This is the beginning of a lifetime of essential bone eating exercise.

A pup that eats and rips and tears at bones from its earliest days develops a strong, strong lean muscular body with healthy bones and joints. This is in stark contrast to a pup raised without bones. Both the muscles and the bones are thinner and weaker and the joints are looser. This lack of eating exercise ensures such pups are much more prone to skeletal problems such as Hip and Elbow Dysplasia.

At five weeks the young pup is spending much of its waking time in some form of exercise. Either eating or play. Play is the key word for the rest of that puppy's puppyhood.

This is important. **Pups do not, should not, indeed must not, undergo any long periods of running or walking until their bones have ceased to grow and have begun to harden. Playing pups stop when they are tired.** No 'endless' tiring walks on a lead. The importance of play as the major form of exercise is that a young pup can stop as soon as it starts to hurt or become tired. In that way, no excessive strain is placed on young growing bones. **If pups do too much or are exercised too hard or with jarring exercise of any type, the stress placed on those young bones can be sufficient to permanently damage their bones.**

What about different breeds and exercise? The rule of thumb is that the smaller and lighter the breed, the sooner it can begin to stress those bones with longer walks and rougher exercise. Maybe as young as ten months for one of the robust and healthy smaller breeds, although twelve months would be safer.

With the Giant breeds however, please wait until they are fifteen to eighteen months old at the very least, but preferably wait until they two years of age before really pushing them.

Modifying the BARF diet for skeletal disease

Where a pup develops problems of pain and lameness - that is OCD or worse - the simple modifications to this diet are as follows ...

1] **Increase the vegetables** in the patties to between 75% and 90% of the basic mix. That is, before the additives are thrown in. The percentage of vegetables chosen will depend on the severity of the problem.

2] **Increase the patties** to between 75% and 90% of the over-all diet, again depending on the severity of the problem.

3] **Do not add** any other food scraps to these patties.

4] **If the pup is really hungry - add more vegetables**

This is so simple isn't it!

Modifying the BARF programme of exercise for skeletal disease in pups

The programme is one of no exercise.

Unless the jaw bones are affected, eating exercise - the eating of raw meaty bones - should be continued. If the disease is affecting the bones of the jaws, the raw meaty bones will have to be minced until such time as the dog can crunch through them.

With regards to whole body exercise, your pup or young dog will require what vets call 'cage rest' with the only exercise allowed being leash walking. And only then to go to the toilet. After that it is back to that cage or its equivalent for continued rest. The total reduction of damaging pressures on bones and joints when OCD [or worse] strikes - is absolutely essential.

How long for? That one is difficult to say. Usually a minimum of two weeks to a month in mild cases, but in severe cases it may be several months or even longer, depending on the response to treatment. As a general rule of thumb, after a pup has become pain free, which means the pup no longer limps - if not sure about the pain check with your vet - wait a week and then gradually phase in the increased activity.

This whole question of exercise is something that will need to be discussed with your vet. Many factors are involved including the diagnosis and the stage to which the disease process has progressed, and whether surgical intervention has become necessary.

Between your vet's expertise, and your close observations, you will be able to work out when the bones and joints are becoming strong enough, healthy enough, and sufficiently free of pain to be allowed more exercise. Any return to normal exercise should be phased in gradually over several weeks to a month. The longer the dog has been resting, the longer it will take to make that return to normal playing exercise.

For more information, do read Chapter Twenty Three together with the chapters which deal with the individual diseases, and remember that any difficulties and extra effort that have to be surmounted or expended now are worth it, because the result will be a maximally sound pup for the rest of its life.

CHAPTER TWENTY THREE

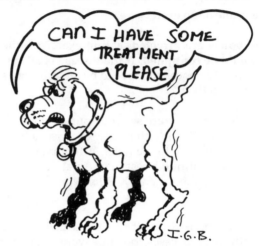

TREATING THE PUPPY
WITH SKELETAL DISEASE

What to do if you suspect your pup has a problem

If you suspect your pup has a problem - you must seek professional help - particularly as regards making a diagnosis. However, with or without that help ...

The general plan is as follows ...

1] Severe restriction of exercise
2] Severe restriction of food
3] Weight loss
4] No more commercial dog food and no more calcium supplements
5] Switch to the BARF programme of diet and exercise for skeletal disease which is low in calories, protein, fat and exercise, and will include various supplements such as mega vitamins, flax seed oil, cod liver oil, cartilage, etc..

Important points to keep in mind

1] Learn and understand the basic rules of sound management.

2] **WATCH THOSE PUPS. Your vigilance is their greatest safeguard. NEVER IGNORE A LAME PUPPY!** Pain and lameness are one and the same thing. If a limp persists for more than a day or two, or it keeps returning after apparently improving, that pup has a problem. Do not ignore it.

3] **There is ALMOST ALWAYS a background of incorrect nutrition** associated with skeletal problems in pups.

4] **Some form of trauma is the major inciting cause** of most lamenesses seen in young growing dogs, so do be careful with them, particularly as regards exercise.

5] **Pups with bone disease usually have more than one bone problem.** So expect more than one part of your pup to be sore.

6] **Treatment must be individualised**. It will depend on the age of the pup, and the severity of the condition.In severe cases, surgery may be necessary.

To give you an idea of how these cases may be approached, I now want to take you through a number of case histories involving young pups that have been brought to me because of skeletal problems. We shall be looking at seven pups, all of different breeds and all having different problems.

Case Histories - the common background

When I questioned the owners of these pups, I found that every single pup was suffering from the results of excesses of food and exercise. The exercise usually consisted of long and boring walks, or situations where the pup was forced to be active for long periods on most days, when for much of that time what it really wanted to do was lie down and sleep. On a number of occasions, these pups had been subjected to trauma from a larger more boisterous or older dog, or possibly a child.

On the diet side of things it was invariably found that the pup was being fed too much food in general, usually with excessively high levels of calories and protein. Some of these pups were being supplemented with extra meat, some were receiving extra calcium, and some were receiving both.

The food being fed was usually a processed food. If the pup was not being supplemented, it was usually being allowed to eat as much of that processed - usually dry - food, as it wanted. The end result was an excessive growth rate, and in some cases obesity, depending on the breed.

Almost every type of processed food has been involved in these problems, including the ordinary supermarket brands, but more often they were one of the super premium brands, or a brand designed to promote a healthy coat, both of which contain high levels of heat damaged polyunsaturates.

Occasionally we find an owner that has been over-feeding their damaging version of the BARF diet. Their version is usually found to be way too rich in both calories and protein, and very lacking in minerals and vegetable matter. This is usually achieved by feeding as much as the pup will eat of very fatty raw meaty bones. The product they feed usually contains only a small percentage of bone, and therefore lots of meat and fat. Not much else is being fed at all. This situation often arises when the pup takes charge and trains the owner to feed it only what it wants.

The general approach to treatment

When deciding how best to treat these problems, a major consideration is that when pups are managed correctly, skeletal problems rarely occur. This means that because these diseases are preventable, the sort of diet and exercise programme that will prevent them will also be a major part of the treatment. That means the BARF programme.

Another important fact related to treatment is that the earlier we can detect skeletal problems, the greater chance we have of turning these problems around before they become more serious and produce permanent damage.

Having decided that a given bone or joint system is abnormal or diseased, our first task is to make a diagnosis. In other words to name the disease process that is occurring. The only reason we want to do that is so that we can decide on the best course of treatment for that particular disease.

Our first aim when managing these problems, must be to stop - as best we are able - the further progression of the disease. That means instituting a specific form of the BARF programme consisting of a very stringent dietary regime together with severely reduced exercise or enforced rest.

At the same time we have to begin a programme of treatment to undo what damage can be undone, and alleviate any pain those pups might be suffering. Once again that involves that specific stringent BARF programme of diet and exercise together with whatever special treatment is required for particular problems.

We also have to institute an on-going prevention programme. A programme that will not only arrest and prevent any further damage, but will also positively promote good general health. That is, not only skeletal health, but all round health, involving every system in that pup including its further reproductive health - if applicable. What we are looking at promoting here, is a puppy with no future degenerative diseases such as cancer, diabetes, kidney disease, heart disease, pancreatitis, and no Osteoarthritis or degenerative joint disease either.

How do we do that ? Very simple. Once again it involves switching them to the BARF programme. I must stress at this point that many people will use a dry dog food in limited amounts to grow their pup slowly and thus avoid most of these problems. However, because they are using processed food, they are setting their pup up for a lifetime of other problems.

As you can see, every treatment aim involves switching these pups to a modified version of the BARF programme.

That programme will vary depending on three factors ...

Firstly, it depends on what exactly is wrong with the pup's skeletal system.

Secondly, we need fairly exact details of the pup's dietary history to that point.

And thirdly we need some idea of the role that overly exuberant exercise or trauma may have played in producing the problem.

Based on that information, we will choose a suitable BARF diet.

That means we are going to put them on the protein and energy restricted version of the BARF diet. That is because we need to drastically reduce their growth rate. Almost invariably, pups with these conditions are growing too fast and are being fed an excess of both protein and energy rich fat.

In practical terms this means feeding those pups a whole heap of crushed raw vegetables, and not too much of anything else, except that between ten and twenty percent of what they eat should consist of raw meaty bones. Just how low the bone component of the diet becomes depends on how overweight and how excessively the pup is growing and how severe the problem is.

So far as exercise is concerned, with any of these juvenile skeletal problems, rest becomes of paramount importance in every case.

From that point onwards, the whole growth process and what the pup is fed and how it is exercised needs very close monitoring. For the first month it needs weekly checks at the very least. This often works in well with weekly injections of pentosan polysulphate - if such a drug is required.

Each week there must be a review of the weight [gain or loss] of the pup, the diet fed and how that diet is being accepted, and the state of the pup in terms of general health and most particularly bone and joint health.

Quite often the older pups have to lose weight. Mostly the very young pup has to continue growing without gaining any more weight. The older pups may have to lose a substantial amount of weight over several weeks to months.

In the case of a young pup we most certainly do not want to stunt the pup, but in most cases we do have to severely reduce its rate of growth. It is also imperative that when comes the time to increase the levels of calories and/or protein, the increase is made slowly to avoid any compensatory growth spurts which would be disastrous.

Many of these pups have also been fed excessive calcium. This is either because the commercial diet contains excessive levels of calcium, or the owners are supplementing with calcium - "just to be sure."

Some of these pups are not receiving enough calcium. These are usually the ones being supplemented with excessive meat and no bones. To make matters worse, some of this meat is very fatty meat which raises the calorie content way too high.

In some cases the pup is not actually eating the bone. This happens when the pup is ripping and chewing the fat and meat off the bone but not eating the bone. The net result of this is that the pup is being fed what is essentially a calcium deficient, high calorie, high protein diet. Disaster!

In yet other cases, pups are fed way too much meat and fat and not enough bone on the pieces of raw meaty bones that people are choosing to feed to their pups. A common example of this would be a Saint Bernard being raised on fatty legs of lamb and fatty lamb breasts.

That is why I like to recommend chicken wings as part of the BARF programme. These have have a high bone to fat and meat ratio - which in most cases is ideal.

If a pup requires calcium supplementation, the preferred method is more bones. However, in most of these cases we need to also reduce the level of calories and protein. Unfortunately, bones happen to be high in both calories and protein as well as calcium, so that rules them out. In that case the supplement of choice will usually be dolomite, because it contains magnesium as well as calcium and has no phosphorus. Magnesium is the mineral next in importance after calcium and phosphorus when it comes to bone mineralisation.

The Case Histories

Bernice the Saint Bernard

The first pup I want to talk about is a female Saint Bernard named Bernice. Bernice was five months old when we met. She was very much down on her front paws. She was somewhat overweight, and seemed reluctant to walk very much, preferring just to flop.

A thorough examination of all her joints revealed that Bernice had all the early signs of OCD or Osteochondrosis. She had been raised on a diet of super premium foods supplemented with loads of fatty meat. This dog was suffering from a rapid growth rate, from the effects of heat affected fatty acids and also a possible calcium deficiency with a phosphorus excess. She was also suffering from excessive walking syndrome.

We slowed her growth rate with the restricted BARF diet, and gave her a calcium supplement as well as some raw meaty bones. The calcium supplement we chose was dolomite.

As Bernice lost weight over the next three weeks, her pasterns straightened, and after a month she was taken off the dolomite. She was kept on a BARF diet of thirty percent chicken wings and necks with the rest being the vegetable mix including flax seed oil. By the time she was twelve months old, the level of raw meaty bones in her diet had risen to about fifty percent. Bernice now has a reasonably straight and upright stance with no obvious skeletal problems. She is twenty months old.

Bernice may in the very late stages of her life develop Osteoarthritis. However, by remaining on the BARF programme, she has every chance of keeping that problem to an absolute minimum.

Gus the Labrador Retriever

The second pup is a male Labrador Retriever named Gus. Gus was six months of age with a funny bunny hopping motion as he walked or ran when we first met.

My examination of Gus revealed that his wrists, elbows, shoulders, hips, stifles and hock joints were all sore. He could not move freely. He was very restricted in his ability to stretch out and run. He had short mincing steps, an arched back and a bunny hopping motion. In addition, Gus was a very fat pup - even for a Labrador.

The major focus of soreness was in the hips. Gus had the beginnings of Hip Dysplasia. But more than that, Gus the Labrador had the beginnings of multiple joint problems. Unfortunately, by the time Gus's owners decided to seek help, the hip problem was well advanced. It had progressed to the point where it would cause lifelong problems.

It took a while but eventually the owners were convinced to radically change the diet by adopting the BARF diet for skeletal disease, and reduce the exercise to almost zero. This radical change in diet and exercise together with injections of pentosan polysulphate saw most of the problems owned by Gus come to a halt.

Gus lost weight, and over time, the soreness in the joints quietly disappeared. Gus continued to improve slowly over the next several months. He is now 15 months old and is able to exercise freely. His motion is still restricted to some degree. We are confident that with time he will continue to improve, although his hips may need some surgery in the future. We are hopeful that we have halted the progression of the OCD and largely reduced the impact of OCD and OCDIS on all of the joints mentioned, including the hips.

Annie the Beagle

The third pup I want to talk about is Annie. I first met Annie when she was eight weeks old. Annie was a wound up spring of a Beagle with front legs that were letting her down badly. They bowed over at the wrists when she walked, ran or simply stood up.

Annie had only been at her new home for about ten days. Upon arrival, she had been found to be quite slim. Perhaps 'skinny' would be a more adequate expression. Over the ten days she had been at her new home, Annie had put on an inordinate amount of weight and been highly active. Over the last couple of days she had become severely incapacitated.

It did not take long to diagnose Annie as having Carpal Instability and Flexion Syndrome. This was great, because if treated properly she had every chance of making a full recovery. We splinted the legs with plaster, the owners reduced the exercise drastically, and switched her to the restricted version of the BARF diet. We had to splint the legs on three occasions.

Annie is now four years old, beautifully slim and very very healthy. She is still kept strictly on the BARF diet. The owners had much difficulty accepting the diagnosis and the treatment - at first - but are now very pleased that Annie had this problem as a pup because it has ensured her present and future excellent health.

Danny the Great Dane

The fourth pup was a four month old male Great Dane called Danny. Danny was presented with severely swollen wrists. Danny was able to walk only with great difficulty. He was refusing food when presented, was running a high temperature and in great pain.

There was no doubting the diagnosis. Danny had Hypertrophic Osteodystrophy or HOD. We struggled with Danny for nearly a month. In the end, it was too painful for any of us to go on, least of all Danny. He heaved a great sigh of relief as he was finally put to sleep. This poor soul needed a lot more help than either a change of diet or all the regalia of modern veterinary science could offer.

After dealing with a number of these cases, and only one of them successfully in that it is still alive, I have come to the conclusion that it is far kinder in some instances to put the poor creatures down rather than let them go through months of suffering. However, if the pup can be made comfortable and does begin to improve in a fairly short period of time, then it may be worthwhile carrying on. Chapter Seventeen which deals with this condition should be consulted for more details on the treatment regime we use.

Which version of the BARF diet is used for this condition will depend very much on the dietary history of the animal in question, together with its general condition. In Danny's case, the diet he was on when the condition first appeared was a super premium food. I feel most strongly that the heat damaged fats in these products which are so inflammation producing contribute in no small way to this problem in susceptible animals.

At the time of presentation, Danny looked great in most respects. We did not have to restrict the food intake, he was already doing that - he was not eating. We just put him on the standard BARF diet - put through a blender until completely 'juiced.'

Emma the Newfoundland

The fifth pup was a seven month female Newfoundland called Emma whose front legs instead of being nice and straight were deviating - again at the wrists - out to the side. She too had some difficulty walking and bunny hopped as she ran.

By the time I saw her, Emma the Newfoundland had many of the advanced signs of OCD and OCDIS, being sore in many joints. She too was way too heavy for her age and size. She had been grown much too rapidly. Emma had been fed a diet of supermarket dry food - as much as she wanted, lean mince, porridge and huge calcium supplements. She lived with an enormous male Saint Bernard and spent much of her time rough and tumbling with him. I judged her to be suffering from excesses of exercise, protein, calories and calcium. We switched her to the severely restricted BARF diet which included reduced exercise and only fifteen percent raw meaty bones.

Emma made steady improvement with respect to the soreness in most of her joints. We did not see much improvement in her deviated legs. In addition she did develop Hip Dysplasia which had its impact reduced by removing both pectineus muscles. She underwent various surgical procedures in an effort to reduce her problems. We did manage to ward off the ultimate or final solution until she was about nine years of age.

At that time Emma developed severe Degenerative Joint Disease. She was put to sleep at the age of nine on humanitarian grounds.

Meetie the Shar-Pei

The sixth pup was an imported male Shar-Pei called Meetie. He was having some difficulties with his hind legs. The owner noticed that his hips seemed to click as he walked. This was an expensive imported pup.

How it came about exactly, we are not entirely sure, but the unfortunate diagnosis was Hip Dysplasia - severe Hip Dysplasia. We did not know too much about Meeti's early history. Whether he had started life on slippery newspaper or not. Whether he had been raised on processed food or not. Whether he was given calcium supplements or not. We suspect he had been raised on processed food, having been imported from Japan.

Meetie had spent some time in Quarantine where he had not fared well physically. He had grown poorly. On arriving at his new home in Australia we suspect he may have undergone a compensatory growth spurt as his new owners, who had paid a lot of money for him, tried to correct his somewhat small stature. He had certainly grown at an alarming rate - being fed since arriving, on masses of chicken wings.

He had also been put in with a pack of other pups to get him to run and play and socialise. Sadly, we feel the combined effect of that compensatory growth spurt, together with excessive exercise which he had not been used to, had pushed his bones well beyond what they were capable of withstanding. Meetie's bones were so badly deformed he had to be put to sleep.

Jed the Rottweiler

The last pup I want to talk about is Jed, a huge male Rottweiler who weighed close to 50 kg at about seven months of age. Jed came to see me because his owner had noticed a vague but persistent lameness in one or possibly both front legs. Jed had had the problem for about two weeks.

Jed was robust, mean and active. His owner is a health freak, working out daily in the gym, and spending several hours each day jogging and running with this pup. The pup was fed a super premium dry food - as much as he wanted - plus calcium supplements.

An examination of the elbows, shoulders and wrists of this dog showed that he was sore in every one of these joints. In both front legs. Jed's left front leg, the one the owner said he was favouring, showed more muscular spasms than the right. He was also sore in the hips and perhaps the hocks. Pressure on his lower back produced a pain reaction of abdominal tensing. This was one sore unhappy wound up dog - that now hated me. Jed was convinced that my only aim in life was to bring him pain.

Jed was diagnosed as having the beginnings of OCD [Osteochondrosis] which as you will remember is overly thickened under mineralised cartilage in the growing points of the bones. This is the basic underlying disease or condition from which can spring any one of the other skeletal problems. That is - if it is allowed to continue unchecked. The next stage may be OCDIS [Osteochondritis Dissecans] in the shoulders, elbows, wrists and hips. You will remember that is when the overly thickened non calcified cartilage of OCD begins to break up or fissure - usually due to the effects of trauma - which in this case was due to being excessively exercised.

If Jed's condition had been allowed to continue, he may well have gone on to develop Elbow Dysplasia, Hip Dysplasia, and possibly Shoulder, Stifle and Hock Dysplasia, as well as similar problems in his wrists. Later on in life he would almost certainly have developed degenerative joint disease or Osteoarthritis in all these joints.

As it happens, Jed's owner who was fanatic about the dog brought him to me at the first sign of problems. He did not take long to understand the gravity of Jed's condition, and undertook to feed him as I directed.

Jed was to have a diet consisting of approximately ninety five percent vegetables to start with plus a total cessation of exercise until further notice. Jed came to see me weekly, receiving an injection of pentosan polysulphate on each of these visits for the next month, then one a month later.

Jed lost weight, and gradually his pain receded. Over time he went on to make a complete recovery. He was able to resume his jogging career after a break of some five months. Jed's owner has continued to feed him properly with the BARF diet, and he is now a magnificently healthy three year old dog. He has even started to like me! Well perhaps tolerate me might be closer to the truth.

Jed is typical of so many dogs in that his skeletal problems started in this insidious way. Had his owner ignored those early tell tale signs and allowed him to continue on his destructive path of excessive food and calcium, obesity and excessive exercise, Jed would have ended up a cripple. However, Jed was fortunate.

He, like numerous other dogs made a full recovery because he was diagnosed early and treated properly with the BARF programme modified for skeletal disease.

Let me finish this book by wishing you well with your breeding programme and with your pups. May your dogs be fertile, free of skeletal disease and healthy in all other respects.

Ian Billinghurst
August 1998